AGING ISSUES, HEALTH AND FINANCIAL ALTERNATIVES SERIES

MENOPAUSE: VASOMOTOR SYMPTOMS, SYSTEMATIC TREATMENTS AND SELF-CARE MEASURES

AGING ISSUES, HEALTH AND FINANCIAL ALTERNATIVES SERIES

AGING ISSUES, HEALTH AND FINANCIAL ALTERNATIVES SERIES

MENOPAUSE: VASOMOTOR SYMPTOMS, SYSTEMATIC TREATMENTS AND SELF-CARE MEASURES

Jacek Michalski
and
Isabela Nowak
EDITORS

Nova Biomedical Books
New York

Library of Congress Cataloging-in-Publication Data

Menopause : vasomotor symptoms, systematic treatments, and self-care measures / editors, Jacek Michalski and Isabela Nowak.
     p. ; cm.
 Includes bibliographical references and index.
 ISBN 978-1-60876-930-8 (hardcover : alk. paper)
 1. Menopause. 2. Menopause--Hormone therapy. 3. Estrogen--Therapeutic use. I. Michalski, Jacek. II. Nowak, Isabela.
 [DNLM: 1. Menopause--physiology. 2. Estrogen Replacement Therapy. 3. Vasomotor System--physiopathology. WP 580 M5487 2009]
 RG186.M4853 2009
 618.1'75--dc22   2009045548

Published by Nova Science Publishers, Inc. ✣ *New York*

Contents

Preface

By 2030, an estimated 47 million women will be undergoing menopause each year. With the progressive increase in life expectancy, the number of women older than 50, and consequently in menopause, is much higher today than in previous decades. In the United States, the average life expectancy for women is about eighty years, indicating not only a greater number of postmenopausal women but also that these women will live more than one third of their lives deprived of estrogen. The authors investigate the levels of the two important hormones, FSH and E2 during perimenopause. Levels of thyrotropin (TSH) in association with reproductive hormone are examined as well. Moreover, the physiopathogenesis of the sex- and menopause-associated differences in chronic liver disease are discussed, which are important to developing new approaches to prevention, diagnosis and treatment. The authors of this book also analyze the gender differences in the epidemiology, symptoms and progression of cardiovascular disease, which increases most markedly in women at the time of menopause. Furthermore, the management of the vasomotor symptoms, including hormonal replacement therapy (HRT) that constitutes the basis of the treatment of menopause symptoms are discussed.

Chapter I - Chronic hepatitis B and C appear to progress more rapidly in males than in females. Liver cancer is predominant in men and postmenopausal women. Almost anyone may "feel," but not recognize the sex-associated difference in liver cancer as a fact. A large body of evidence has been accumulated suggesting that increased oxidative stress is an essential step in the development of hepatic fibrosis to the end-stage cirrhosis and its complication liver cancer. Environmental and lifestyle risk factors such as hepatitis B/C virus infection, obesity, and heavy alcohol intake lead to increased oxidative stress, which in general occurs more frequently in males. In contrast, biological female sex factors such as estrogen, hepatic iron storage status, and growth hormone, which change a lot after menopause, play antioxidative and cytoprotective roles in the functional and morphological modulation of the liver physiopathology.

Currently, metabolic disorders such as being overweight and diabetes are emerging as cofactors of hepatic fibrosis. Fatty liver is considered the hepatic manifestation of the metabolic syndrome. The transition from premenopause to postmenopause is associated with the emergence of many features of the metabolic syndrome, including increased intra-abdominal body fat. Intra-abdominal fat accumulation is a predictor of fatty liver.

Females are more resistant to certain infections. Indeed, females, particularly before menopause, can produce antibodies against hepatitis B virus at a higher frequency than males with hepatitis B virus infection. The decline in ovarian function with menopause is associated with spontaneous increase in proinflammatory cytokines.

Being female or male is an important basic human variable that affects health and liver disease throughout the life span. Sex is defined as female or male according to their biological functions, while gender is shaped by environment and experience. A better understanding the physiopathogenesis of the sex- and menopause-associated differences in chronic liver disease is important to developing new approaches to prevention, diagnosis, and treatment.

Three hundred fifty million and 170 million people worldwide are persistently infected with hepatitis B virus (HBV) and hepatitis C virus (HCV), respectively. Chronic HBV infection is the most common cause of cirrhosis and hepatocellular carcinoma (HCC) in the world. Clinical observations and death statistics support the view that chronic hepatitis B and C appear to progress more rapidly in males than in females, and that cirrhosis is largely a disease of men and postmenopausal women, with the exception of classically autoimmune liver diseases. Biological female sex factors such as estrogen, hepatic iron storage status, and growth hormone, which change a lot after menopause, play antioxidative and cytoprotective roles in the functional and morphological modulation of the liver physiopathology. A better understanding the biological mechanisms underlying the sex- and menopause-associated differences in chronic liver disease would provide valuable information to design care of health and liver disease more effectively for individuals, both females and males.

Chapter II - The loss of circulating hormones (estrogens) that occur during the menopausal transition manifests itself through a variety of symptoms, including those related to changes in the cardiovascular system. Cardiovascular disease is often regarded as a problem that only men face, since most women do not consider cardiovascular disease as a serious health problem and in fact report that they are not well informed about their risks. This is despite the fact that, over their life span, women are more likely to experience cardiovascular disease and disability than men and will require intervention to improve survival. The Framingham Heart Study revealed that there is a gradual increase in the incidence of cardiovascular morbidity and mortality between the ages of 40 and 55 years in premenopausal women, which were significantly elevated in postmenopausal women of all age groups. Furthermore, at any age, the incidence of cardiovascular disease was significantly higher in postmenopausal compared to premenopausal women, suggesting that cessation of ovarian function and the consequent ovarian hormone deficiency exacerbates the impact of cardiovascular risk factors.

Chapter III - Since women's life expectancy is increasing all over the world, most of them are expected to live a significant part of their life in menopausal status. This period marks the end of the reproductive status and, in addition to bringing about negative feelings about this, might be accompanied by many complaints due to the decline of circulating estrogen levels. The most common complaint during this period is related to vasomotor symptoms such as hot flashes and night sweats. Although not all women are bothered by them, vasomotor symptoms represent a very frequent and distressing occurrence. The mechanism by which vasomotor symptoms are triggered has not been fully clarified but the link with low estrogen concentrations has been well established. Low estrogen levels result in disturbance of the temperature regulating mechanism situated in the anterior-preoptic hypothalamus, where there is a thermoneutral zone that is reduced after menopause, becoming hypersensitive to hot stimuli and abnormally inducing hot flashes. In this way the sweating threshold seems to be *reduced to a greater level* and the shivering threshold is increased. Also, estrogen is known to influence serotonin, endorphin, noradrenalin and dopamine levels, and neurotransmitters that have been associated with regulatory mechanisms in body temperature control. Additionally, hypoestrogenism may interfere with vascular reactivity to the inputs from this altered thermoneutral zone. This culminates with symptoms including sudden feelings of warmth and skin redness that begin in the chest and spread to the neck and face, accompanied by sweating, palpitations, anxiety and sleeping disturbance that potentially impair the quality of life of women. The management of these symptoms includes hormonal replacement therapy (HRT) that constitutes the basis of the treatment of menopause symptoms especially regarding hot flashes. Some measures including lifestyle changes are useful to reduce vasomotor symptoms and should be considered in all cases. The efficacy of complementary alternative medicine therapies remains inconclusive due to the lack of evidence.

Chapter IV - Background: Among Caucasian populations, it is reported that changes in hormone levels (decreased E2 and increased FSH) occur within one to two years on each side of the final menstrual period, and that variations of hormone levels between individuals are large.

Objective: To investigate the levels of the two important hormones, FSH and E2, during perimenopause in a Japanese cohort.

Method: The Adult Health Study (AHS) is a longitudinal population-based study. Non-menopausal women, aged 47-54 years, were measured in terms of FSH and E2 levels every six months. For 89 women whose FSH and E2 levels were measured within three months from their final menstrual period (FMP), the trends of FSH and E2 within 21 months of FMP were investigated at six-month intervals. For 17 women whose hormone levels were measured for a period of more than 50 months, the individual trends of FSH and E2 were observed.

Results: The FSH and E2 levels within three months of FMP exhibited a wide range. Although FSH increased and E2 decreased during perimenopause, FSH and E2 levels at individual time points were found to not be a reliable marker of biological menopause, since the trends for the combination of FSH and E2 displayed such wide variations longitudinally. Temporal fluctuations in a single individual exhibited various patterns, and the trends of the hormone levels were not uni-directional during perimenopause, displaying remarkably increased E2 levels in some case. Longitudinal hormone changes within 21 months of FMP in this study are compatible with previous studies in which the length of perimenopausal transition was estimated to be approximately four years.

Conclusions: Among Japanese women who had natural menopause around the age of 50, hormone levels in and between individuals exhibited a wide variation throughout perimenopause, with a convergence of the biochemical menopausal pattern characterized by high FSH and low E2 by approximately two years after the FMP.

Chapter V - Objective: Climacteric symptoms resemble those of thyroid dysfunction, raising the possibility of changes in thyrotropin (TSH) during the perimenopause. The objective of the study was to investigate TSH levels in association with reproductive hormone.

Methods: Non-menopausal women of the Adult Health Study of the Radiation Effects Research Foundation, aged 47-54 years, were followed between 1993 and 2003 for changes in reproductive hormonal levels during the perimenopause. The TSH levels of 35 perimenopausal women whose frozen sera had been preserved after the measurements of follicle stimulating hormone (FSH), and estradiol (E2), were measured in 2008.

Results: Although FSH increased and E2 decreased, there was no uniform pattern in individual trend of TSH. Two cases developed hyperthyroidism during the perimenopause without specific onset of symptoms or reproductive hormone changes.

Conclusions: Although there was no association between TSH and reproductive hormone found, it is suggested that caution is required in diagnosing thyroid dysfunction during the perimenopause.

Chapter VI - Objectives: To address the many symptoms of menopause experienced by women as a result of treatment for their cancer.

Discussion: There is a relationship of premature ovarian failure with atherosclerosis and osteoporosis. Options for treating vasomotor symptoms may include environmental factors, physical activity, paced respiration, herbal and botanical, phytoestrogens, non-hormonal and hormonal therapy. Management of sleep disturbances will be reviewed. Risk factors for a depressed mood and management including conventional modalities and estrogen will be discussed. Vulvo-vaginal symptoms, joint pain and stiffness and sexuality concerns will be reviewed.

Conclusion: With increasing numbers of cancer patients living longer, quality of survivorship becomes an important issue. Menopausal symptoms are important for women and treatment options need to be made available.

Chapter VII - Breast cancer is a common malignancy and remains a major health issue with significant morbitiy and mortality. Surveillance, Epidemiology and End Results (SEER) data shows that white women in the US have a 13.1% lifetime risk of developing breast cancer, while African American women have a 9.6% lifetime incidence. The lifetime risk of dying of breast cancer is 3.4% in both groups. It has been known for over 100 years that breast tissue is sensitive to endogenous hormones. However, it has only become clear in recent decades that prolonged exposure to endogenous and exogenous sex steroids, particularly estrogens can lead to the development of breast cancer.

In view of the hormone dependent nature of breast cancers, issues around the management of cancer treatment related menopausal symptoms are particularly pertinent. The reasons that women with breast cancer are more prone to both the short and long term consequences of menopause are as follows:

- The average age of diagnosis with breast cancer in women is 62, making most women peri- or post-menopausal at the time of their diagnosis.

- At diagnosis, many women are taking an estrogen replacement which they are conventionally instructed to discontinue. This may result in an abrupt recurrence of menopause-associated symptoms.
- For post-menopausal women, therapeutic hormonal manipulation with agents such as tamoxifen and the aromatase inhibitors, leads to an adjustment of a woman's endogenous estrogen state and consequently menopausal symptoms are a common consequence.
- For pre-menopausal women receiving either endocrine or chemotherapy premature and permanent menopause is common. Chemotherapy and endocrine therapy with aromatase inhibitors also have additional adverse effects on bone health.
- As a consequence of improved therapy and/or earlier detection more women are surviving breast cancer and living longer. As a result patients are living longer with their menopausal symptoms.

Based on the above factors, the management of menopause and its complications in breast cancer survivors is becoming an increasingly concerning issue – both in the short and long term. While estrogens and hormone replacement therapy has been studied extensively for the treatment and prevention of post-menopausal symptoms, their use in breast cancer patients is questionable. Current guidelines state that the use of hormone replacement therapies in breast cancer patients is not recommended. Alternatives to this therapy include several non-hormonal agents and lifestyle modifications which will be discussed further. These therapies and recommendations may help improve the general health and quality of life in post-menopausal women with breast cancer.

In: Menopause: Vasomotor Symptoms, Systematic… ISBN: 978-1-60876-930-8
Editors: J. Michalski, I. Nowak, pp. 1-54 © 2010 Nova Science Publishers, Inc.

Chapter I

Menopause-Associated Difference in Chronic Liver Disease

Ichiro Shimizu[*]

Department of Gastroenterology, Seirei Yokohama Hospital, 215 Iwai-cho, Hodogaya-ku,
Yokohama, Kanagawa 240-8521, Japan

Abstract

Chronic hepatitis B and C appear to progress more rapidly in males than in females. Liver cancer is predominant in men and postmenopausal women. Almost anyone may "feel," but not recognize the sex-associated difference in liver cancer as a fact. A large body of evidence has been accumulated suggesting that increased oxidative stress is an essential step in the development of hepatic fibrosis to the end-stage cirrhosis and its complication liver cancer. Environmental and lifestyle risk factors such as hepatitis B/C virus infection, obesity, and heavy alcohol intake lead to increased oxidative stress, which in general occurs more frequently in males. In contrast, biological female sex factors such as estrogen, hepatic iron storage status, and growth hormone, which change a lot after menopause, play antioxidative and cytoprotective roles in the functional and morphological modulation of the liver physiopathology.

Currently, metabolic disorders such as being overweight and diabetes are emerging as cofactors of hepatic fibrosis. Fatty liver is considered the hepatic manifestation of the metabolic syndrome. The transition from premenopause to postmenopause is associated with the emergence of many features of the metabolic syndrome, including increased intra-abdominal body fat. Intra-abdominal fat accumulation is a predictor of fatty liver.

Females are more resistant to certain infections. Indeed, females, particularly before menopause, can produce antibodies against hepatitis B virus at a higher frequency than males with hepatitis B virus infection. The decline in ovarian function with menopause is associated with spontaneous increase in proinflammatory cytokines.

---

[*] Corresponding author: Department of Gastroenterology, *Seirei Yokohama Hospital,* 215 Iwai-cho, Hodogaya-ku, *Yokohama,* Kanagawa 240-8521, Japan, Phone: 81-45-715-3111, Fax: 81-45-715-3387, E-mail: ichiro.shimizu@sis.seirei.or.jp

Being female or male is an important basic human variable that affects health and liver disease throughout the life span. Sex is defined as female or male according to their biological functions, while gender is shaped by environment and experience. A better understanding the physiopathogenesis of the sex- and menopause-associated differences in chronic liver disease is important to developing new approaches to prevention, diagnosis, and treatment.

Three hundred fifty million and 170 million people worldwide are persistently infected with hepatitis B virus (HBV) [1] and hepatitis C virus (HCV) [2], respectively. Chronic HBV infection is the most common cause of cirrhosis and hepatocellular carcinoma (HCC) in the world. Clinical observations and death statistics support the view that chronic hepatitis B and C appear to progress more rapidly in males than in females [3, 4], and that cirrhosis is largely a disease of men and postmenopausal women, with the exception of classically autoimmune liver diseases [5]. Biological female sex factors such as estrogen, hepatic iron storage status, and growth hormone, which change a lot after menopause, play antioxidative and cytoprotective roles in the functional and morphological modulation of the liver physiopathology. A better understanding the biological mechanisms underlying the sex- and menopause-associated differences in chronic liver disease would provide valuable information to design care of health and liver disease more effectively for individuals, both females and males.

1. Increase of HCC Incidence Rates among Females Aged over 50 Years

Male sex, older age and cirrhosis are important host-related risk factors for the development of HCC (Table 1-1). The large majority of liver cancer cases occur in individuals with chronic HBV or HCV infection. Among patients with chronic hepatitis C or HCV-related cirrhosis, male sex and older age at diagnosis (>55 years) increase a 2- to 3-fold and a 2- to 4-fold risks of developing HCC, respectively [6-8]. Among patients with chronic hepatitis B or HBV-related cirrhosis, male sex and older age at diagnosis (>50 years) are also independent factors affecting progression to HCC [8, 9].

The areas of high incidence of HCC are Middle (sub-Saharan) Africa and Eastern (China, Taiwan, Korea, and Japan) and South-Eastern Asia. The incidence is low in developed areas (only in Southern Europe is there any substantial risk), South America, and South-Central Asia (Figure 1-1). Based on the age-adjusted incidence rates of liver cancer registered in different countries in the world, male cases have higher liver cancer rates than female cases in most populations [10]. In high-risk countries, sex ratios of HCC incidence tend to be higher, and the male excess is more pronounced below 50 years of age. Immigrant populations also show a shift in the sex ratio values. Japanese populations in the United States show a fairly stable sex ratio between 2 and 3 in the age groups above 50 years. Among Japanese-American females below age 50 years, however, the HCC incidence is too rare, and the sex ratio calculations are unreliable [11]. In Japan, Japanese populations show the male-to-female ratios of age-adjusted HCC incidence rates ranging from 6 to 7 in the age groups 40 to 55 years, whereas, in the age groups above 55 years, the incidence rates among females markedly increase with the less male excess and the sex ratios range between 2 and 5 [10].

These data suggest that Japanese females aged below 50 or 55 years are less vulnerable to HCC.

Table 1.1. Host-related major risk factors for development of HCC in cases with chronic HBV or HCV infection

Male sex	Up to 3-fold increased risk
Older age at diagnosis (>50 or 55 years)	Up to 4-fold increased risk
Cirrhosis	Up to 4-fold increased risk; 80%-90% of HCC cases in most populations

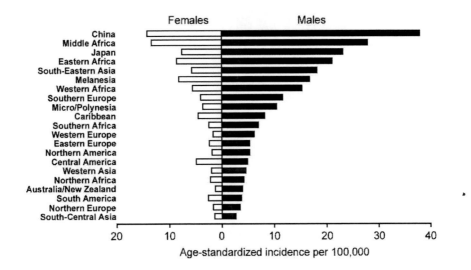

Figure 1.1. Age-standardized incidence per 100,000 of liver cancer by sex in different geographic regions worldwide in the year 2002 [12].

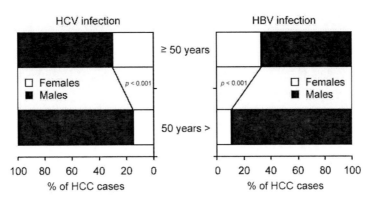

Figure 1-2. Comparison of sex ratios between younger (<50 years) and older (≥50 years) groups of HCV-related HCC patients (left panel) and HBV-related HCC patients (right panel). Japanese individuals with HCV-related HCC were seropositive for anti-HCV and seronegative for HBsAg, and HBV-related individuals were seropositive for HBsAg and seronegative for anti-HCV. HCC was detected for the period 1993 to 2000 for HCV-related individuals [13] and 1994 to 2006 for HBV-related individuals [14] in Tokushima in Japan.

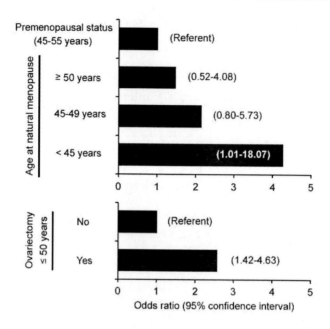

Figure 1-3. Relationship between natural or artificial menopause and HCC among Taiwanese female persons [15].

In Tokushima of my hometown in Japan, a study on the age-specific sex ratios among Japanese HCC patients with HCV-related cirrhosis (n=1199) and chronic HBV infection (n=901) also confirmed the marked increase of HCC incidence rates among females aged 50 years and older. When the HCC patients were divided at diagnosis into two age groups, based on whether they are younger or older than the average menopausal age of 50 years, the older groups (≥50 years) with HCV (30.0%) and HBV (32.8%) infections had a 2- to 3-fold higher proportion of females than the younger groups (<50 years) with HCV (15.0%) and HBV (10.5%) infections [13, 14] (Figure 1-2). These data show that cases of female sex and under 50 years old, namely "premenopausal women" are least vulnerable to HCC.

In Taiwan, where HBV infectin is hyper-endemic, a study of female persons on associations between natural or artificial menopause and HCC showed that the HCC risk was inversely related to the age at natural menopause. Ovariectomy performed at age 50 years or younger during premenopausal years was also a risk factor for HCC [15] (Figure 1-3). These data show that HCC incidence of female persons increase after menopause, suggesting that biological factors including estrogen-related sex hormone may play some role in the development of HCC and sex difference in HCC risk [5].

2. "Mona Lisa Smile"

In general, males have a greater risk of exposure to hepatitis viruses. Moreover, they have a greater opportunity for drinking, and they may fall into alcoholic liver injure easily, although alcoholism is increasing among females, owing to a decline in the social stigma attached to drinking and to the ready availability of alcohol in supermarkets. Factors of social environment and lifestyles may result in a higher preponderance of nutritional and exercise-associated problems in males, and these factors may promote intra-abdominal (visceral) fat accumulation, causing fatty liver in males. Fatty liver histologically results from the deposition of triglycerides via the accumulation of fatty acids in hepatocytes (liver cells), playing a role in the progression of hepatic fibrosis [14].

"Sex" is defined as female or male according to their reproductive organs and biological functions, and "gender" as a person's self-representation as female or male, or how that person is responded to by social institutions on the basis of the individual's gender presentation. Gender is shaped by environment and experience [16]. Environment factors different between the genders are one of the mechanisms underlying the sex-associated differences in hepatic fibrogenesis and carciogenesis. However, there are the clinical and experimental data which cannot be completely explained by the difference in exposure to environmental factors. Female individuals, especially before menopause, produce antibodies against hepatitis B surface antigen (HBsAg) and HBV e antigen (HBeAg) at higher frequency than males [17]. In chronic infection with HCV, the clearance rate of blood HCV RNA appears to be higher in females [18]. Most asymptomatic carriers of HCV with persistent normal liver function tests such as alanine aminotransferase (ALT) in the blood are females [19-21] (Figure 2-1) and have a good prognosis with a low risk of progression of hepatic fibrosis to the end-stage cirrhosis and its complications such as HCC. Hepatic fibrosis in chronic hepatitis B and C progresses more slowly in females than in males [14, 22]. The menopause is associated with accelerated progression of hepatic fibrosis, and the HCC risk is inversely related to the age at natural menopause. Chronic HBV- and HCV-infected patients of female sex and under 50 years old, namely premenopausal women are less vulnerable to HCC.

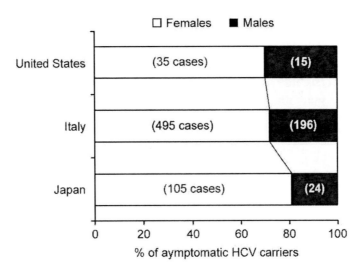

Figure 2-1. Female predominance among asymptomatic HCV carriers. Asymptomatic HCV carriers are defined as persistently HCV RNA positive persons with normal blood ALT levels over a 6- to 36-month period. The definitions of "normal" ALT levels are different among studies: < 40 IU/L in Italy [19]; ≤ 30 IU/L in Japan [20]; no available information on the definition in the above study from the United States [21].

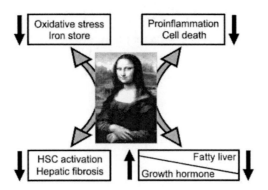

Figure 2-2. Mysterious forces of the Mona Lisa (by Leonardo da Vinci) as a symbol of eternal femininity [22]. Females have four major kinds of abilities against oxidative stress, inflammation and apoptosis, hepatic fibrosis, and intra-abdominal (visceral) fat accumulation and fatty liver formation via estrogen, hepatic iron storage status and growth hormone. There is no sharp outline separating the female person (female sex factors) from the background (environmental factors).

It is difficult to clearly distinguish the biological "female sex" factors and the environmental factors in individuals. In practice, both factors are considered to have influence each other mutually, resulting in protection of the female liver from the attacks of inflammatory and oxidative stimuli and cell death. With regard to the female sex factors, four major kinds of abilities can be mentioned as follows (Figure 2-2): (1) Females have the antioxidant ability against oxidative stress. Estrogen inhibits reactive oxygen species (ROS) production processes. Iron is a potent inducer of the production of highly reactive ROS that are harmful to the liver. Females have lower iron stores in the liver, possibly because of iron loss during menstruation and increased requirements during pregnancy; (2) Females have the anti-inflammatory and antiapoptotic force. Estrogen inhibits the accumulation of monocytes-macrophages and the production of proinflammatory cytokines as well as early apoptosis; (3) Females have the antifibrogenic force. Estrogen inhibits the activation of hepatic stellate cells (HSCs); and (4) Females have the inhibitory ability against intra-abdominal (visceral) fat accumulation. Visceral fat is an independent predictor of fatty liver, and fatty liver is a risk factor of the progression of hepatic fibrosi. Estrogen lowers the visceral fat accumulation and induce the hepatocellular fatty acid β-oxidation (degradation), leading to reduction of fatty liver formation. Growth hormone also inhibits the hepatocellular fat accumulation via fat transport. Likely clinical manifestation of growth hormone deficiency in adults is increased visceral fat accumulation. Growth hormone secretion is greater in females and is stimulated by estrogen.

3. Liver Plays a Major Role in Iron Homeostasis in the Body

Iron is an essential nutrient required for a variety of biochemical processes. It is a vital component of the heme in hemoglobin of red blood cells, myoglobin and cytochromes, and is also an essential cofactor for non-heme enzymes such as ribonucleotide reductase, the limiting enzyme for DNA synthesis. The average daily dietary iron intake of an adult person is approximately 11-15 mg, and 6-12% of that amount (nearly 1 mg per day) is absorbed (Figure 3-1). Adults have a total of 3-5 g of iron. Approximately 65-75% is found in the heme. The liver stores 10-20% in the form of ferritin, which can be mobilized easily when needed. There is no regulated pathway for the excretion of iron in the body except by blood loss or desquamated intestinal cells. The amount of iron loss is nearly 1 mg per day. When in excess iron is toxic because it produces ROS such as hydroxyl radicals that react readily with biological molecules, including proteins, lipids and DNA, leading to cell death and DNA mutagenesis [23] (Figure 3-2).

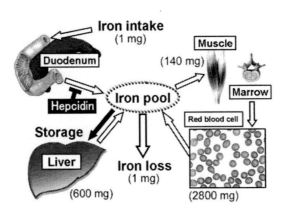

Figure 3-1. Liver plays a major role in iron homeostasis in the body [22]. Both the iron amount of uptake in the duodenum and loss by blood loss and desquamated intestinal cells are about 1 mg per day. Hepcidin, a circulatory peptide synthesized by the liver, regulates iron homeostasis by inhibiting the uptake of dietary iron in the duodenum.

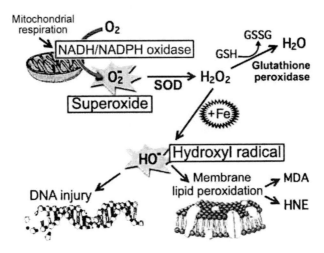

Figure 3-2. Oxidative stress and hepatocyte damage [22]. A primary source of ROS production is mitochondrial NADH/NADPH oxidase. Hydrogen peroxide (H_2O_2) is converted to a highly reactive ROS, the hydroxyl radical, in the presence of iron (+Fe). The hydroxyl radical induces DNA cleavage and lipid peroxidation in the structure of membrane phospholipids, leading to cell death and discharge of products of lipid peroxidation, malondialdehyde (MDA) and 4-hydroxynonenal (HNE) into the space of Disse. Cells have comprehensive antioxidant protective systems, including superoxide dismutase (SOD), glutathione peroxidase and glutathione (GSH). Upon oxidation, GSH forms glutathione disulfide (GSSG).

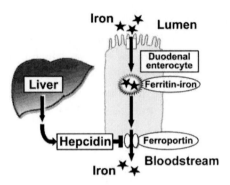

Figure 3-3. Hepcidin binds to the iron exporter, ferroportin, and inhibits iron influx into blood [22]. The rate of iron flux into the blood depends primarily on hepcidin levels. When blood iron levels are high, the hepcidin synthesis by the liver increases, diminishing the release of iron from duodenal enterocytes. When blood iron levels drop, the hepcidin synthesis is down-regulated, allowing enterocytes to release increased amounts of iron.

Iron uptake and transport is tightly controlled. Liver plays an important role in iron homeostasis in the body, while liver is particularly susceptible to excess iron levels. Hepcidin, a circulatory antimicrobial peptide synthesized by the liver, regulates iron homeostasis by inhibiting the uptake of dietary iron in the duodenum and the export of iron from reticuloendothelial cells. The reticuloendothelial cell system is part of the immune system, including all phagocytic cells such as monocytes- macrophages and Kupffer cells except the granular white blood cells. Reticuloendothelial cells filter out and destroy viruses, bacteria, foreign substances, and worn-out or abnormal cells. In particular, reticuloendothelial cells in the spleen destroy old red blood cells and recycle their hemoglobin.

Unlike humans or rats, mice have 2 hepcidin genes, hepcidin1 and hepcidin2. The C-terminal 25 amino acid mature peptide region of mouse hepcidin1 shares higher homology with human hepcidin than mouse hepcidin2. Targeted disruption of hepcidin1 gene results in severe iron overload, demonstrating increased blood iron and ferritin levels as compared with controls [24], whereas mice overexpressing hepcidin1, but not hepcidin2, display anemia [25]. These data suggest a role for hepcidin1 but not hepcidin2 in the regulation of iron metabolism. It is noteworthy that female mice express higher levels of both hepcidin1 and hepcidin2 in the liver than males [26]. An increase in hepcidin levels would lead to a decrease in duodenal iron absorption and the mobilization of reticuloendothelial iron stores. This is achieved by hepcidin binding to the iron exporter, ferroportin, and inducing its internalization and degradation (Figure 3-3). It is not known whether female and male persons differ in the level of human hepcidin expression in the liver.

Iron deficiency is prevalent in females of reproductive age mainly due to the physiological loss of blood by menstruation and pregnancy throughout the world. Based on the differences between the amount of iron available for absorption and the increased requirement for iron, most females before menopause do not have adequate iron stores. Females experience iron deficiency anemia more commonly than males [27].

In the absence of hepatic inflammation, blood ferritin is a reliable marker of iron stores in the liver. In a study from Japan, blood ferritin levels were examined by sex and age in healthy individuals [14] (Figure 3-4). In males, the blood ferritin values reached the maximum level in the age group of 40 to 49 years and declined thereafter. By contrast, in females the blood ferritin remained relatively low until menopause, at a level which was one-fifth of that for males of comparable age, and reached the maximum level after menopause to approximately one-half of that for males of comparable age. These data correlate with the data obtained from the third National Health and Nutrition Examination Survey (NHANES III) in the United States [28], and indicate that females, especially before menopause, have lower iron stores in the liver.

Oxidative stress induced by HCV proteins and alcohol is suggested to be one of the mechanisms responsible for the down-regulation of hepcidin expression [29, 30]. Ethanol produces ROS via the alcohol dehydrogenase (ADH)- and cytochrome P450 2E1 (CYP2E1)-metabolizing system. In addition, inflammation is a dominant and robust inducer of hepcidin gene transcription regardless of body iron levels [31]. Interleukin-6 (IL-6) and possibly other proinflammatory cytokines such as interleukin-1 (IL-1) are the major players in this process. Estradiol is a strong endogenous antioxidant that inhibits ROS production processes and stimulates antioxidant enzyme activities. There is a large body of evidence indicating that the decline in ovarian function with menopause is associated with spontaneous increase in proinflammatory cytokines, tumor necrosis factor-α (TNF-α) as well as IL-1 and IL-6 [32]. Estradiol, at physiological concentrations, inhibits the spontaneous secretion of proinflammatory cytokines in murine peritoneal macrophages [33] and human peripheral blood mononuclear cells [34, 35]. Furthermore, male mice display lower hepcidin expression compared to female mice following treatment with ethanol [29]. The more pronounced down-regulation of hepcidin among males is abrogated by antioxidants. In a preliminary report, concomitant administration of estradiol resulted in a reduction in blood levels of liver enzyme (ALT) and ferritin and hepatic iron stores in a young male patient with chronic hepatitis C and irradiation-induced testicular dysfunction, in whom testosterone replacement therapy was initiated at puberty [36] (Figure 3-5). Taken together, these data suggest that, besides iron, hepcidin may be also regulated by female sex-specific factors including estrogen.

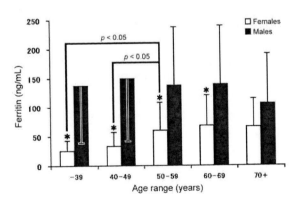

Figure 3-4. Age-specific blood ferritin levels among females and males in 305 healthy Japanese individuals (mean age 50.6 years, 52.8% females) [14]. Blood ferritin levels reflect the iron stores in the liver. Premenopausal females have a one-fifth level of the blood ferritin for males of comparable age. *$P < 0.05$ compared with males of comparable age.

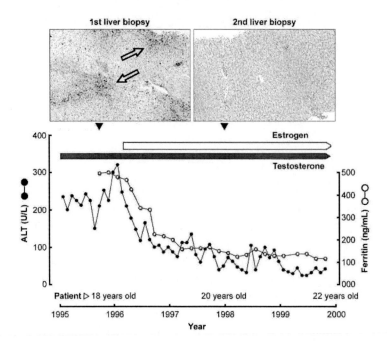

Figure 3-5. Serial levels of blood ALT and ferritin in the male patient with chronic hepatitis C and irradiation-induced testicular dysfunction [36]. Estrogen (□) and testosterone (■) therapies were started in January 1995 and February 1996, respectively. Two needle liver biopsies (▼) were performed in July 1995 (1st) and January 1998 (2nd), and liver sections were stained with Prussian blue for hepatic iron. Stainable iron (darkness) decreased from 35-50% (1st, arrow) to less than 10% (2nd) of the hepatocytes.

An analysis of the NHANES III data in the United States showed that patients with chronic hepatitis C have higher blood levels of iron and ferritin compared to healthy subjects [37]. The lobular and cellular distributions of the stainable iron in the liver of chronic hepatitis C patients are correlated with hepatitis severity [38], although most patients with chronic hepatitis C do not have an elevated hepatic iron concentration despite the abnormal blood iron parameters [39].

Genetic hemochromatosis, a prevalent iron overload disorder among the Caucasian population, is the abnormalities of genes such as *HFE* [40]. The clinical expression of genetic hemochromatosis is 5 to 10 times more frequent in males than in females. Male patients with genetic hemochromatosis accumulate more iron and have a higher incidence of the liver injury [41]. Moreover, iron overload induces mitochondrial injury and increases the risk of HCC development in transgenic mice expression the HCV polyprotein [42]. Iron reduction therapy by repeated phlebotomy improves hepatocyte injury in patients with HCV infection [43]. Phlebotomy is the opening of a vein to remove blood.

It is widely recognized that hepatic iron overload develops in a significant portion of individuals who consume alcohol on a chronic basis. Chronic alcohol consumption in moderate to excess quantities results in increased blood ferritin, which may thus result in increased hepatic iron stores [44]. As noted above, ethanol-treated mice showed a sex difference with a greater suppression of hepcidin gene expression among males. Females drink less alcohol and have fewer alcohol-related problems than males [45]. The data demonstrate that chronic alcohol consumption-related hepatic iron stores are less likely in females than in males.

There is growing concern in clinical practice with regard to the development of non-alcoholic fatty liver disease (NAFLD). Its name implies a histological picture that is indistinguishable from alcoholic liver disease. Although in most cases, fatty liver does not progress to more severe liver disease, approximately 15-20% of patients have histological signs of hepatic fibrosis and necroinflammation, indicating the presence of non-alcoholic steatohepatitis (NASH). These patients are at a higher risk of developing cirrhosis and HCC [46]. NAFLD is more prevalent in males, and there is a male predominance for NASH as well [47]. The pathogenesis of NAFLD and NASH is associated with insulin resistance and metabolic syndrome via oxidative stress and inflammation [48]. Although the data regarding actual hepatic iron overload in HAFLD has been somewhat conflicting, NASH patients have increased hepatic iron accumulation [49, 50].

As a target organ, the liver is particularly susceptible to excess iron levels. Females have less total body storage iron and lower iron stores in the liver, possibly because of iron loss during menstruation and increased requirements during pregnancy. Sex-related differences in body iron storage and metabolism may be a potential candidate to explain in part the observed sex-related differences in many chronic liver diseases. The lower hepatic iron stores provide help to females by protecting the liver against chronic liver injury.

4. Hepatic Fibrosis and Oxidative Stress

Hepatic fibrosis is a complex dynamic process which is mediated by death of hepatocytes and activation of hepatic stellate cells (HSCs). Damage of any etiology (HBV or HCV infection, heavy alcohol intake, or iron overload) to hepatocytes can produce oxygen-derived free radicals and other ROS derived from lipid peroxidative processes [51]. Persistent production of ROS constitutes a general feature of a sustained inflammatory response and liver injury, once antioxidant mechanisms have been depleted. The major source of ROS production in hepatocytes is NADH and NADPH oxidases (respiratory chain-linked enzymes) localized in mitochondria. NADH and NADPH oxidases leak ROS as part of its operation. Kupffer cells (hepatic resident macrophages), infiltrating inflammatory cells such as macrophages and neutrophils, and HSCs (Figure 4-1) also produce ROS in the injured liver. ROS include the free radicals superoxide (O_2^-) and hydroxyl radical (HO^-) and non-radicals such as hydrogen peroxide (H_2O_2). A number of reactive nitrogen species including nitric oxide (NO) and peroxynitrite ($ONOO^-$) are also ROS. Superoxide production is mediated mainly by NADH oxidase. Hydrogen peroxide is more stable and membrane permeable in comparison to other ROS. Thus, hydrogen peroxide plays an important role in the intracellular signaling under physiological conditions. With respect to pathological actions, ROS participate in the development of liver disease. In this regard, hydrogen peroxide is converted into the hydroxyl radical, a harmful and highly reactive ROS, in the presence of transition metals such as iron (see Figure 3-2). The hydroxyl radical is able to induce not only lipid peroxidation in the structure of membrane phospholipids, which results in irreversible modifications of cell membrane structure and function (membrane injury), but

DNA cleavage (DNA injury) as well. Such a chain of events due to increased ROS production exceeding cellular antioxidant defense systems are called oxidative stress, inducing cell death.

At the cellular levels, origin of hepatic fibrosis is initiated by the damage of hepatocytes, followed by the accumulation of neutrophils and macrophages including Kupffer cells on the sites of injury and inflammation in the liver. When hepatocytes are continuously damaged, leading to cell death, production of extracellular matrix proteins such as collagens predominates over hepatocellular regeneration. Collagen types 1 and III are major components of the extracellular matrix, which is principally produced by cells known as HSCs. HSCs are located in the space of Disse in close contact with hepatocytes and sinusoidal endothelial cells. Overproduced collagens are deposited in injured areas instead of destroyed hepatocytes. In other words, hepatic fibrosis is fibrous scarring of the liver in which excessive collagens build up along with the duration and extent of persistence of liver injury. The trigger is oxidative stress as noted above. Hepatic fibrosis itself causes no symptoms but can lead to the end-stage cirrhosis.

In the injured liver, HSCs are regarded as the primary target cells for inflammatory and oxidative stimuli, and they are proliferated, enlarged and transformed into myofibroblast-like cells. These HSCs are referred to as activated cells and are responsible for the overproduction of collagens during hepatic fibrosis to cirrhosis. HSCs are activated mainly by ROS, products of lipid peroxidation, malondialdehyde (MDA) and 4-hydroxynonenal (HNE) [53, 54], and transforming growth factor-β (TGF-β), •which are released from destroyed hepatocytes, activated Kupffer cells and infiltrating macrophages and neutrophils in the injured liver (Figure 4-2). In addition to ROS, exogenous TGF-β increases the production of ROS, particularly hydrogen peroxide, by HSCs, whereas the addition of hydrogen peroxide induces ROS and TGF-β production and secretion by HSCs [55]. This so-called autocrine loop of ROS by HSCs is regarded as mechanism corresponding to the autocrine loop of TGF-β which HSCs produce in response to this cytokine with an increased collagen expression in the injured liver [56].

The female sex hormones estradiol and progesterone have opposing effects on production of ROS and activity of antioxidant enzymes. When production of ROS is enhanced and/or their metabolism by antioxidant enzymes is impaired, a condition called oxidative stress can develop. The production of ROS and decrease of antioxidant enzymes superoxide dismutase (SOD) and glutathione peroxidase (see Figure 3-2) are inhibited by estradiol, and then they are further stimulated by progesterone both in cultured rat HSCs and human hepatoma cells [56, 57]. The major source of ROS production is mitochondrial NADH and NADPH oxidases in the liver. Estradiol inhibits the activation of mitogen activated protein kinase (MAPK) intracellular signaling pathways and transcriptional factors of activator protein-1 (AP-1) and nuclear factor κB (NF-κB) [58] via the suppression of NADH/NADPH oxidase activity, and inactivates the downstream transcription processes involved in TGF-β expression and HSC proliferation and transformation into the principal matrix-producing cell type [56]. Moreover, TNF-α expression in cultured rat HSCs is inhibited by estradiol. In addition to HSCs, estradiol inhibits the activation of AP-1 and NF-κB in cultured rat hepatocytes in a state of oxidative stress [59, 60]. In contrast, progesterone acts in opposition to the favorable effects of estradiol [56] (Figure 4-2).

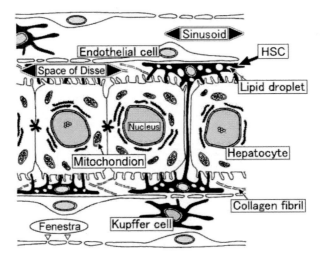

Figure 4-1. Schema of the sinusoidal wall of the liver. Kupffer cells rest on fenestrated endothelial cells (white arrowhead shows a fenestra) [52]. Hepatic stellate cells (HSCs) are located in the space of Disse in close contact with endothelial cells and hepatocytes, functioning as the primary retinoid storage area. Retinoids, a group of chemical compound associated with vitamin A, are occupied in the cytoplasmic space by numerous lipid droplets. Collagen fibrils course through the space of Disse between endothelial cells and the cords of hepatocytes.

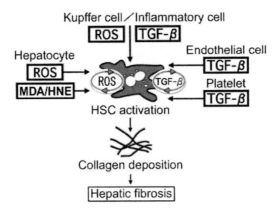

Figure 4-2. Activation of HSCs [22]. HSCs are activated by such factors as ROS, lipid peroxidation products (MDA and HNE), and TGF-β released when adjacent cells including hepatocyte, Kupffer cells, and endothelial cells are injured. ROS and TGF-β are also produced by HSCs in response to exogenous ROS and TGF-β in an autocrine manner.

The activation processes to HSCs, which are regarded as the principal matrix-producing cells, are inhibited by estradiol, and are further stimulated by progesterone. Such prooxidative and fibrogenic effects via the induction of NADH/NADPH oxidase activity by progesterone are blocked by estradiol at a one hundredth and one tenth dose of progesterone in cultured rat HSCs. These occur at physiological relevant concentration of estradiol (10^{-9} - 10^{-7} mol/L) and progesterone (10^{-8} - 10^{-6} mol/L), equivalent to blood levels of estradiol (10^{-10} - 10^{-8} mol/L) and progesterone (10^{-9} - 10^{-7} mol/L) measured in female persons during their reproductive years [61], and tissue levels of steroid sex hormones may actually be greater [62].

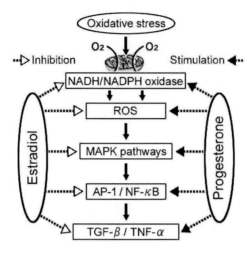

Figure 4-3. Estradiol and progesterone have opposing effects on the activation of ROS production processes, MAPK pathways, transcriptional factors of AP-1 and NF-κB, and downstream transcription processes involved in TGF-β and TFN-α in the injured liver [56, 57].

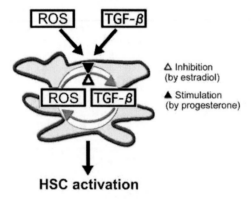

Figure 4-4. The autocrine loop of ROS and TGF-β in HSCs is prevented by estradiol and induced by progesterone, leading to inhibition and stimulation of HSC activation, respectively [22].

As illustrated in Figure 4-2, ROS and TGF-β are produced by HSCs in response to exogenous ROS and TGF-β in an autocrine manner. ROS increase the production of TGF-β and are produced by TGF-β from HSCs, and vice versa. The autocrine loop of ROS and TGF-β in HSCs is prevented by estradiol and induced by progesterone through the regulation of NADH/NADPH oxidase activity (Figure 4-4). These data suggest that estradiol and progesterone may work together with the resultant suppression of hepatic fibrosis in female individuals.

5. Innate Immune Response and Sex Hormones

In inflammatory and oxidative liver injury, the accumulation of neutrophils, lymphocytes, monocytes and macrophages including Kupffer cells to sites of inflammation and injury is thought to be mediated by chemokines, such as monocyte chemoattractant protein-1 (MCP-1) and interleukin-8 (IL-8). Chemokines are a subset of cytokines, which attract and activate immune cells. Monocytes develop into macrophages when they migrate into the tissues. The inflammatory cells such as neutrophils, monocytes and macrophages are in turn able to release proinflammatory cytokines, including TNF-α, IL-1 and IL-6, as well as ROS, leading to cell death and persistent liver injury (Figure 5-1). Hepatocyte destruction derives from such actions as lipid peroxidation and DNA injury by ROS, apoptosis by TNF-α, and phagocytosis by inflammatory cells.

Neutrophils are the first cells recruited from the bloodstream to sites of infection. The function of neutrophils is mainly phagocytosis. Neutrophils respond to chemotactic stimuli and produce factors, such as ROS, in order to kill the phagocytosed cells. It is reported that estrogen decreases chemotactic activity of neutrophils, while another female sex hormone, progesterone enhances this activity [63]. Several studies showed inhibitory effects of estrogen on monocyte MCP-1 production and the MCP-1-induced migration of monocytes [64-66]. The principal estrogen and the most potent naturally occurring estrogen is estradiol. In general, estradiol seems to have anti-inflammatory effects on neutrophils, whereas progesterone seems to have proinflammatory effects on these cells.

Natural killer (NK) cells are capable of killing virus-infected cells or tumour cells in the absence of prior immunization and without MHC restriction. They lyse target cells by direct contact with them in the absence of antibody or by antibody dependent cellular cytotoxicity (ADCC). Increased potency to lyse other cells is found in postmenopausal females and in males as compared to females with a regular menstrual cycle [67, 67]. This is in line with the fact that NK cell activity is also decreased in postmenopausal females using hormone replacement therapy (HRT) [68]. For HRT, estrogen is combined with progestin for women with a uterus to prevent endometrial hyperplasia and endometrial cancer. *In vitro* estrogen appears to suppresse NK cell activity [67, 68].

Dendritic cells are specialist antigen presenting cells, which are derived from monocytes and immature dendritic cells reside in the tissues. They serve as a link between innate and adaptive immune responses and are essential for activation and regulation of immune responses against infections. The innate immune response is the first line of defence against infections. The adaptive immune system is activated by the innate immune response. Both innate and adaptive immunity depend on the ability of the immune system to distinguish between "self" and "non-self" molecules. Studies on the different subpopulations of dendritic cells have shown that progesterone inhibits interferon-γ (IFN-γ) production by plasmacoid dendritic cells. These plasmacoid dendritic cells are circulating and tissue-based dendritic cells that produce large amounts of IFN-γ after encountering viruses. Since IFN-γ induces an antiviral state and primes antiviral response in the adaptive immune response, via this mechanisms, progesterone seems to inhibit antiviral responses [69]. In contrast, estradiol induces the production of IFN-γ in lymphocytes [70].

The effects of sex and the reproductive condition upon monocyte cytokine production are obvious. The most important and consistent effects are as follows. Blood IL-6 levels appear to be decreased by estrogen, stimulated TNF-α and IL-1 production is increased in males as compared to females, and also increased in the luteal phase as compared to the follicular phase of the ovarian cycle [71]. Hormonal fluctuations in the menstrual cycle include increasing estradiol, but low progesterone blood concentrations in the follicular phase, and high blood concentrations of estradiol and progesterone in the luteal phase (Figure 5-2). During the luteal phase, however, the blood concentration of progesterone rises up to a maximum, which is ten to a hundred times higher than that of estradiol [72].

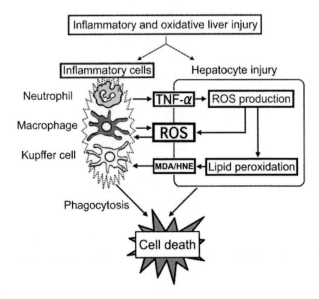

Figure 5-1. In inflammatory and oxidative liver injury, hepatocyte (liver cell) destruction derives from such actions as lipid peroxidation and DNA injury by ROS, apoptosis by TNF-α, and phagocytosis by inflammatory cells (neutrophils, macrophages and Kupffer cells) [22]. Destructed hepatocytes release ROS and end products of lipid peroxidation, MDA) and HNE, which also activate inflammatory cells. Activated inflammatory cells produce TNF-α and ROS.

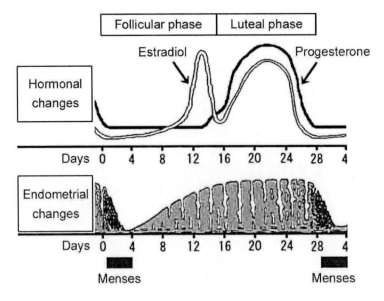

Figure 5-2. The hormonal and endometrial changes and relationship through the normal menstrual cycle.

There is large body of evidence indicating that the decline in ovarian function with menopause is associated with spontaneous increases in proinflammatory cytokines TNF-α, IL-1 and IL-6 [32]. During menopause and in males an increase in blood monocyte number is demonstrated as compared to females in the follicular phase [73]. Moreover, during menopause the monocyte counts decline following estrogen replacement therapy [74]. A very important function of monocytes is to direct immune responses by the production of cytokines including TNF-α, IL-1 and IL-6. Endotoxin-stimulated monocytes in males produce more TNF-α as compared to females [75]. Endotoxins, bacterial lipopolysaccharides in gastrointestinal tract, are detoxified in the reticuloendothelial system, particularly in monocytes-macrophages and Kupffer cells. These cells stimulated by endotoxin induce proinflammatory cytokines. Whether the sex difference of TNF-α response to endotoxin is due to direct effects of high levels of testosterone in males remains uncertain since *in vitro* studies showed no effect of testosterone upon monocyte TNF-α production [76]. Higher blood levels of TNF-α and IL-1 are reported during the luteal phase as compared with the follicular phase, while endotoxin-stimulated monocytes from the luteal phase produce more TNF-α and IL-1 as compared with the follicular phase [77, 78]. Increased blood IL-6 levels after menopause are also decreased by HRT [79, 80]. Further evaluation indicates that the decrease in blood IL-6 levels is due to the estrogenic component in HRT [79, 81]. Whereas one study showes that the prostagens in the HRT up-regulate stimulated IL-6 production [82].

As far as the *in vitro* studies with female sex hormones on the proinflammatory cytokine production by monocytes are concerned, however, conflicting data have been published [83], varying from some [84-86] to no [75, 87] effect of estradiol or progesterone on the cytokine production. Estradiol, at physiological concentrations, has been shown to inhibit the spontaneous secretion of these proinflammatory cytokines in whole blood cultures [87] and peripheral blood mononuclear cells (PBMCs) [34]. The spontaneous production of TNF-α and IL-1 by PBMCs is higher in patients with chronic hepatitis C than in healthy subjects [88]. Endotoxin-stimulated TNF-α production by PBMCs is also higher in HBsAg carriers with elevated ALT levels than in HBsAg carriers with normal ALT levels [89]. Moreover, TNF-α production by hepatocytes from patients with chronic HBV infection is reported to be transcriptionally up-regulated by HBx protein [90, 91]. Treatment with estradiol transdermally in postmenopausal females decreases spontaneous IL-6 production by PBMCs after 12 months of the therapy [34]. Recent studies also show inhibitory effects of estradiol on the unstimulated and hydrogen peroxide-stimulated production of TNF-α, IL-1, IL-8, and MCP-1 in PBMCs from patients with chronic hepatitis C and in murine peritoneal macrophages, whereas progesterone counteract the estradiol effects by enhancing the accumulation of inflammatory cells and their cytokine production [33, 35] (Figure 5-3).

In general, the data suggest an inhibition of the innate immune response in females as compared to males. Although a suppression of innate immune responses may inhibit the clearance of the virus in the acute liver infection, decreased production of proinflammatory cytokines may be beneficial in the progression of the liver disease. Judging from these findings and the previous data showing that the action for ROS production processes is completely opposite to estradiol (antioxidant) with progesterone (pro-oxidant), estradiol may exert a hepatoprotective action against inflammation and oxidative stress in the course of persistent liver injury by preventing the accumulation of neutrophils, monocytes and macrophages and by inhibiting the production of proinflammatory cytokines and ROS, whereas progesterone may counteract the favorable estradiol effects (Figure 5-4). Progesterone also resembles testosterone in the part of the structure and function. Therefore, the sex hormones estrogen, progesterone and testosterone may affect innate immune responses by modulating inflammatory cell numbers and function as well as ROS production.

Total lymphocyte count in males is similar to females [73], while the percentage of T cells within the total lymphocyte population in males is lower as compared to females [73]. The decreased T-cell counts in males as compared to females may be due to the increased testosterone concentrations, since testosterone may increase apoptosis in T cells [92].

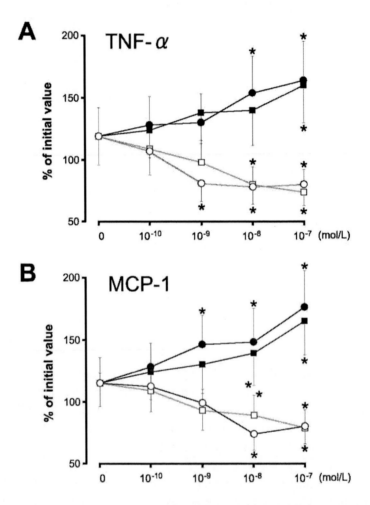

Figure 5-3. Estradiol (open) inhibits and progesterone (solid) stimulates spontaneous production of TNF-α (A) and MCP-1 (B) by unstimulated peripheral blood mononuclear cells (PBMCs) from age-matched older male (square) and postmenopausal female (circle) patients with chronic hepatitis C [35]. The unstimulated PBMCs were cultured with and without estradiol (10^{-10}-10^{-7} mol/L) or progesterone (10^{-10}-10^{-7} mol/L). The results are expressed as the percentages of each initial value for the cytokine production in the absence of the female sex hormones. The values are the mean ± SD ($n = 18$). *$P < 0.05$ in comparison with the cultures in the absence of the female sex hormones.

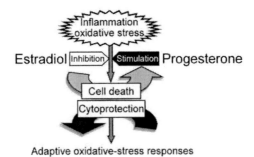

Figure 5-4. Adaptive oxidative-stress responses to inflammatory and oxidative stimuli by estradiol and progesterone [22]. For neutrophils, monocytes and macrophages, estradiol exerts anti-inflammatory and antioxidative effects, while progesterone exerts proinflammatory and pro-oxidative effects [33, 71, 71]. The decrease in immune responses by estradiol limits tissue destruction during the inflammatory and oxidative liver injury and thus relatively protects females against the progression of liver disease.

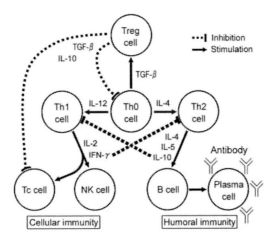

Figure 5-5. Adaptive immune responses [22]. Uncommitted helper T lymphocytes (Th0 cells) become activated and, according to the presence in the microenvironment of IL-12 or IL-4 and the nature of the antigen, differentiate into Th1 or Th2 and initiate a series of immune reactions determined by the cytokines they produce: Th2 secrete mainly IL-4, IL-5 and IL-10, and direct antibody production by B lymphocytes; Th1 secrete IL-2 and IFN-γ, which stimulate cytotoxic T lymphocytes (Tc cells), enhance expression of class I and induce expression of class II MHC molecules on hepatocytes and activate macrophages; activated macrophages release TNF-α and IL-1 as well as ROS. The major function of regulatory T lymphocytes (Treg cells) is the suppression of Th and Tc cells via secretion of TGF-β and IL-10.

Many studies both *in vitro* and *in vivo* have shown that estrogen and progesterone suppress cell-mediated immune response [93]. Estrogen or progesterone inhibit proliferation of T cells (or T lymphocyte cell lines) after stimulation with mitogenic substances [94]. Estrogen decreases TNF-α-induced cytotoxicity in peripheral T cells [95], and it enhances secretion of interleukin-10 (IL-10) in T cells isolated from females [96]. IL-10 is an inhibitory cytokine serving to limit cell-mediated responses. The inhibitory effect of sex hormones on cytotoxic T lymphocyte (Tc cell) function may play a role in the differences in progression of liver disease between males and females, since, as suggested for neutrophils, monocytes and macrophages, decreased Tc cell cytotoxicity in females as compared to males could limit tissue destruction following acute infection and thereby progression of liver disease.

Moreover, females have a higher number of helper T lymphocytes (Th cells) than males [97]. Uncommitted Th cells (Th0 cells) become activated and, according to the presence in the microenvironment of interleukin-12 (IL-12) or interleukin-4 (IL-4) and the nature of the antigen, differentiate into Th1 or Th2 and initiate a series of immune reactions determined by the cytokines they produce (Figure 5-5): Th2 secrete mainly IL-4, interleukin-5 (IL-5) and IL-10, and direct antibody production by B lymphocytes; Th1 secrete interleukin-2 (IL-2) and IFN-γ, which stimulate Tc cells. Estrogen is also reported to enhance humoral immune responses [98]. Such effects of estrogen on humoral and cell-mediated immune responses may be modulated by their effects on Th1 and Th2 cytokine production.

The main function of B cells is the production of antibodies. B cells have two subsets. The first set is the conventional B cell subset (B2 cells), which present internalised antigens to T cells through which they get activated and develop into antibody-producing blood cells (plasma cells) [99]. The second subset is the B1 cell subset, which produce antibodies in a T cell independent manner and are suggested to be responsible for autoantibody production [100]. B1 subsets appear to remaine stable after menopause, while the B2 subset appear to decrease after menopause and to increase after HRT [101]. Studies in animals have shown that estrogen increases bone marrow progenitor B cells in mice by protecting the progenitor cells from apoptosis, and increase survival in splenic B cells [102]. Females, particularly before menopause, can produce antibodies against HBeAg and HBsAg at a higher frequency than males with chronic HBV infection. In addition to the inhibitory effect of estrogen on the cell-mediated immune response, estrogen also enhances B cell development (Figure 5-6), while androgen appears to inhibit humoral immunity [103]. These may be involved in the higher incidence of autoimmune diseases in females. Indeed, estrogen increased and testosterone decreased autoantibody production of PBMC in patients with systemic lupus erythematosus (SLE) [104], which is one of common autoimmune diseases predominat in females.

Regulatory T cells (Treg cells), formerly known as suppressor T cells, are now thought to be a central mechanism of immune regulation [105]. The major function of Treg cells is the suppression of Th and Tc cells via secretion of TGF-β and IL-10 (see Figure 5-5). The number of Treg cells increase during the late follicular phase, concomitantly with high estradiol concentrations, compared to early follicular phase or luteal phase, while during the luteal phase with high progesterone concentrations there are no changes in numbers of Treg cells between these phases of the ovarian cycle [106, 107]. This suggests that high concentrations of estradiol is involved in the increase in numbers of Treg cells. Therefore, estrogen induces the suppressive function of Treg cells for immune responses to self or foreign antigens [106]. It has been shown in mice that estrogen increases expression of Foxp3 present in Treg cells together with Treg cell function [108]. Foxp3 is a transcription factor that controls the development and function of Treg cells [108]. Since Treg cells may inhibit the adaptive immune response during the progression phase and thereby limit tissue destruction and progression of the liver disease, estrogen may also suppress the disease progression via affecting adaptive immune responses in the liver.

Studies on the effects of sex hormones on Treg cells are limited at the moment, especially the effects on Treg cell subsets and function. Further studies are needed to substantiate this hypothesis [71].

6. Non-Alcoholic Fatty Liver Disease in Females

Non-alcoholic fatty liver disease (NAFLD) is currently recognized as the most common form of chronic liver disease in many parts of the world. There is a growing concern regarding the development of NAFLD in clinical hepatology. Its name implies a histological picture that is indistinguishable from alcoholic liver disease. Fatty liver, which is also histologically called hepatic steatosis, is the result of the deposition of triglycerides via the accumulation of fatty acids in hepatocytes. Increased echogenicity ("bright" scan) with ultrasonography or increased radiolucency with computerized tomography (CT) compared with kidney provide supportive evidence of fatty liver [109] (Figure 6-1). Although in most cases, fatty liver does not progress to more severe liver diseases, approximately 15-20% of patients have histological signs of hepatic fibrosis and necroinflammation, indicating the presence of non-alcoholic steatohepatitis (NASH). In a "two hit" theory of NASH pathogenesis [110], the "first hit" of hepatic steatosis is followed by the "second hit" of oxidative stress and endotoxin (bacterial lipopolysaccharides)-induced proinflammatory stimuli, leading to cell death and progression to hepatic fibrosis and NASH. Hepatic fat accumulation leads to ROS production caused by mitochondrial respiratory chain dysfunction and/or CYP2E1 in the microsomes. CYP2E1 has a very high NADPH oxidase activity and extensively produces ROS. Endotoxins, one of the components of the outer wall of gram-negative bacteria in gastrointestinal tract, are detoxified in the reticuloendothelial system, particularly in macrophages and Kupffer cells in the liver. Kupffer cells stimulated by gut-derived endotoxin via the portal vein produce proinflammatory cytokines such as TNF-α. Patients with NASH are at higher risk for developing cirrhosis and its complications such as HCC [46]. Therefore, NAFLD refers to a spectrum of histopathology, ranging from simple hepatic steatosis to NASH and the end-stage cirrhosis, all occurring in the absence of history of alcohol abuse defined as an alcohol intake of more than 20 g per day.

Earlier impressions that NAFLD/NASH was a female-predominate condition have been dispelled; it actually appears to be more prevalent in males [47, 111, 112]. Data from the NHANES III in the United States were estimated that 16% of adult females and 31% of adult males have NAFLD [47, 113]. NAFLD has a very high prevalence in much of Europe, the Middle East (spanning southwestern Asia and northeastern Africa), Asia-Pacific (including Australia and New Zealand), and the United States. In most regions, ultrasonographic surveys of the general population indicate that almost one-quarter of the adult population has fatty liver [113, 114]. NAFLD is more common in males than females, particularly in Asians [115]. In support of the sex difference in NAFLD among Asians, the incidence of ultrasonographic NAFLD was examined by sex and age in 3,229 Japanese adults from 2005 to 2006 in a health checkup center in Tokushima, Japan. NAFLD was 2.5-fold more prevalent in males (31.5%) than in females (12.4%). Although NAFLD was more prevalent in females over the age of 70 years, the biggest difference in the prevalence of NAFLD between females and males was found in individuals of less than 50 years old [14] (Figure 6-2). Furthermore, among 3,175 Shanghai adults, the peak incidence of fatty liver in males occurred earlier (40-49 years) than in females (over 50 years) [116].

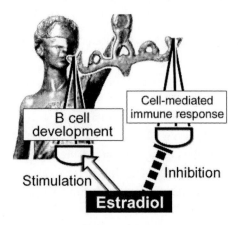

Figure 5-6. Estradiol inhibits cell-mediated immune response, and it stimulates B cell development [22]. The scales of adaptive immune responses are carried by "Lady Justice." She is known as a goddess of divine justice, but she appers here as a symbol of powerful femininity.

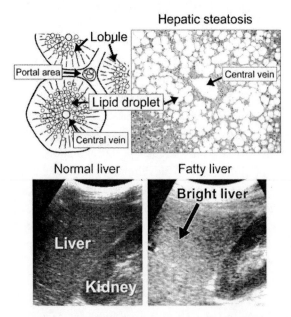

Figure 6-1. Histological and ultrasonographic findings of fatty liver [22]. Fats containing triglycerides are occupied in hepatocytes mainly around central vein by numerous lipid droplets (Hepatic steatosis). Fatty liver is detected by ultrasonography based on the comparative assessment of image brightness of the liver relative to the kidney.

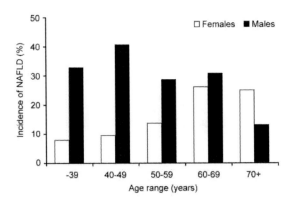

Figure 6-2. Incidence of NAFLD by sex and age [14]. NAFLD incidence was determined ultrasonographically in 3,229 Japanese subjects (mean age 52.4 years, 54.1% females) in the Tokushima Health Checkup Center in Japan. The subjects had no history of alcohol abuse, defined as an alcohol intake >20 g/day, and were seronegative for HBsAg and anti-HCV. The overall incidence of NAFLD was 25.6%.

Currently, metabolic disorders such as being overweight and diabetes are emerging as cofactors of hepatic fibrosis. Fatty liver is considered the hepatic manifestation of the metabolic syndrome. The transition from premenopause to postmenopause is associated with the emergence of many features of the metabolic syndrome, including increased visceral body fat, a shift towards a more atherogenic lipid profile and increased glucose and insulin levels (these conditions are known as peripheral insulin resistance). Visceral fat accumulation is a predictor of fatty liver. In fact, coronary heart disease and stroke are rare before the menopause [117]. Obesity and diabetes, conditions associated with insulin resistance, are frequently observed in patients with NAFLD [118]. As depicted in **Figure 6-3**, the incidence of increased visceral fat accumulation was quite low in females, particularly, aged less than 60 years old in a cohort study of local residents in Japan [119]. Increased fat accumulation areas ($\geq$100cm^2) were measured by CT. Visceral fat areas from a single CT scan obtained at the level of the umbilicus are correlated with the total visceral fat volume [120].

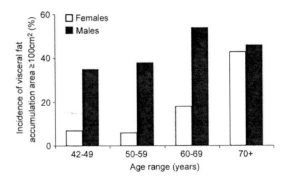

Figure 6-3. Incidence of increased visceral fat accumulation (visceral obesity) by sex and age [119]. Increased fat accumulation areas ($\geq$100cm^2) were measured by CT in a population-based cohort study of 504 local residents (ages of 42 to 82 years old; 244 females and 260 males) in Aichi prefecture in Japan.

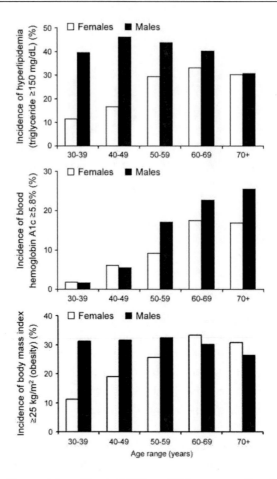

Figure 6-4. Incidence of hypertriglyceridemia (≥150 mg/dl) (upper panel) and increased blood hemoglobin A1c (≥5.8%) (lower panel) and obese individuals (body mass index ≥ 25 kg/m²) based on data from the National Nutrition Survey in Japan [22].

Based on data in 2002 from the National Nutrition Survey in Japan, increased blood levels of triglycerides (≥150 mg/dL) and hemoglobin A1c (≥5.8%) and obese individuals (body mass index ≥25 kg/m², see below) were more frequently observed in postmenopausal females and males (Figure 6-4). However, there was no significant difference of the incidences of abnormatily of hemoglobin A1c between female and male persons aged less than 50 yerars old. Hemoglobin A1c is used for screening and identification of impaired glucose tolerance and diabetes. A hemoglobin A1c of 5.8% shows the high sensitivity and specificity for diagnosing diabetes (fasting blood glucose >126 mg/dL) [121]. Hemoglobin A1c and fasting blood glucose are found to be similarly effective in diagnosing diabetes.

However, obesity prevalence data in Japan indicate the tendency of females to be more obese than males, which is almost similar to those in other different parts of the world [122]. In Japanese females, the prevalence rate gradually increases to 30% in their 60s, and thereafter remains higher than in males. These differences are probably biologically based and relate to male's ability to deposit more lean (muscle) than fat tissue when energy imbalance occurs with weight gain. Females have more fat mass and less lean mass than males.

Table 6-1. Definitions of terms on BMI

Formula of BMI	BMI = body weight (in kg) ÷ height (in meters) squared
Normal weight	BMI ≥ 18.5 to 24.9 kg/m²
Overweight	BMI ≥ 25.0 to 29.9 kg/m²
Obesity	BMI ≥ 30 kg/m²

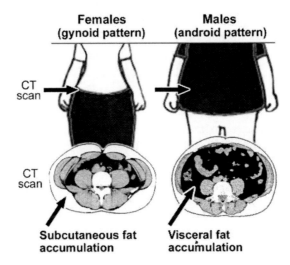

Figure 6-5.   Difference of regional fat distribution between females (pear shape, gynoid pattern) and males (apple shape, android pattern) [22]. Males generally have larger visceral fat areas than females. Visceral fat areas from a single CT scan obtained at the level of the umbilicus are correlated with the total visceral fat volume.

Visceral fat accumulation, or visceral (central) obesity, is an independent predictor of hepatic steatosis, even in persons with a normal body mass index (BMI). BMI is the most practical way to evaluate the overall degree of excess weight (Table 6-1), which mainly reflects total body fat accumulation, or subcutaneous fat accumulation. Overweight and obesity are defined as BMI ≥ 25 to 29.9 kg/m² and ≥30 kg/m², respectively. Visceral fat accumulation is a more important factor for hepatic steatosis than BMI. It should be noted that regional fat distribution differs between females and males. After correction for total body fat mass, males generally have larger visceral fat areas than females [123] (Figure 6-5). Visceral fat accumulation (android pattern) is much more harmful than subcutaneous fat accumulation (gynoid pattern) [124, 125]. Menopause is associated with a shift toward relatively more fat as well as toward the deposition of more fat in the abdominal region. In fact, starting within the first year from the menopause, females tend to gain weight and have a redistribution of body fat from a gynoid to an android pattern [126].

Increased lipid peroxidation and accumulation of end products of lipid peroxidation are commonly observed in NAFLD and alcoholic liver disease based on studies of human alcohol-related liver injury and animal models of diet-induced hepatic steatosis and drug-induced steatohepatitis [127-129]. Fatty liver is the result of the deposition of triglycerides via the accumulation of fatty acids in hepatocytes. In the progression of fatty liver disease, lipid peroxidation products are generated because of impaired β-oxidation of the accumulated fatty acids. The major site for fatty acid β-oxidation (degradation of fatty acids) in the liver is hepatocyte mitochondria (Figure 6-6). Key mediators of impaired fatty acid β-oxidation include a reduced mitochondrial electron transport (respiratory chain dysfunction). In addition to impaired mitochondrial β-oxidation of fatty acids, an activity of CYP2E1 in the microsomes is increased. Increased activity of CYP2E1 is found in the livers of obese animals [130] and NASH patients [131]. CYP2E1 catalyzes fatty acid ω-hydroxylations (microsomal ω-oxidation of fatty acids). Elevated CYP2E1 and mitochondrial defects result in an increase in the ROS formation and lipid peroxidation products. ROS and lipid peroxidation in turn cause further mitochondrial dysfunction and oxidative stress, thus contributing to cell death via ROS-induced DNA injury and membrane lipid peroxidation and discharge of products of lipid peroxidation, MDA and HNE, into the space of Disse (see Figure 3-2). MDA and HNE besides ROS are able to activate inflammatory cells (neutrophils, macrophages and Kupffer cells) (see Figure 5-1) and HSCs. Activated HSCs are responsible for much of the collagen synthesis observed during fibrosis development to the end-stage cirrhosis. Activated inflammatory cells in turn produce chemokines as well as TNF-α and ROS. Chemokines such as MCP-1 and IL-8 attract neutrophils, lymphocytes, monocytes, macrophages, and Kupffer cells to inflammatory sites, leading to the persistent liver injury.

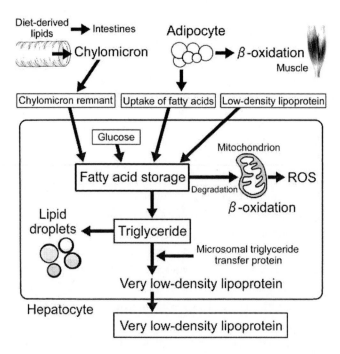

Figure 6-6. Increased hepatic uptake of free fatty acids, increased triglyceride synthesis, and impaired transport of very low-density lipoprotein (triglyceride-rich lipoprotein) into the blood mainly contribute to the accumulation of hepatocellular triglycerides. Microsomal trigyceride transfer protein is essential for the secretion of very low-density lipoprotein. Excess triglycerides are stored as lipid droplets in hepatocytes, which in turn results in a preferential shift to fatty acid degradation (β-oxidation), leading to the formation of ROS and lipid peroxidation products.

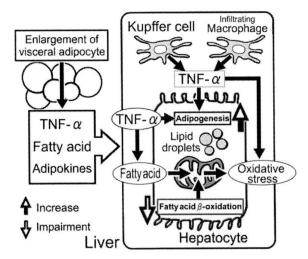

Figure 6-7. Working hypothesis regarding the disrupted balance between fat formation (adipogenesis) and fatty acid degradation (β-oxidation) in inducing hepatic steatosis [22]. Hepatic steatosis is characterized by lipid deposition in hepatocytes. Enlargement of visceral adipocytes is an essential factor for hepatic steatosis, which is principally induced by the increased adipogenesis and impaired fatty acid β-oxidation.

Mitochondrial defects may possibly have a genetic basis [132] and are likely worsened by aging and environmental factors such as high saturated fats [133, 134]. Visceral fat accumulation arises through enlarged adipocytes (Figure 6-7). Adipocytes in visceral fat tissue release fatty acids and so called adipokines including adiponectin, leptin and TNF-α [135]. These adipokines and fatty acids flow directly into the liver via the portal vein, and they are involved in the development of metabolic syndrome and NAFLD. Mitochondrial dysfunction and oxidative stress are reported in the livers of patients with NASH [136]. Production of TNF-α and ROS by activated Kupffer cells and accumulated macrophages in the liver is also thought to play an important role in NASH-associated cirrhosis. Kupffer cells and macrophages are stimulated by gut-derived endotoxin via the portal vein, and produce a variety of cytokines such as TNF-α and IL-6. TNF-α is responsible, at least in part, for a number of pathophysiological responses in the liver, including ROS production, fat formation, insulin resistance, and hepatic fibrogenesis.

Adiponectin decreases in obese states, particularly with visceral obesity [137]. Blood adiponectin levels correlate inversely with visceral fat, fasting insulin concentrations and blood triglycerides [138]. Importantly, adiponectin levels are consistently higher in females than in males, independent of age and body fat [139]. These results are validated in adult populations inclusive of multiple ethnic groups such as Caucasians [139], Maoris [140], African Americans and Hispanics [141]. Adiponectin stimulates peroxisome proliferator-activated receptor α (PPARα) which has a number of beneficial effects including increased fatty acid β-oxidation, a reduction in hepatic triglycerides and inhibition of cytokines such as IL-6 [142]. Further anti-inflammatory effects of adiponectin are mediated via inhibition of macrophages and direct blockade of TNF-α release [143]. Such anti-steatotic and anti-inflammatory properties of adiponectin [144] may, in part, explain the decreased visceral fat accumulation and lower prevalence of fatty liver in females.

However, adiponectin levels in the older (> 51 years) group in a cohort in the United States were higher than in the younger (≤51 years) group, although the older individuals had greater visceral fat accumulation [139]. Two population studies demonstrated an inverse correlation between estrogen and adiponectin levels [145]. In addition, blood levels of total testosterone appear to correlate positively with blood adiponectin levels in both females and males, independent of measures of body fat [146]. Thus, estrogen alone is not responsible and may in fact have a negative rather than positive influence on circulating adiponectin levels.

Leptin plays a key role in the regulation of appetite and body weight. It also acts on the hypothalamus, altering energy intake by decreasing appetite and increasing energy expenditure via sympathetic stimulation of several tissues [144]. Blood leptin levels correlate well with body fat mass; this correlation is strongest for subcutaneous fat which secretes more leptin [147]. Although leptin levels are higher in premenopausal and postmenopausal females than in males even after adjustment for age and BMI [148], most studies show no difference of leptin levels between premenopausal and postmenopausal females when matched for BMI [149, 150]. In contrast, testosterone inhibits leptin production by human adipocytes [149, 151], and hypogonadal males (defined as the failure to produce androgen) have elevated leptin levels which are reduced by testosterone substitution [152]. These data suggest that sex differences in blood leptin levels appear to be due to an interaction between sex hormones and differences in body composition [142].

Chronic hepatitis B and C are both frequently associated with hepatic steatosis. The frequency of hepatic steatosis in chronic hepatitis B ranges from 27 to 51%, while in chronic hepatitis C it is between 31 and 72% [153-156]. Hepatic steatosis is a characteristic feature of chronic HBV and HCV infections, suggesting that hepatic steatosis may reflect a direct cytopathic effect of hepatitis viruses and may play a role in the progression of the disease. In fact, a transgenic mouse model, which expressed the HCV core gene, develops progressive hepatic steatosis and HCC [157, 158]. Chronic hepatitis C is commonly associated with hepatic steatosis [159], insulin resistance and diabetes [160]. A meta-analysis of over 3000 patients with hepatitis C shows that hepatic steatosis is a strong predictor of advanced disease [161]. It is conceivable that following hepatocyte injury, hepatic steatosis leads to an increase in lipid peroxidation, which may contribute to HSC activation by releasing soluble mediators [162] such as lipid peroxidation products, TNF-α and ROS, and thereby inducing hepatic fibrosis.

In contrast to HCV, there is little information on the correlation between HBV-associated hepatic steatosis and fibrosis. The molecular mechanism by which HBV mediates hepatic steatosis has not yet been clearly studied. Although a cross-sectional study in Australia failed to confirm the impact of hepatic steatosis on fibrosis in chronic hepatitis B, but not C [163], another cross-sectional analysis in Taiwanese adults revealed that HBV carrier status, ultrasonographic fatty liver and male sex are independently associated with liver damage evaluated by a conventional marker, blood ALT level [164]. Moreover, HBx protein induces hepatic fat accumulation mediated by sterol regulatory element binding protein 1 (SREBP-1) and peroxisome proliferator-activated receptor γ (PPARγ), leading to hepatic steatosis [165]. Increasing evidence indicates that hepatic fat accumulation is related to hepatic fibrosis, inflammation, apoptosis, and cancer [166, 167].

In animal and *in vitro* studies, when incubated with adiponectin, HSCs undergo a number of antifibrogenic changes such as decreased the potent profibrogenic cytokine TGF-β [168]. In obese leptin deficient mice, adiponectin treatment is associated with improvement in hepatic steatosis, liver enzyme levels and hepatic inflammation [169], while adiponectin knockout mice demonstrate enhanced hepatic fibrosis [168]. Currently, however, there is insufficient evidence to suggest that differential expression of adiponectin is enough to explain the better prognosis seen in females with chronic liver disease. Activated HSCs produce leptin [170], which is reported to up-regulate TNF-α, TGF-β and the expression of collagen type I [171]. Thus, leptin may play a role in the development of hepatic fibrosis. However, there is no evidence that the higher levels of leptin found in females may contribute to modulation of disease severity in NAFLD and chronic hepatitis B and C [142].

Fat accumulation is much more harmful in the visceral adipose tissue than in the subcutaneous adipose tissue [124, 125]. Adipokines and fatty acids, derived from enlarged visceral adipcytes, flow directly into the liver via the portal vein, and they are involved in the development of metabolic syndrome and NAFLD. Human adipose tissue contains estrogen receptor α and estrogen receptor β. Low estrogen levels in females with menopause are associated with a loss in subcutaneous fat and a gain in visceral fat [172]. In fact, starting within the first year from the menopause, females tend to have a redistribution of body fat from a gynoid to an android pattern (see Figure 6-5). Estrogen treatment of male-to-female transsexuals can increase the amount of subcutaneous adipose tissue; thus, estrogen changes the male type of visceral fat distribution into a female type of fat accumulation [173]. Postmenopausal females treated with estrogen replacement are reported to have a lower visceral fat accumulation of adipose tissue in comparison to controls [174].

Patients with Turner's syndrome, which is characterized by estrogen deficiency, are associated with visceral obesity, increased liver enzyme ALT levels, and histologically proven NAFLD in up to 40% of cases [175-177]. Furthermore, a man with estrogen deficiency due to the aromatase gene inactivating mutation is reported to develop both steatohepatitis and insulin resistance, which are reversible with estradiol treatment [178]. Interestingly, polycystic ovary syndrome (PCOS) is associated with the development of NAFLD [179]. PCOS is a leading cause of infertility in premenopausal females. PCOS is a syndrome of ovarian dysfunction along with the cardinal features hyperandrogenism and polycystic ovary morphology. Its clinical manifestations may include menstrual irregularities, signs of androgen excess, and obesity [180, 181]. In addition of the inhibitory role of estrogen in visceral fat accumulation and NAFLD development, androgen levels may also impact the NAFLD.

Microsomal triglyceride transfer protein (MTP) (see Figure 6-6) is essential and rate limiting for the assembly and secretion of very low-density lipoprotein (triglyceride-rich lipoprotein). Decreased hepatic expression of MTP contributes to the accumulation of hepatocellular triglycerides. Excess triglycerides are stored as lipid droplets in hepatocytes, leading to hepatic steatosis. Hepatic MTP expression is higher in females than in males, and this sex difference is regulated by the sexually dimorphic secretory pattern of growth hormone [182]. A continuous infusion of growth hormone increases MTP expression. Likely clinical manifestations of growth hormone deficiency in adults are increased visceral fat mass with a decrease in lean body mass. The profile of growth hormone secretion pattern shows clear sex dimorphism [182]. In female rats, the growth hormone is continuously secreted, and the hormone levels are always detectable in the circulation, while, in male rats, it is secreted by episodic bursts every several hours with low or undetectable levels between peaks [183]. Integrated 24-hour growth hormone secretion [184] and fasting blood growth hormone levels (Figure 6-8) are higher in female individuals than in male individuals. Growth hormone secretion is stimulated by estrogen [182]. Oral and high-dose transdermal estrogen administration in menopausal females increases integrated 24-hour growth hormone secretion [185].

An experimental animal study showed that hepatic steatosis spontaneously becomes evident in an aromatase-deficient mouse, which lacks the intrinsic ability to produce estrogen and is impaired with respect to hepatic fatty acid β-oxidation. Estradiol replacement reduces hepatic steatosis and restores the impairment in mitochondrial and peroxisomal fatty acid β-oxidation to a wild-type level [186]. Moreover, tamoxifen is a potent antagonist of estrogen, and it is used in the hormone treatment of estrogen receptor-positive breast cancer. Tamoxifen has been shown to be associated with an increased risk of developing hepatic steatosis and NASH in non-obese female patients with breast cncer [187, 188]. In a clinical study from Japan, the frequency of tamoxifen-induced hepatic steatosis and NASH had increased to 36% [189]. These suggest that tamoxifen, as an antiestrogen, could suppress hepatic fatty acid β-oxidation and accelerate fat accumulation in hepatocytes. Therefore, the greater progression of liver injury with steatosis regardless of the etiology in males may be due, at least in part, to the decreased production of estradiol.

Over the last two decades, lifestyle changes have resulted in a dramatic increase in the prevalence of obesity in economically developed countries [190]. Organized physical activities, or purposeful exercise, such as walking, sport and physical play are now less popular than sedentary or 'spectator' activities, like television watching and internet surfing. More importantly, the minute-by-minute, hour-by-hour physical activities of everyday living (incidental activity) are dramatically reduced by modern lifestyle based on cars, household and building conveniences, and computer-based workstations [191]. Energy imbalance is responsible for excessive fat deposition. The increasing prevalence of obesity has also led to a higher incidence of metabolic syndrome including visceral obesity, hyperglycemia, hyperlipidemia and hypertension. The rising incidence of obesity and metabolic syndrome has occurred in paralleled with a dramatic increase of NAFLD.

Cirrhosis is 6 times more prevalent in obese individuals than in the general population [192]. Obesity, especially visceral obesity, is an independent risk factor in the development of NASH and HCC [193, 194]. Visceral obesity is no longer a predictor of NAFLD/NASH, but rather is considered to be an essential risk factor for HCC. Higher risks associated with increased incidence and death rates for liver cancer are observed among obese males than among obese females [193, 195]. Oxidative stress, proinflammatory cytokines, and other proinflammatory mediators as well as lipotoxicity may each play a role in transition of hepatic steatosis to NASH [196]. Patients with NASH who progress to cirrhosis are at increased risk of HCC. The second hit capable of inducing oxidative stress and proinflammatory stimuli in the first hit of hepatic steatosis is required for NASH, leading to cell death and progression to hepatic fibrosis and HCC [197].

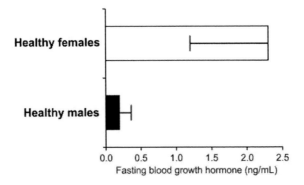

Figure 6-8.   Fasting mean blood levels of growth hormone in 15 premenopausal females (mean age 41.3 years) and 15 age-matched males (mean age 41.1 years) of healthy non-obese (BMI ≥ 18.5 to 24.9 kg/m²) individuals [22]. The subjects had no history of alcohol abuse (defined as an alcohol intake >20 g/day).

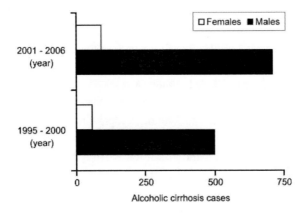

Figure 7-1. Male-to-female ratio in Japanese patients with alcoholic cirrhosis [22]. Male-to-female ratio in alcoholic cirrhosis was examined from 1995 to 2000 and from 2001 to 2006 in 1,005 Japanese patients (mean age 59.5 years, 10.4% females) hospitalized in Tokushima, Japan. The subjects were seronegative for HBsAg and anti-HCV.

It is important not only to diagnosis NASH in daily clinical practice but also to perform appropriate treatment taking into consideration the sex difference and influence of menopause in females. Understanding the sex-associated difference is necessary to inform the rational design of treatment strategies directed at visceral obese individuals who may develop from hepatic steatosis to cirrhosis and HCC.

7. "Female Paradox" in Alcoholic Liver Disease

Alcoholic liver disease occurs after prolonged heavy drinking, particularly among persons who are physically dependent on alcohol. Alcoholic liver disease is pathologically classified into three forms: fatty liver (hepatic steatosis), alcoholic hepatitis, and cirrhosis. There is considerable overlap among these conditions. The incidence of alcoholic liver disease increases in a dose-dependent manner proportionally to the cumulative alcoholic intake. Alcoholism is increasing among females, owing to a decline in the social stigma attached to drinking and to the ready availability of alcohol in supermarkets. In general, however, males have a greater opportunity for drinking. Despite the male predominance for alcoholism, chronic alcohol consumption induces more rapid and more severe liver injury in females than males. As already mentioned, the progression of hepatic fibrosis in chronic hepatitis B and C is slower in females. The "female paradox" observed in patients with alcoholic liver disease in comparison with chronic viral hepatitis is based on susceptibility by females to liver damage from smaller quantities of ethanol.

The amount of alcohol required producing hepatitis or cirrhosis varies among individuals, but as little as 40 g/day for 10 years is associated with an increased incidence of cirrhosis. There is considerable evidence to suggest that females require less total alcohol consumption (20 g ethanol/day) to produce clinically significant liver disease. Indeed, it is reported that the lowest point of weekly alcohol intake that helps to develop liver disease was higher in males (168-324 g) than in females (84-156 g), and that, in the case of heavy drinkers with a weekly consumption of 336-492 g, the relative risk for alcoholic liver disease was 3.7 in males and 7.3 in females, while it was 1.0 in the group with a weekly consumption of 12-72 g [198]. Thus, safe drinking guidelines recommend that females do not drink more than 20 g ethanol per day, and males not more than 40 g ethanol. A common, reasonable recommendation is not to exceed 70 g of ethanol a week.

Ethanol is metabolized by hepatic alcohol dehydrogenase (ADH) and the hepatic microsomal ethanol oxidizing system to acetaldehyde, which is subsequently converted by aldehyde dehydrogenase (ALDH) to acetate. The accumulation of acetaldehyde leads to the clinical syndrome of flushing, nausea and vomiting. Isoenzymes of ALDH with low activities are common among Asian populations and are associated with lower rates of alcoholism. These persons experience a similar flushing syndrome after consuming ethanol. This inhibits Asian populations from taking alcohol and is a negative risk for the development of alcoholic liver disease [199].

Indeed, in a study on the sex difference in Japanese patients hospitalized in Tokushima, Japan, the incidence of alcoholic cirrhosis was 9-fold higher in males than females (Figure 7-1). However, females develop higher blood ethanol levels following a standard dose, possibly because of a smaller mean apparent volume of ethanol distribution. Moreover, sex differences in hepatic metabolism with increased production of acetaldehyde may contribute to vulnerability of females to alcohol consumption [200], suggesting that chronic alcohol consumption may induce more rapid and more severe liver injury in females than males. Females with alcoholic cirrhosis survive a shorter time than males [201].

Alcoholic liver injury is mainly due to ethanol hepatotoxicity linked to its metabolism by means of the ADH and CYP2E1 pathways and the resulting production of toxic acetaldehyde (Figure 7-2). CYP2E1 is the key enzyme of the microsomal ethanol oxidizing system (MEOS), and it is involved in the oxygenation of substrates such as ethanol and fatty acids. Although most ethanol is oxidized by ADH, CYP2E1 assumes a more important role in ethanol oxidation at elevated levels of ethanol or after chronic consumption of ethanol. CYP2E1 has a very high NADPH oxidase activity. Therefore, excess of ethanol and fatty acids and their metabolism by means of CYP2E1 pathway produce extensively ROS, which cause oxidative stress with lipid peroxidation and membrane damage, leading to cell death.

ROS and products of lipid peroxidation (such as MDA and HNE) activate not only inflammatory cells (including neutrophils, macrophages and Kupffer cells) but HSCs as well. As already noted, excess fatty acids lead to hepatic steatosis (see Figure 6-6), and activated HSCs are accountable for hepatofibrogenesis (see Figure 4-2).

Oxidation of ethanol through the ADH and CYP2E1 pathways produces acetaldehyde which is also toxic to the hepatocyte mitochondria. Acetaldehyde aggravates oxidative stress by binding to reduced glutathione, an antioxidant, and promoting its leakage, which triggers an inflammatory response of the host. This involves the activation of Kupffer cells and the attraction of inflammatory cells to injured sites. The inflammatory cells in the liver produce TGF-β and proinflammatory mediators including TNF-α and ROS, leading to oxidative tress and hepatic fibrosis. Thus, TNF-α mediates not only the early stages of NAFLD but also the transition to more advanced stages of liver damage. Acetaldehyde is converted by ALDH to acetate. Reactions of ethanol converted to acetaldehyde and subsequently acetate reduce nicotinamide adenine dinucleotide (NAD) to its reduced form (NADH). Excess NADH causes a number of metabolic disorders, including stimulation of the fatty acid synthesis and inhibition of the Krebs cycle and of its fatty acid oxidation [202]. The stimulation of the fatty acid synthesis and inhibition of fatty acid oxidation favor fat accumulation (hepatic steatosis) and hyperlipidemia.

Alcohol ingestion disrupts gastrointestinal barrier function and subsequently induces the diffusion of luminal bacterial products including bacterial lipopolysaccharides (endotoxins) into the portal vein. Experiments using animals show direct evidence of increased translocation of endotoxin from the gut lumen into the portal bloodstream caused by ethanol [203]. Acute ethanol ingestion, especially at high concentrations, facilitates the absorption of endotoxin from rat small intestine via an increase in intestinal permeability, which may play an important role in endotoxemia observed in alcoholic liver injury [204]. Increased endotoxin levels in the portal blood are essential for initiation and progression of alcoholic liver disease [205].

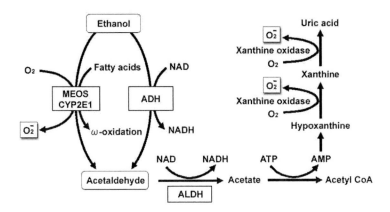

Figure 7-2. Ethanol oxidation by alcohol dehydrogenase (ADH) and the hepatic microsomal ethanol oxidizing system (MEOS), which involves cytochrome P450 2E1 (CYP2E1), produces acetaldehyde. CYP2E1 produces ROS (superoxide, O_2^-) [22]. Acetaldehyde is converted by aldehyde dehydrogenase (ALDH) to acetate. Both reactions of ethanol to acetaldehyde and then acetate reduce nicotinamide adenine dinucleotide (NAD) to its reduced form (NADH). Excess NADH causes inhibition of fatty acid oxidation, leading to fat accumulation (hepatic steatosis).

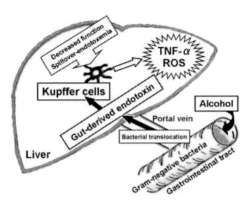

Figure 7-3.   Activation of Kupffer cells by gut-derived endotoxin plays a pivotal role in alcoholic liver injury [22]. Following chronic alcohol ingestion, endotoxin, also called lipopolysaccharide, released from intestinal gram-negative bacteria moves from gastrointestinal tract (gut) into the liver via the portal bloodstream.

Bacterial translocation from the gastrointestinal tract, namely spillover endotoxemia, is important in the relationship between endotoxin and hepatotoxicity in the reticuloendothelial system such as monocytes-macrophages and Kupffer cells. Gut-derived endotoxin activates Kupffer cells, which produce proinflammatory mediators such as TNF-α and ROS. The ability of Kupffer cells to eliminate and detoxify various exogenous and endogenous substances including endotoxin is an important physiological regulatory function (Figure 7-3).

The profile of growth hormone secretion pattern shows clear sex dimorphism [182]. Integrated 24-hour growth hormone secretion [184] and fasting blood growth hormone levels (see Figure 6-8) are higher in female individuals than in male individuals. Growth hormone secretion is stimulated by estrogen [182]. Oral and high-dose transdermal estrogen administration in menopausal females increases integrated 24-hour growth hormone secretion [185]. Interestingly, growth hormone increases ADH activity in the liver. The steady exposure of hepatocytes in cultures to growth hormone resulting in increased ADH activity resembles the female pattern of growth hormone secretion [206]. ADH activity is higher in female rats and mice than in their male counterparts [207]. Thus, increased rates of the resulting production of toxic acetaldehyde in females compared with males may be responsible for the known increased susceptibility to alcohol-induced liver injury by females. Females are more likely to progress from alcoholic hepatitis to cirrhosis even if they abstain.

Endotoxin-stimulated monocytes in males produce more TNF-α as compared to females [75]. Like Kupffer cells (hepatic resident macrophages), monocytes stimulated by endotoxin induce proinflammatory cytokines and ROS. In studies using animals, however, the stimulation of Kupffer cells by estrogen increased sensitivity to endotoxin after ethanol [208]. It appears that monocytes-macrophages respond differently to endotoxins compared to Kupffer cells as far as the signaling pathways are concerned [209]. The estrogen addition to ethanol ingestion enhanced TNF-α production in Kupffer cells via elevation of the blood endotoxin level and hepatic endotoxin receptor (CD14) expression, resulting in increased inflammatory activity in the liver [210]. The administration of ethanol in female rats induced the hepatic activity of CYP2E1, and the ethanol-induced CYP2E1 activity was reduced by the treatment with antiestrogen [211]. Because activity of cytochrome P-450 (CYP) isoenzymes is regulated by circulating growth hormone, sex differences in growth hormone secretion profiles account for a different expression pattern of hepatic CYP isoenzymes between females and males [212].

8. Sex and Gender Specific Medicine in Chronic Liver Disease

Premenopausal females have favorable factors against hepatic fibrogenesis, hepatic iron overload, hetatocyte death, and visceral fat accumulation (central obesity). Males generally have a greater risk of exposure to hepatitis viruses as well as greater opportunities for drinking and smoking. However, chronic alcohol consumption induces more rapid and more severe liver injury in females than males. Hepatitis C is a major health problem. About one-third of chronic hepatitis C patients have an asymptomatic disease with persistently normal liver enzyme ALT. Premenopausal females are predominant among asymptomatic HCV carriers, in whom liver histology shows minimal to mild chronic hepatitis, and levels of blood HCV RNA are lower than in those with a raised ALT. Most asymptomatic HCV carriers have a good prognosis with a low risk of progression of hepatic fibrosis to the end-stage cirrhosis and its complications such as HCC. In contrast to premenopausal females, males and postmenopausal females may need to consider not only their own environmental and lifestyle risk factors, such as nutritional and exercise-associated problems including obesity and iron overload, heavy alcohol intake, and smoking, which in general occur more frequently in males, but also biological risk factors including loss of estrogen, which may give some unfavorable change to females. Obesity, iron overload, heavy alcohol intake, and smoking lead to increased oxidative stress. Cigarette smoke is a major source of carcinogens, some of which, after absorption into the bloodstream, will remain chemically inert until metabolically activated into a short-lived DNA-damaging form by partial oxidation in hepatocytes [213]. Smoking is also associated with increased risks for infertility and premature menopause [214]. Smoking cessation can reduce the increased risk of developing early menopause associated with smoking. On the other hand, female sex factors such as estrogen, hepatic iron storage status, and growth hormone play antioxidative and cytoprotective roles in the functional and morphological modulation of the liver physiopathology. The interaction of biological factors with environmental and lifestyle factors affects the progression of chronic liver disease (Figure 8-1).

The combination of pegylated interferon-α with ribavirin is the current standard of care for chronic hepatitis C. The goal of antiviral therapy with interferon and ribavirin is to achieve a permanent eradication of the virus, or a sustained virologic response (SVR). SVR is defined as the absence of detectable HCV RNA in the blood at the end of treatment and at least 6 months after the cessation of therapy.In the United States, the SVR rate to the combination therapy in patients with chronic hepatitis C was higher in females than in males, whereas, in Japan, the SVR rate showed no sex differences among patients under 50 years of age, and was higher in males than in females among patients aged 50 years and older. However, elderly female patients (> 60 years) with chronic hepatitis C after interferon therapy had a reduced risk of HCC appearance and achieved prolonged survival compared with elderly male patients [215].

The extremes of nutritional or energy balance, obesity and starvation (for example, with bulimia or prolonged fasting), can either cause or worsen liver disease [216]. For patients with chronic hepatitis C, all that are required are simple advice to eat a well-balanced diet, to limit alcohol intake and smoking, and to exercise regularly so as to maintain body mass, correct lipid disorders and prevent metabolic bone disease. Dietary guidelines for patients with chronic hepatitis C are similar to those for patients with diabetes. As modifying diet and lifestyle is one of the things that HCV-infected persons can do for themselves, it is important that doctors take more interest in this subject [191]. Doctors should try to know how patients live a life and what they eat. What are their dietary habits? How are their physical activities? Are they drinking or smoking? In cases of female patients, doctors conform whether they went through the menopause. If they complain of menopausal disorders, doctors may try HRT for a few years based on the course and degree of chronic hepatitis C. Recently, drospirenone, a novel compound of progesterone with antiandorogenic and antimineralocorticoid properties has been developed [217], and it may be a candidate as a component of oral contraceptives or HRT. Postmenopausal females, along with age after menopause, tend likely to grow central obesity, fatty liver, dyslipidemia (raised blood triglycerides, high low-density lipoprotein, and low high-density lipoprotein levels), and osteoporosis compared with males of comparable age. To eat food containing calcium is particularly important for middle-aged and older females in order to help prevent bone thinning (osteoporosis). Osteoporosis is also a complication of cirrhosis. Raloxifene, a tissue-specific selective estrogen receptor modulator (SERM), may be a prescription medicine for postmenopausal osteoporosis in patients with minimal to mild chronic hepatitis. However, it should be noted that the medicine may produce harmful side effects on liver function.

Combined infection with HCV and HBV conveys a higher chance of cirrhosis, and a greater risk of HCC. In addition, there is a poor response to antiviral therapy directed at either HCV or HBV. Antiviral therapy of chronic HBV infection is interferon-α and oral nucleoside analogues such as lamivudine and entecavir. The most effective approach to prevent HBV infection is HBV vaccination. A community-wide HBV vaccination program directed at the newborn has already been shown to reduce the rate of HCC among children in Taiwan [218]. Females can produce higher levels of anti-HBs after HBV vaccination.

Energy imbalance leading to excessive fat deposition appears epidemic in economically developed countries, including parts of North America, Europe, Asia, and Australia. Importantly, incidental physical-activities of everyday living are dramatically reduced by modern lifestyle based on cars, household and building conveniences, and computer-based workstations. The nutritional problem is a consequence of dietary intake of energy in excess of metabolic need, an imbalance that results from both changes in diet and falling levels of physical activity. After correction for total body fat mass, males generally have larger visceral fat areas (apple shape, android morphology) than females (pear shape, gynoid morphology) (see Figure 6-5). Visceral fat accumulation, or central obesity, correlates with metabolic disorders, rather than deposition of fat in limbs. Thus, central obesity is much more harmful than subcutaneous fat accumulation. Central obesity as well as heavy alcohol intake and hepatic iron overload, which may more often exist for male patients with chronic hepatitis C, are risk factors for the progression of hepatic fibrosis (Figure 8-2). Obesity also correlates with fibrotic severity in chronic hepatitis B, alcoholic liver disease and NAFLD/NASH. If a person in a state of energy imbalance has fatty liver, a low-fat, weight-reducing diet coupled with lifestyle changes to increase energy output can reduce the amount of fat in the liver. In obese patients with chronic hepatitis C, in fact, weight reduction was shown to improve hepatic steatosis and fibrosis as well as liver function tests such as ALT in the blood [219]. Doctors need to appreciate how to give practical advice about modifying energy intake, food composition and exercise levels, when appropriate.

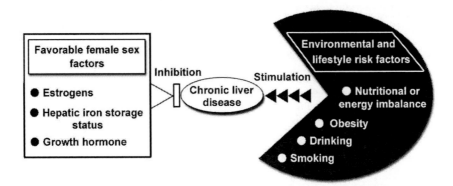

Figure 8-1. The interaction of biological factors with environmental and lifestyle factors affects the progression of chronic liver disease to cirrhosis and HCC [22]. Obesity, iron overload, heavy alcohol intake, and smoking lead to increased oxidative stress, while favorable female sex factors play antioxidative and cytoprotective roles in hepatic fibrogenesis and carcinogenesis.

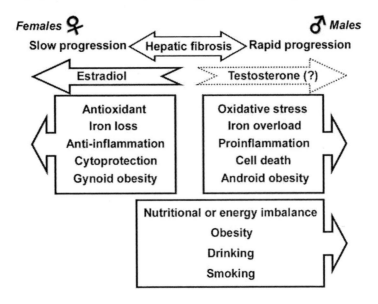

Figure 8-2. Hepatic fibrosis in chronic hepatitis C and B appears to progress to end-stage cirrhosis more slowly in females than in males [22]. Premenopausal females have favorable factors against hepatic iron overload and central obesity (android morphology) as well as hepatic fibrosis. Female sex factors show antioxidative, cytoprotectant, and anti-inflammatory properties. In general, males have more frequently nutritional and exercise-associated problems including obesity and iron overload, heavy alcohol intake, and smoking.

Table 8-2. Sex and gender specific treatment of chronic hepatitis C

	Approaches to prevent the liver disease	Comments
HCV infection	●Antiviral therapy with pegylated interferon-α and ribavirin ●Monitor carefully hemoglobin level in patients who are female and old (≥50 years) during combination therapy	●Asymptomatic HCV carriers are predominant in premenopausal females ●Premenopausal females have a favorable response to the antiviral therapy
Iron overload	●Iron reduction therapy by repeated phlebotomy improves hepatocyte injury mainly in males, but not in premenopausal females	●Males especially need to take precautions against iron overload ●Females usually have less total body storage iron and lower iron stores
Obesity	●Weight reduction improves liver function, hepatic steatosis and fibrosis ●Maintain a healthy body weight by balancing physical activity and food intake; dietary guidelines are similar to those for diabetes	●Obesity is associated with increased incidence rates and increased death rates for HCC ●Males induce more frequently central obesity
Drinking	●Females do not drink more than 20 g ethanol/day; males not more than 40 g ethanol/day ●Some alcohol-free days each week ●For persons with a pattern of binge drinking, abstinence is essential because of their inability to abstain after the first drink	●Females are more susceptible to alcoholic liver disease ●Most HCC cases with alcoholic cirrhosis are in males
Smoking	●The reduction in male smokers is a public health achievement ●Stop smoking especially in premenopausal females to prevent the increased risks for infertility and early menopause	●Early menopause plays some role in the development of HCC
Nutritional disorder	●Enjoy a wide variety of nutritious food including seafoods, soybeans, grains, vegetables, and fruits ●Eat a diet low in fat, particularly saturated fat	●Phytoestrogens are present in common foods such as soybeans, grains, vegetables, and fruits
Osteoporosis	●Raloxifene is a prescription medicine for postmenopausal osteoporosis (note the harmful side effects on liver function) ●Administration of vitamin K(2) in cirrhosis	●Menopause and smoking are important osteoporosis risk factors ●Vitamin K(2) may reduce the risk of HCC

Excessive alcohol intake is the most important controllable co-morbid factor that accelerates the progression of hepatic fibrosis in chronic hepatitis C. Excess of ethanol by means of CYP2E1 pathway produce extensively ROS, which cause oxidative stress with lipid peroxidation and membrane damage, leading to cell death. It is necessary to stop or reduce excessive alcohol intake. In particular, for persons with a pattern of binge drinking, abstinence is essential because of their inability to abstain after the first drink. Females are more susceptible to alcoholic liver disease than males, partly because of differences in the rate of alcohol metabolism but possibly also for other biological reasons. Thus, safe drinking guidelines recommend that females do not drink more than 20 g ethanol per day, and males not more than 40 g ethanol. A common, reasonable recommendation is not to exceed 70 g of ethanol a week. Moreover, some alcohol-free days each week are advisable because recovery from the metabolic effects of alcohol is slow [191].

Attention to iron over intake is required for chronic liver disease. Iron is essential for life, but is toxic in excess. Males especially need to take precautions against iron overload. Females usually have less total body storage iron and lower iron stores in the liver than males possibly due to the physiological loss of blood. The low iron stores in the liver are helpful in protecting the liver against inflammatory and oxidative stimuli and cell death.

Being female or male is an important basic human variable that affects health and liver disease throughout the life span. A better understanding the biological mechanisms underlying the sex- and menopause-associated differences in chronic liver disease would provide valuable information to design care of health and liver disease more effectively for individuals, both females and males (Table 8-2).

References

[1]   Lee, W. M. (1997). Hepatitis B virus infection. *N Engl J Med*, *337*, 1733-1745.

[2]   WHO (1997). Hepatitis C: global prevalence. *Wkly Epidemiol Rec*, *72*, 341-344.

[3]   McMahon, B. J., Alberts, S. R., Wainwright, R. B., Bulkow, L. & Lanier, A. P. (1990). Hepatitis B-related sequelae: prospective study in 1400 hepatitis B surface antigen-positive Alaska native carriers. *Arch Intern Med*, *150*, 1051-1054.

[4]   Poynard, T., Ratziu, V., Charlotte, F., Goodman, Z., McHutchison, J. & Albrecht, J. (2001). Rates and risk factors of liver fibrosis progression in patients with chronic hepatitis C. *J Hepatol*, *34*, 730-739.

[5]   Shimizu, I. (2003). Impact of estrogens on the progression of liver disease. *Liver Int*, *23*, 63-69.

[6]   Velazquez, R. F., Rodriguez, M., Navascues, C. A., Linares, A., Perez, R., Sotorrios, N. G., Martinez, I. & Rodrigo, L. (2003). Prospective analysis of risk factors for hepatocellular carcinoma in patients with liver cirrhosis. *Hepatology*, *37*, 520-527.

[7]   Iwasaki, Y., Takaguchi, K., Ikeda, H., Makino, Y., Araki, Y., Ando, M., Kobashi, H., Kobatake, T., Tanaka, R., Tomita, M., Senoh, T., Kawaguchi, M., Shimoe, T., Manabe, K., Kita, K., Shimamura, J., Sakaguchi, K. & Shiratori, Y. (2004). Risk factors for hepatocellular carcinoma in Hepatitis C patients with sustained virologic response to interferon therapy. *Liver Int*, *24*, 603-610.

[8]   Fattovich, G., Stroffolini, T., Zagni, I. & Donato, F. (2004). Hepatocellular carcinoma in cirrhosis: incidence and risk factors. *Gastroenterology*, *127*, S35-S50.

[9]   Tanaka, Y., Mukaide, M., Orito, E., Yuen, M. F., Ito, K., Kurbanov, F., Sugauchi, F., Asahina, Y., Izumi, N., Kato, M., Lai, C. L., Ueda, R. & Mizokami, M. (2006). Specific mutations in enhancer II/core promoter of hepatitis B virus subgenotypes C1/C2 increase the risk of hepatocellular carcinoma. *J Hepatol*, *45*, 646-653.

[10]   (2002). Cancer incidence in five continents. Vol. VIII. IARC Scientific Publications No. 155 edited by D. M., Parkin, S. L., Whelan, J., Ferlay, L., Teppo, & D. B., Thomas, Lyon, France: IARC; International Association of Cancer Registries.

[11]   Bosch, F. X., Ribes, J., Diaz, M. & Cleries, R. (2004). Primary liver cancer: worldwide incidence and trends. *Gastroenterology*, *127*, S5-S16.

[12]   Ferlay, J., Bray, F., Pisani, P. & Parkin, D. M. (2004). GLOBOCAN 2002: Cancer incidence, mortality and prevalence worldwide, IARC Cancer Base No. 5 Version 2.0. Lyon, France: IARC Press.

[13]   Shimizu, I., Inoue, H., Yano, M., Shinomiya, H., Wada, S., Tsuji, Y., Tsutsui, A., Okamura, S., Shibata, H. & Ito S (2001). Estrogen receptor levels and lipid peroxidation in hepatocellular carcinoma with hepatitis C virus infection. *Liver*, *21*, 342-349.

[14]   Shimizu, I., Kohno, N., Tamaki, K., Shono, M., Huang, H. W., He, J. H. & Yao, D. F. (2007). Female hepatology: favorable role of estrogen in chronic liver disease with hepatitis B virus infection. *World J Gastroenterol*, *13*, 4295-4305.

[15]   Yu, M. W., Chang, H. C., Chang, S. C., Liaw, Y. F., Lin, S. M., Liu, C. J., Lee, S. D., Lin, C. L., Chen, P. J., Lin, S. C. & Chen, C. J. (2003). Role of reproductive factors in hepatocellular carcinoma: Impact on hepatitis B- and C-related risk. *Hepatology*, *38*, 1393-1400.

[16]   (2001). Exploring the biological contributions to human health: does sex matter? Washington: National Academy Press.

[17]   Zacharakis, G. H., Koskinas, J., Kotsiou, S., Papoutselis, M., Tzara, F., Vafeiadis, N., Archimandritis, A. J. & Papoutselis, K. (2005). Natural history of chronic HBV infection: a cohort study with up to 12 years follow-up in North Greece (part of the Interreg I-II/EC-project). *J Med Virol*, *77*, 173-179.

[18]   Bakr, I., Rekacewicz, C., El, H. M., Ismail, S., El, D. M., El-Kafrawy, S., Esmat, G., Hamid, M. A., Mohamed, M. K. & Fontanet, A. (2006). Higher clearance of hepatitis C virus infection in females compared with males. *Gut*, *55*, 1183-1187.

[19]   Puoti, C., Castellacci, R., Montagnese, F., Zaltron, S., Stornaiuolo, G., Bergami, N., Bellis, L., Precone, D. F., Corvisieri, P., Puoti, M., Minola, E. & Gaeta, G. B. (2002). Histological and virological features and follow-up of hepatitis C virus carriers with normal aminotransferase levels: the Italian prospective study of the asymptomatic C carriers (ISACC). *J Hepatol*, *37*, 117-123.

[20]   Okanoue, T., Makiyama, A., Nakayama, M., Sumida, Y., Mitsuyoshi, H., Nakajima, T., Yasui, K., Minami, M. & Itoh, Y. (2005). A follow-up study to determine the value of liver biopsy and need for antiviral therapy for hepatitis C virus carriers with persistently normal serum aminotransferase. *J Hepatol*, *43*, 599-605.

[21]   Gholson, C. F., Morgan, K., Catinis, G., Favrot, D., Taylor, B., Gonzalez, E. & Balart, L. (1997). Chronic hepatitis C with normal aminotransferase levels: a clinical histologic study. *Am J Gastroenterol*, *92*, 1788-1792.

[22] Shimizu, I. (2009). Female Hepatology: favorable role of female factors in chronic liver disease. Hauppauge, New York: Nova Science.

[23] Berger, M., de Hazen, M., Nejjari, A., Fournier, J., Guignard, J., Pezerat, H. & Cadet, J. (1993). Radical oxidation reactions of the purine moiety of 2'- deoxyribonucleosides and DNA by iron-containing minerals. *Carcinogenesis, 14*, 41-46.

[24] Lesbordes-Brion, J. C., Viatte, L., Bennoun, M., Lou, D. Q., Ramey, G., Houbron, C., Hamard, G., Kahn, A. & Vaulont, S. (2006). Targeted disruption of the hepcidin 1 gene results in severe hemochromatosis. *Blood, 108*, 1402-1405.

[25] Lou, D. Q., Nicolas, G., Lesbordes, J. C., Viatte, L., Grimber, G., Szajnert, M. F., Kahn, A. & Vaulont, S. (2004). Functional differences between hepcidin 1 and 2 in transgenic mice. *Blood, 103*, 2816-2821.

[26] Courselaud, B., Troadec, M. B., Fruchon, S., Ilyin, G., Borot, N., Leroyer, P., Coppin, H., Brissot, P., Roth, M. P. & Loreal, O. (2004). Strain and gender modulate hepatic hepcidin 1 and 2 mRNA expression in mice. *Blood Cells Mol Dis, 32*, 283-289.

[27] Looker, A. C., Dallman, P. R., Carroll, M. D., Gunter, E. W. & Johnson, C. L. (1997). Prevalence of iron deficiency in the United States. *JAMA, 277*, 973-976.

[28] Zacharski, L. R., Ornstein, D. L., Woloshin, S. & Schwartz, L. M. (2000). Association of age, sex, and race with body iron stores in adults: analysis of NHANES III data. *Am Heart J, 140*, 98-104.

[29] Harrison-Findik, D. D., Schafer, D., Klein, E., Timchenko, N. A., Kulaksiz, H., Clemens, D., Fein, E., Andriopoulos, B., Pantopoulos, K. & Gollan, J. (2006). Alcohol metabolism-mediated oxidative stress down-regulates hepcidin transcription and leads to increased duodenal iron transporter expression. *J Biol Chem, 281*, 22974-22982.

[30] Nishina, S., Hino, K., Korenaga, M., Vecchi, C., Pietrangelo, A., Mizukami, Y., Furutani, T., Sakai, A., Okuda, M., Hidaka, I., Okita, K. & Sakaida, I. (2008). Hepatitis C virus-induced reactive oxygen species raise hepatic iron level in mice by reducing hepcidin transcription. *Gastroenterology, 134*, 226-238.

[31] Zhang, A. S. & Enns, C. A. (2009). Iron homeostasis: recently identified proteins provide insight into novel control mechanisms. *J Biol Chem, 284*, 711-715.

[32] Pfeilschifter, J., Koditz, R., Pfohl, M. & Schatz, H. (2002). Changes in Proinflammatory Cytokine Activity after Menopause. *Endocr Rev, 23*, 90-119.

[33] Huang, H., He, J., Yuan, Y., Aoyagi, E., Takenaka, H., Itagaki, T., Sannomiya, K., Tamaki, K., Harada, N., Shono, M., Shimizu, I. & Takayama, T. (2008). Opposing effects of estradiol and progesterone on the oxidative stress-induced production of chemokine and proinflammatory cytokines in murine peritoneal macrophages. *J Med Invest, 55*, 133-141.

[34] Rachon, D., Mysliwska, J., Suchecka-Rachon, K., Wieckiewicz, J. & Mysliwski, A. (2002). Effects of oestrogen deprivation on interleukin-6 production by peripheral blood mononuclear cells of postmenopausal women. *J Endocrinol, 172*, 387-395.

[35] Yuan, Y., Shimizu, I., Shen, M., Aoyagi, E., Takenaka, H., Itagaki, T., Urata, M., Sannomiya, K., Kohno, N., Tamaki, K., Shono, M. & Takayama, T. (2008). Effects of estradiol and progesterone on the proinflammatory cytokine production by mononuclear cells from patients with chronic hepatitis C. *World J Gastroenterol, 14*, 2200-2207.

[36] Shimizu, I., Omoya, T., Kondo, Y., Kusaka, Y., Tsutsui, A., Shibata, H., Honda, H., Sano, N. & Ito, S. (2001). Estrogen therapy in a male patient with chronic hepatitis C and irradiation-induced testicular dysfunction. *Intern Med, 40*, 100-104.

[37] Shan, Y., Lambrecht, R. W. & Bonkovsky, H. L. (2005). Association of hepatitis C virus infection with serum iron status: analysis of data from the third National Health and Nutrition Examination Survey. *Clin Infect Dis, 40*, 834-841.

[38] Barton, A. L., Banner, B. F., Cable, E. E. & Bonkovsky, H. L. (1995). Distribution of iron in the liver predicts the response of chronic hepatitis C infection to interferon therapy. *Am J Clin Pathol, 103*, 419-424.

[39] Arber, N., Konikoff, F. M., Moshkowitz, M., Baratz, M., Hallak, A., Santo, M., Halpern, Z., Weiss, H. & Gilat, T. (1994). Increased serum iron and iron saturation without liver iron accumulation distinguish chronic hepatitis C from other chronic liver diseases. *Dig Dis Sci, 39*, 2656-2659.

[40] Eijkelkamp, E. J., Yapp, T. R. & Powell, L. W. (2000). HFE-associated hereditary hemochromatosis. *Can J Gastroenterol, 14*, 121-125.

[41] Siemons, L. J. & Mahler, C. H. (1987). Hypogonadotropic hypogonadism in hemochromatosis: recovery of reproductive function after iron depletion. J Clin *Endocrinol Metab, 65*, 585-587.

[42] Furutani, T., Hino, K., Okuda, M., Gondo, T., Nishina, S., Kitase, A., Korenaga, M., Xiao, S. Y., Weinman, S. A., Lemon, S. M., Sakaida, I. & Okita, K. (2006). Hepatic iron overload induces hepatocellular carcinoma in transgenic mice expressing the hepatitis C virus polyprotein. *Gastroenterology, 130*, 2087-2098.

[43] Yano, M., Hayashi, H., Yoshioka, K., Kohgo, Y., Saito, H., Niitsu, Y., Kato, J., Iino, S., Yotsuyanagi, H., Kobayashi, Y., Kawamura, K., Kakumu, S., Kaito, M., Ikoma, J., Wakusawa, S., Okanoue, T., Sumida, Y., Kimura, F., Kajiwara, E., Sata, M. & Ogata, K. (2004). A significant reduction in serum alanine aminotransferase levels after 3-month iron reduction therapy for chronic hepatitis C: a multicenter, prospective, randomized, controlled trial in Japan. *J Gastroenterol, 39*, 570-574.

[44] Rouault, T. A. (2003). Hepatic iron overload in alcoholic liver disease: why does it occur and what is its role in pathogenesis? *Alcohol, 30*, 103-106.

[45] Nolen-Hoeksema, S. (2004). Gender differences in risk factors and consequences for alcohol use and problems. *Clin Psychol Rev, 24*, 981-1010.

[46] Harrison, S. A., Kadakia, S., Lang, K. A. & Schenker, S. (2002). Nonalcoholic steatohepatitis: what we know in the new millennium. *Am J Gastroenterol, 97*, 2714-2724.

[47] Clark, J. M., Brancati, F. L. & Diehl, A. M. (2002). Nonalcoholic fatty liver disease. *Gastroenterology, 122*, 1649-1657.

[48] Cortez-Pinto, H., de Moura, M. C. & Day, C. P. (2006). Non-alcoholic steatohepatitis: from cell biology to clinical practice. *J Hepatol, 44*, 197-208.

[49] George, D. K., Goldwurm, S., MacDonald, G. A., Cowley, L. L., Walker, N. I., Ward, P. J., Jazwinska, E. C. & Powell, L. W. (1998). Increased hepatic iron concentration in nonalcoholic steatohepatitis is associated with increased fibrosis. *Gastroenterology, 114*, 311-318.

[50]   Bonkovsky, H. L., Jawaid, Q., Tortorelli, K., LeClair, P., Cobb, J., Lambrecht, R. W. & Banner, B. F. (1999). Non-alcoholic steatohepatitis and iron: increased prevalence of mutations of the HFE gene in non-alcoholic steatohepatitis. *J Hepatol, 31*, 421-429.

[51]   Poli, G. (2000). Pathogenesis of liver fibrosis: role of oxidative stress. *Mol Aspects Med, 21*, 49-98.

[52]   Shimizu, I. (2001). Antifibrogenic therapies in chronic HCV infection. *Curr Drug Targets Infect Disord, 1*, 227-240.

[53]   Lee, K. S., Buck, M., Houglum, K. & Chojkier, M. (1995). Activation of hepatic stellate cells by TGF alpha and collagen type I is mediated by oxidative stress through c-myb expression. *J Clin Invest, 96*, 2461-2468.

[54]   Parola, M., Pinzani, M., Casini, A., Albano, E., Poli, G., Gentilini, P. & Dianzani, M. U. (1993). Stimulation of lipid peroxidation or 4-hydroxynonenal treatment increases procollagen (I) gene expression in human liver fat-storing cells. *Biochem Biophys Res Commun, 194*, 1044-1050.

[55]   De Bleser, P. J., Xu, G., Rombouts, K., Rogiers, V. & Geerts, A. (1999). Glutathione levels discriminate between oxidative stress and transforming growth factor-beta signaling in activated rat hepatic stellate cells. *J Biol Chem, 274*, 33881-33887.

[56]   Itagaki, T., Shimizu, I., Cheng, X., Yuan, Y., Oshio, A., Tamaki, K., Fukuno, H., Honda, H., Okamura, Y. & Ito, S. (2005). Opposing effects of oestradiol and progesterone on intracellular pathways and activation processes in the oxidative stress induced activation of cultured rat hepatic stellate cells. *Gut, 54*, 1782-1789.

[57]   Cheng, X., Shimizu, I., Yuan, Y., Wei, M., Shen, M., Huang, H., Urata, M., Sannomiya, K., Fukuno, H., Hashimoto-Tamaoki, T. & Ito, S. (2006). Effects of estradiol and progesterone on tumor necrosis factor alpha-induced apoptosis in human hepatoma HuH-7 cells. *Life Sci, 79*, 1988-1994.

[58]   Pinkus, R., Weiner, L. M. & Daniel, V. (1996). Role of oxidants and antioxidants in the induction of AP-1, NF-kappaB, and glutathione S-transferase gene expression. *J Biol Chem, 271*, 13422-13429.

[59]   Omoya, T., Shimizu, I., Zhou, Y., Okamura, Y., Inoue, H., Lu, G., Itonaga, M., Honda, H., Nomura, M. & Ito, S. (2001). Effects of idoxifene and estradiol on NF-κB activation in cultured rat hepatocytes undergoing oxidative stress. *Liver, 21*, 183-191.

[60]   Inoue, H., Shimizu, I., Lu, G., Itonaga, M., Cui, X., Okamura, Y., Shono, M., Honda, H., Inoue, S., Muramatsu, M. & Ito, S. (2003). Idoxifene and estradiol enhance antiapoptotic activity through the estrogen receptor-beta in cultured rat hepatocytes. *Dig Dis Sci, 48*, 570-580.

[61]   White, M. M., Zamudio, S., Stevens, T., Tyler, R., Lindenfeld, J., Leslie, K. & Moore, L. G. (1995). Estrogen, progesterone, and vascular reactivity: potential cellular mechanisms. *Endocr Rev, 16*, 739-751.

[62]   Meizel, S. & Turner, K. O. (1991). Progesterone acts at the plasma membrane of human sperm. *Mol Cell Endocrinol, 11,* R1-R5.

[63]   Miyagi, M., Aoyama, H., Morishita, M. & Iwamoto, Y. (1992). Effects of sex hormones on chemotaxis of human peripheral polymorphonuclear leukocytes and monocytes. *J Periodontol, 63,* 28-32.

[64] Okada, M., Suzuki, A., Mizuno, K., Asada, Y., Ino, Y., Kuwayama, T., Tamakoshi, K., Mizutani, S. & Tomoda, Y. (1997). Effects of 17 beta-estradiol and progesterone on migration of human monocytic THP-1 cells stimulated by minimally oxidized low-density lipoprotein in vitro. *Cardiovasc Res*, *34*, 529-535.

[65] Janis, K., Hoeltke, J., Nazareth, M., Fanti, P., Poppenberg, K. & Aronica, S. M. (2004). Estrogen decreases expression of chemokine receptors, and suppresses chemokine bioactivity in murine monocytes. *Am J Reprod Immunol*, *51*, 22-31.

[66] Yada-Hashimoto, N., Nishio, Y., Ohmichi, M., Hayakawa, J., Mabuchi, S., Hisamoto, K., Nakatsuji, Y., Sasaki, H., Seino-Noda, H., Sakata, M., Tasaka, K. & Murata, Y. (2006). Estrogen and raloxifene inhibit the monocytic chemoattractant protein-1-induced migration of human monocytic cells via nongenomic estrogen receptor alpha. *Menopause*, *13*, 935-941.

[67] Yovel, G., Shakhar, K. & Ben-Eliyahu, S. (2001). The effects of sex, menstrual cycle, and oral contraceptives on the number and activity of natural killer cells. *Gynecol Oncol*, *81*, 254-262.

[68] Stopinska-Gluszak, U., Waligora, J., Grzela, T., Gluszak, M., Jozwiak, J., Radomski, D., Roszkowski, P. I. & Malejczyk, J. (2006). Effect of estrogen/progesterone hormone replacement therapy on natural killer cell cytotoxicity and immunoregulatory cytokine release by peripheral blood mononuclear cells of postmenopausal women. *J Reprod Immunol*, *69*, 65-75.

[69] Hughes, G. C., Thomas, S., Li, C., Kaja, M. K. & Clark, E. A. (2008). Cutting edge: progesterone regulates IFN-alpha production by plasmacytoid dendritic cells. *J Immunol*, *180*, 2029-2033.

[70] Fox, H. S., Bond, B. L. & Parslow, T. G. (1991). Estrogen regulates the IFN-gamma promoter. *J Immunol*, *146*, 4362-4367.

[71] Faas, M. M., Bouman, A. & de Vos, P. (2009). The immune response in humans is affected by the sex hormones estrogens, progesterone and testosterone, Female Hepatology: Impact of female sex against progression of liver disease, edited by I. Shimizu, Kerala, India: Research Signpost.

[72] Clayton, R. N., Royston, J. P., Chapman, J., Wilson, M., Obhrai, M., Sawers, R. S. & Lynch, S. S. (1987). Is changing hypothalamic activity important for control of ovulation? *Br Med J* (Clin Res Ed), *295*, 7-12.

[73] Bouman, A., Schipper, M., Heineman, M. J. & Faas, M. M. (2004). Gender difference in the non-specific and specific immune response in humans. *Am J Reprod Immunol*, *52*, 19-26.

[74] Ben-Hur, H., Mor, G., Insler, V., Blickstein, I., mir-Zaltsman, Y., Sharp, A., Globerson, A. & Kohen, F. (1995). Menopause is associated with a significant increase in blood monocyte number and a relative decrease in the expression of estrogen receptors in human peripheral monocytes. *Am J Reprod Immunol*, *34*, 363-369.

[75] Bouman, A., Schipper, M., Heineman, M. J. & Faas, M. (2004). 17beta-estradiol and progesterone do not influence the production of cytokines from lipopolysaccharide-stimulated monocytes in humans. *Fertil Steril 82 Suppl*, *3*, 1212-1219.

[76]   Posma, E., Moes, H., Heineman, M. J. & Faas, M. M. (2004). The effect of testosterone on cytokine production in the specific and non-specific immune response. *Am J Reprod Immunol*, *52*, 237-243.

[77]   Bouman, A., Moes, H., Heineman, M. J., de Leij, L. F. & Faas, M. M. (2001). The immune response during the luteal phase of the ovarian cycle: increasing sensitivity of human monocytes to endotoxin. *Fertil Steril*, *76*, 555-559.

[78]   Marino, M., Galluzzo, P. & Ascenzi, P. (2006). Estrogen signaling multiple pathways to impact gene transcription. *Curr Genomics*, *7*, 497-508.

[79]   Komi, J. & Lassila, O. (2000). Nonsteroidal anti-estrogens inhibit the functional differentiation of human monocyte-derived dendritic cells. *Blood*, *95*, 2875-2882.

[80]   Rachon, D., Mysliwska, J., Suchecka-Rachon, K., Wieckiewicz, J. & Mysliwski, A. (2002). Effects of oestrogen deprivation on interleukin-6 production by peripheral blood mononuclear cells of postmenopausal women. *J Endocrinol*, *172*, 387-395.

[81]   Komi, J. & Lassila, O. (2000). Nonsteroidal anti-estrogens inhibit the functional differentiation of human monocyte-derived dendritic cells. *Blood*, *95*, 2875-2882.

[82]   Brooks-Asplund, E. M., Tupper, C. E., Daun, J. M., Kenney, W. L. & Cannon, J. G. (2002). Hormonal modulation of interleukin-6, tumor necrosis factor and associated receptor secretion in postmenopausal women. *Cytokine*, *19*, 193-200.

[83]   Bouman, A., Heineman, M. J. & Faas, M. M. (2005). Sex hormones and the immune response in humans. *Hum Reprod Update*, *11*, 411-423.

[84]   Loy, R. A., Loukides, J. A. & Polan, M. L. (1992). Ovarian steroids modulate human monocyte tumor necrosis factor alpha messenger ribonucleic acid levels in cultured human peripheral monocytes. *Fertil Steril*, *58*, 733-739.

[85]   Konecna, L., Yan, M. S., Miller, L. E., Scholmerich, J., Falk, W. & Straub, R. H. (2000). Modulation of IL-6 production during the menstrual cycle in vivo and in vitro. *Brain Behav Immun*, *14*, 49-61.

[86]   Schwarz, E., Schafer, C., Bode, J. C. & Bode, C. (2000). Influence of the menstrual cycle on the LPS-induced cytokine response of monocytes. *Cytokine*, *12*, 413-416.

[87]   Rogers, A. & Eastell, R. (2001). The effect of 17beta-estradiol on production of cytokines in cultures of peripheral blood. *Bone*, *29*, 30-34.

[88]   Kishihara, Y., Hayashi, J., Yoshimura, E., Yamaji, K., Nakashima, K. & Kashiwagi, S. (1996). IL-1 beta and TNF-alpha produced by peripheral blood mononuclear cells before and during interferon therapy in patients with chronic hepatitis C. *Dig Dis Sci*, *41*, 315-321.

[89]   Hsu, H. Y., Chang, M. H., Ni, Y. H. & Lee, P. I. (1999). Cytokine release of peripheral blood mononuclear cells in children with chronic hepatitis B virus infection. *J Pediatr Gastroenterol Nutr*, *29*, 540-545.

[90]   Gonzalez-Amaro, R., Garcia-Monzon, C., Garcia-Buey, L., Moreno-Otero, R., Alonso, J. L., Yague, E., Pivel, J. P., Lopez-Cabrera, M., Fernandez-Ruiz, E. & Sanchez-Madrid, F. (1994). Induction of tumor necrosis factor alpha production by human hepatocytes in chronic viral hepatitis. *J Exp Med*, *179*, 841-848.

[91]   Lara-Pezzi, E., Majano, P. L., Gomez-Gonzalo, M., Garcia-Monzon, C., Moreno-Otero, R., Levrero, M. & Lopez-Cabrera, M. (1998). The hepatitis B virus X protein up-

regulates tumor necrosis factor alpha gene expression in hepatocytes. *Hepatology*, *28*, 1013-1021.

[92] McMurray, R. W., Suwannaroj, S., Ndebele, K. & Jenkins, J. K. (2001). Differential effects of sex steroids on T and B cells: modulation of cell cycle phase distribution, apoptosis and bcl-2 protein levels. *Pathobiology*, *69*, 44-58.

[93] Grossman, C. J. (1984). Regulation of the immune system by sex steroids. *Endocr Rev*, *5*, 435-455.

[94] Van Voorhis, B. J., Anderson, D. J. & Hill, J. A. (1989). The effects of RU 486 on immune function and steroid-induced immunosuppression in vitro. *J Clin Endocrinol Metab*, *69*, 1195-1199.

[95] Takao, T., Kumagai, C., Hisakawa, N., Matsumoto, R. & Hashimoto, K. (2005). Effect of 17beta-estradiol on tumor necrosis factor-alpha-induced cytotoxicity in the human peripheral T lymphocytes. *J Endocrinol*, *184*, 191-197.

[96] Gilmore, W., Weiner, L. P. & Correale, J. (1997). Effect of estradiol on cytokine secretion by proteolipid protein-specific T cell clones isolated from multiple sclerosis patients and normal control subjects. *J Immunol*, *158*, 446-451.

[97] Amadori, A., Zamarchi, R., De, S. G., Forza, G., Cavatton, G., Danieli, G. A., Clementi, M. & Chieco-Bianchi, L. (1995). Genetic control of the CD4/CD8 T-cell ratio in humans. *Nat Med*, *1*, 1279-1283.

[98] Cutolo, M., Sulli, A., Capellino, S., Villaggio, B., Montagna, P., Seriolo, B. & Straub, R. H. (2004). Sex hormones influence on the immune system: basic and clinical aspects in autoimmunity. *Lupus*, *13*, 635-638.

[99] Fagarasan, S. & Honjo, T. (2000). T-Independent immune response: new aspects of B cell biology. *Science*, *290*, 89-92.

[100] Kasaian, M. T. & Casali, P. (1993). Autoimmunity-prone B-1 (CD5 B) cells, natural antibodies and self recognition. *Autoimmunity*, *15*, 315-329.

[101] Kamada, M., Irahara, M., Maegawa, M., Yasui, T., Yamano, S., Yamada, M., Tezuka, M., Kasai, Y., Deguchi, K., Ohmoto, Y. & Aono, T. (2001). B cell subsets in postmenopausal women and the effect of hormone replacement therapy. *Maturitas*, *37*, 173-179.

[102] Grimaldi, C. M., Cleary, J., Dagtas, A. S., Moussai, D. & Diamond, B. (2002). Estrogen alters thresholds for B cell apoptosis and activation. *J Clin Invest*, *109*, 1625-1633.

[103] Araneo, B. A., Dowell, T., Diegel, M. & Daynes, R. A. (1991). Dihydrotestosterone exerts a depressive influence on the production of interleukin-4 (IL-4), IL-5, and gamma-interferon, but not IL-2 by activated murine T cells. *Blood*, *78*, 688-699.

[104] Kanda, N., Tsuchida, T. & Tamaki, K. (1999). Estrogen enhancement of anti-double-stranded DNA antibody and immunoglobulin G production in peripheral blood mononuclear cells from patients with systemic lupus erythematosus. *Arthritis Rheum*, *42*, 328-337.

[105] Bluestone, J. A. & Abbas, A. K. (2003). Natural versus adaptive regulatory T cells. *Nat Rev Immunol*, *3*, 253-257.

[106] Prieto, G. A. & Rosenstein, Y. (2006). Oestradiol potentiates the suppressive function of human CD4 CD25 regulatory T cells by promoting their proliferation. *Immunology*, *118*, 58-65.

[107] Arruvito, L., Sanz, M., Banham, A. H. & Fainboim, L. (2007). Expansion of CD4+CD25+and FOXP3+ regulatory T cells during the follicular phase of the menstrual cycle: implications for human reproduction. *J Immunol*, *178*, 2572-2578.

[108] Tai, P., Wang, J., Jin, H., Song, X., Yan, J., Kang, Y., Zhao, L., An, X., Du, X., Chen, X., Wang, S., Xia, G. & Wang, B. (2008). Induction of regulatory T cells by physiological level estrogen. *J Cell Physiol*, *214*, 456-464.

[109] Saadeh, S., Younossi, Z. M., Remer, E. M., Gramlich, T., Ong, J. P., Hurley, M., Mullen, K. D., Cooper, J. N. & Sheridan, M. J. (2002). The utility of radiological imaging in nonalcoholic fatty liver disease. *Gastroenterology*, *123*, 745-750.

[110] Brunt, E. M. (2001). Nonalcoholic steatohepatitis: definition and pathology. *Semin Liver Dis*, *21*, 3-16.

[111] Browning, J. D., Szczepaniak, L. S., Dobbins, R., Nuremberg, P., Horton, J. D., Cohen, J. C., Grundy, S. M. & Hobbs, H. H. (2004). Prevalence of hepatic steatosis in an urban population in the United States: impact of ethnicity. *Hepatology*, *40*, 1387-1395.

[112] Browning, J. D., Szczepaniak, L. S., Dobbins, R., Nuremberg, P., Horton, J. D., Cohen, J. C., Grundy, S. M. & Hobbs, H. H. (2004). Prevalence of hepatic steatosis in an urban population in the United States: impact of ethnicity. *Hepatology*, *40*, 1387-1395.

[113] Clark, J. M. & Diehl, A. M. (2003). Defining nonalcoholic fatty liver disease: implications for epidemiologic studies. *Gastroenterology*, *124*, 248-250.

[114] Clark, J. M. & Diehl, A. M. (2003). Defining nonalcoholic fatty liver disease: implications for epidemiologic studies. *Gastroenterology*, *124*, 248-250.

[115] Weston, S. R., Leyden, W., Murphy, R., Bass, N. M., Bell, B. P., Manos, M. M. & Terrault, N. A. (2005). Racial and ethnic distribution of nonalcoholic fatty liver in persons with newly diagnosed chronic liver disease. *Hepatology*, *41*, 372-379.

[116] Fan, J. G., Zhu, J., Li, X. J., Chen, L., Li, L., Dai, F., Li, F. & Chen, S. Y. (2005). Prevalence of and risk factors for fatty liver in a general population of Shanghai, China. *J Hepatol*, *43*, 508-514.

[117] Lerner, D. J. & Kannel, W. B. (1986). Patterns of coronary heart disease morbidity and mortality in the sexes: a 26-year follow-up of the Framingham population. *Am Heart J*, *111*, 383-390.

[118] Kim, H. J., Kim, H. J., Lee, K. E., Kim, D. J., Kim, S. K., Ahn, C. W., Lim, S. K., Kim, K. R., Lee, H. C., Huh, K. B. & Cha, B. S. (2004). Metabolic significance of nonalcoholic fatty liver disease in nonobese, nondiabetic adults. *Arch Intern Med*, *164*, 2169-2175.

[119] Koda, M., Ando, F., Niino, N. & Shimokata, H. (2002). Relationship between age and visceral fat areas in a community-living population in Japan. *J Geriatrics*, *38*, 118.

[120] Sjostrom, L., Kvist, H., Cederblad, A. & Tylen, U. (1986). Determination of total adipose tissue and body fat in women by computed tomography, 40K, and tritium. *Am J Physiol*, *250*, E736-E745.

[121] Buell, C., Kermah, D. & Davidson, M. B. (2007). Utility of A1C for diabetes screening in the 1999 2004 NHANES population. Diabetes Care *30*, 2233-2235.

[122] James, P. T. (2004). Obesity: the worldwide epidemic. *Clin Dermatol*, *22*, 276-280.

[123] Elbers, J. M., Asscheman, H., Seidell, J. C. & Gooren, L. J. (1999). Effects of sex steroid hormones on regional fat depots as assessed by magnetic resonance imaging in transsexuals. *Am J Physiol*, *276*, E317-E325.

[124] Bellentani, S., Saccoccio, G., Masutti, F., Croce, L. S., Brandi, G., Sasso, F., Cristanini, G. & Tiribelli, C. (2000). Prevalence of and risk factors for hepatic steatosis in Northern Italy. *Ann Intern Med*, *132*, 112-117.

[125] Omagari, K., Kadokawa, Y., Masuda, J., Egawa, I., Sawa, T., Hazama, H., Ohba, K., Isomoto, H., Mizuta, Y., Hayashida, K., Murase, K., Kadota, T., Murata, I. & Kohno, S. (2002). Fatty liver in non-alcoholic non-overweight Japanese adults: incidence and clinical characteristics. *J Gastroenterol Hepatol*, *17*, 1098-1105.

[126] Vitale, C., Miceli, M. & Rosano, G. M. (2007). Gender-specific characteristics of atherosclerosis in menopausal women: risk factors, clinical course and strategies for prevention. *Climacteric 10 Suppl*, *2*, 16-20.

[127] Letteron, P., Duchatelle, V., Berson, A., Fromenty, B., Fisch, C., Degott, C., Benhamou, J. P. & Pessayre, D. (1993). Increased ethane exhalation, an in vivo index of lipid peroxidation, in alcohol-abusers. *Gut*, *34*, 409-414.

[128] Letteron, P., Fromenty, B., Terris, B., Degott, C. & Pessayre, D. (1996). Acute and chronic hepatic steatosis lead to in vivo lipid peroxidation in mice. *J Hepatol*, *24*, 200-208.

[129] Berson, A., De, B., V Letteron, P., Robin, M. A., Moreau, C., El Kahwaji, J., Verthier, N., Feldmann, G., Fromenty, B. & Pessayre, D. (1998). Steatohepatitis-inducing drugs cause mitochondrial dysfunction and lipid peroxidation in rat hepatocytes. *Gastroenterology*, *114*, 764-774.

[130] Raucy, J. L., Lasker, J. M., Kraner, J. C., Salazar, D. E., Lieber, C. S. & Corcoran, G. B. (1991). Induction of cytochrome P450IIE1 in the obese overfed rat. *Mol Pharmacol*, *39*, 275-280.

[131] Weltman, M. D., Farrell, G. C., Hall, P., Ingelman-Sundberg, M. & Liddle, C. (1998). Hepatic cytochrome P450 2E1 is increased in patients with nonalcoholic steatohepatitis. *Hepatology*, *27*, 128-133.

[132] Petersen, K. F., Dufour, S., Befroy, D., Garcia, R. & Shulman, G. I. (2004). Impaired mitochondrial activity in the insulin-resistant offspring of patients with type 2 diabetes. *N Engl J Med*, *350*, 664-671.

[133] Petersen, K. F., Befroy, D., Dufour, S., Dziura, J., Ariyan, C., Rothman, D. L., DiPietro, L., Cline, G. W. & Shulman, G. I. (2003). Mitochondrial dysfunction in the elderly: possible role in insulin resistance. *Science*, *300*, 1140-1142.

[134] Lowell, B. B. & Shulman, G. I. (2005). Mitochondrial dysfunction and type 2 diabetes. *Science*, *307*, 384-387.

[135] Czaja, M. J. (2004). Liver injury in the setting of steatosis: crosstalk between adipokine and cytokine. *Hepatology*, *40*, 19-22.

[136] Sanyal, A. J., Campbell-Sargent, C., Mirshahi, F., Rizzo, W. B., Contos, M. J., Sterling, R. K., Luketic, V. A., Shiffman, M. L. & Clore, J. N. (2001). Nonalcoholic steatohepatitis: association of insulin resistance and mitochondrial abnormalities. *Gastroenterology*, *120*, 1183-1192.

[137] Whitehead, J. P., Richards, A. A., Hickman, I. J., MacDonald, G. A. & Prins, J. B. (2006). Adiponectin--a key adipokine in the metabolic syndrome. Diabetes Obes Metab 8, 264-280.

[138] Lihn, A. S., Bruun, J. M., He, G., Pedersen, S. B., Jensen, P. F. & Richelsen, B. (2004). Lower expression of adiponectin mRNA in visceral adipose tissue in lean and obese subjects. Mol Cell Endocrinol, 219, 9-15.

[139] Cnop, M., Havel, P. J., Utzschneider, K. M., Carr, D. B., Sinha, M. K., Boyko, E. J., Retzlaff, B. M., Knopp, R. H., Brunzell, J. D. & Kahn, S. E. (2003). Relationship of adiponectin to body fat distribution, insulin sensitivity and plasma lipoproteins: evidence for independent roles of age and sex. Diabetologia, 46, 459-469.

[140] Shand, B., Elder, P., Scott, R., Poa, N. & Frampton, C. M. (2007). Comparison of plasma adiponectin levels in New Zealand Maori and Caucasian individuals. N Z Med J, 120, U2606.

[141] Hanley, A. J., Bowden, D., Wagenknecht, L. E., Balasubramanyam, A., Langfeld, C. Saad, M. F., Rotter, J. I., Guo, X., Chen, Y. D., Bryer-Ash, M., Norris, J. M. & Haffner, S. M. (2007). Associations of adiponectin with body fat distribution and insulin sensitivity in nondiabetic Hispanics and African-Americans. J Clin Endocrinol Metab, 92, 2665-2671.

[142] van der Poorten, D., Milner, K. L. & George, J. (2009). Effect of adipokines on liver disease in females, Female Hepatology: Impact of female sex against progression of liver disease, edited by I. Shimizu, Kerala, India: Research Signpost.

[143] Ouchi, N., Kihara, S., Arita, Y., Okamoto, Y., Maeda, K., Kuriyama, H., Hotta, K., Nishida, M., Takahashi, M., Muraguchi, M., Ohmoto, Y., Nakamura, T., Yamashita, S., Funahashi, T. & Matsuzawa, Y. (2000). Adiponectin, an adipocyte-derived plasma protein, inhibits endothelial NF-kappaB signaling through a cAMP-dependent pathway. Circulation, 102, 1296-1301.

[144] Kamada, Y. Takehara, T. & Hayashi, N. (2008). Adipocytokines and liver disease. J Gastroenterol, 43, 811-822.

[145] Im, J. A. Lee, J. W. Lee, H. R. & Lee, D. C. (2006). Plasma adiponectin levels in postmenopausal women with or without long-term hormone therapy. Maturitas, 54, 65-71.

[146] Isobe, T., Saitoh, S., Takagi, S., Takeuchi, H., Chiba, Y., Katoh, N. & Shimamoto, K. (2005). Influence of gender, age and renal function on plasma adiponectin level: the Tanno and Sobetsu study. Eur J Endocrinol, 153, 91-98.

[147] Van, H. V, Reynisdottir, S., Eriksson, P., Thorne, A., Hoffstedt, J., Lonnqvist, F. & Arner, P. (1998). Leptin secretion from subcutaneous and visceral adipose tissue in women. Diabetes, 47, 913-917.

[148] Havel, P. J., Kasim-Karakas, S., Dubuc, G. R., Mueller, W. & Phinney, S. D. (1996). Gender differences in plasma leptin concentrations. Nat Med, 2, 949-950.

[149] Haffner, S. M., Mykkanen, L. & Stern, M. P. (1997). Leptin concentrations in women in the San Antonio Heart Study: effect of menopausal status and postmenopausal hormone replacement therapy. Am J Epidemiol, 146, 581-585.

[150] Bennett, P. A., Lindell, K., Karlsson, C., Robinson, I. C., Carlsson, L. M. & Carlsson, B. (1998). Differential expression and regulation of leptin receptor isoforms in the rat brain: effects of fasting and oestrogen. *Neuroendocrinology*, *67*, 29-36.

[151] Wabitsch, M., Blum, W. F., Muche, R., Braun, M., Hube, F., Rascher, W., Heinze, E., Teller, W. & Hauner, H. (1997). Contribution of androgens to the gender difference in leptin production in obese children and adolescents. *J Clin Invest*, *100*, 808-813.

[152] Jockenhovel, F., Blum, W. F., Vogel, E., Englaro, P., Muller-Wieland, D., Reinwein, D., Rascher, W. & Krone, W. (1997). Testosterone substitution normalizes elevated serum leptin levels in hypogonadal men. *J Clin Endocrinol Metab*, *82*, 2510-2513.

[153] Scheuer, P. J., Ashrafzadeh, P., Sherlock, S., Brown, D. & Dusheiko, G. M. (1992). The pathology of hepatitis C. *Hepatology*, *15*, 567-571.

[154] Bach, N., Thung, S. N. & Schaffner, F. (1992). The histological features of chronic hepatitis C and autoimmune chronic hepatitis: a comparative analysis. Hepatology *15*, 572-577.

[155] Lefkowitch, J. H., Schiff, E. R., Davis, G. L., Perrillo, R. P., Lindsay, K., Bodenheimer, H. C., Jr. Balart, L. A., Ortego, T. J., Payne, J. & Dienstag, J. L. (1993). Pathological diagnosis of chronic hepatitis C: a multicenter comparative study with chronic hepatitis B. The Hepatitis Interventional Therapy Group. *Gastroenterology*, *104*, 595-603.

[156] Czaja, A. J. & Carpenter, H. A. (1993). Sensitivity, specificity, and predictability of biopsy interpretations in chronic hepatitis. *Gastroenterology*, *105*, 1824-1832.

[157] Moriya, K., Yotsuyanagi, H., Shintani, Y., Fujie, H., Ishibashi, K., Matsuura, Y., Miyamura, T. & Koike, K. (1997). Hepatitis C virus core protein induces hepatic steatosis in transgenic mice. *J Gen Virol*, 78 (Pt 7), 1527-1531.

[158] Moriya, K., Fujie, H., Shintani, Y., Yotsuyanagi, H., Tsutsumi, T., Ishibashi, K., Matsuura, Y., Kimura, S., Miyamura, T. & Koike, K. (1998). The core protein of hepatitis C virus induces hepatocellular carcinoma in transgenic mice. *Nat Med*, *4*, 1065-1067.

[159] Asselah, T., Rubbia-Brandt, L., Marcellin, P. & Negro, F. (2006). Steatosis in chronic hepatitis C: why does it really matter? *Gut*, *55*, 123-130.

[160] Shintani, Y., Fujie, H., Miyoshi, H., Tsutsumi, T., Tsukamoto, K., Kimura, S., Moriya, K. & Koike, K. (2004). Hepatitis C virus infection and diabetes: direct involvement of the virus in the development of insulin resistance. *Gastroenterology*, *126*, 840-848.

[161] Leandro, G., Mangia, A., Hui, J., Fabris, P., Rubbia-Brandt, L., Colloredo, G., Adinolfi, L. E., Asselah, T., Jonsson, J. R., Smedile, A., Terrault, N., Pazienza, V., Giordani, M. T., Giostra, E., Sonzogni, A., Ruggiero, G., Marcellin, P., Powell, E. E., George, J. & Negro, F. (2006). Relationship between steatosis, inflammation, and fibrosis in chronic hepatitis C: a meta-analysis of individual patient data. *Gastroenterology*, *130*, 1636-1642.

[162] Gressner, A. M., Lotfi, S., Gressner, G. & Lahme, B. (1992). Identification and partial characterization of a hepatocyte-derived factor promoting proliferation of cultured fat-storing cells (parasinusoidal lipocytes). *Hepatology*, *16*, 1250-1266.

[163] Gordon, A., McLean, C. A., Pedersen, J. S., Bailey, M. J. & Roberts, S. K. (2005). Hepatic steatosis in chronic hepatitis B and C: predictors, distribution and effect on fibrosis. *J Hepatol*, *43*, 38-44.

[164] Lin, Y. C., Hsiao, S. T. & Chen, J. D. (2007). Sonographic fatty liver and hepatitis B virus carrier status: synergistic effect on liver damage in Taiwanese adults. *World J Gastroenterol*, *13*, 1805-1810.

[165] Kim, K. H., Shin, H. J., Kim, K., Choi, H. M., Rhee, S. H., Moon, H. B., Kim, H. H., Yang, U. S., Yu, D. Y. & Cheong, J. (2007). Hepatitis B virus X protein induces hepatic steatosis via transcriptional activation of SREBP1 and PPARgamma. *Gastroenterology*, *132*, 1955-1967.

[166] Ohata, K., Hamasaki, K., Toriyama, K., Matsumoto, K., Saeki, A., Yanagi, K., Abiru, S., Nakagawa, Y., Shigeno, M., Miyazoe, S., Ichikawa, T., Ishikawa, H., Nakao, K. & Eguchi, K. (2003). Hepatic steatosis is a risk factor for hepatocellular carcinoma in patients with chronic hepatitis C virus infection. *Cancer*, *97*, 3036-3043.

[167] Powell, E. E., Jonsson, J. R. & Clouston, A. D. (2005). Steatosis: co-factor in other liver diseases. *Hepatology*, *42*, 5-13.

[168] Kamada, Y., Tamura, S., Kiso, S., Matsumoto, H., Saji, Y., Yoshida, Y., Fukui, K., Maeda, N., Nishizawa, H., Nagaretani, H., Okamoto, Y., Kihara, S., Miyagawa, J., Shinomura, Y., Funahashi, T. & Matsuzawa, Y. (2003). Enhanced carbon tetrachloride-induced liver fibrosis in mice lacking adiponectin. *Gastroenterology*, *125*, 1796-1807.

[169] Xu, A., Wang, Y., Keshaw, H., Xu, L. Y., Lam, K. S. & Cooper, G. J. (2003). The fat-derived hormone adiponectin alleviates alcoholic and nonalcoholic fatty liver diseases in mice. *J Clin Invest*, *112*, 91-100.

[170] Potter, J. J., Womack, L., Mezey, E. & Anania, F. A. (1998). Transdifferentiation of rat hepatic stellate cells results in leptin expression. Biochem Biophys Res Commun *244*, 178-182.

[171] Aleffi, S., Petrai, I., Bertolani, C., Parola, M., Colombatto, S., Novo, E., Vizzutti, F., Anania, F. A., Milani, S., Rombouts, K., Laffi, G., Pinzani, M. & Marra, F. (2005). Upregulation of proinflammatory and proangiogenic cytokines by leptin in human hepatic stellate cells. *Hepatology*, *42*, 1339-1348.

[172] Toth, M. J., Tchernof, A. Sites, C. K. & Poehlman, E. T. (2000). Effect of menopausal status on body composition and abdominal fat distribution. *Int J Obes Relat Metab Disord*, *24*, 226-231.

[173] Elbers, J. M., Asscheman, H., Seidell, J. C. & Gooren, L. J. (1999). Effects of sex steroid hormones on regional fat depots as assessed by magnetic resonance imaging in transsexuals. *Am J Physiol*, *276*, E317-E325.

[174] Haarbo, J., Marslew, U., Gotfredsen, A. & Christiansen, C. (1991). Postmenopausal hormone replacement therapy prevents central distribution of body fat after menopause. *Metabolism*, *40*, 1323-1326.

[175] Roulot, D., Degott, C., Chazouilleres, O., Oberti, F., Cales, P., Carbonell, N., Benferhat, S., Bresson-Hadni, S. & Valla, D. (2004). Vascular involvement of the liver in Turner's syndrome. *Hepatology*, *39*, 239-247.

[176] Ostberg, J. E., Thomas, E. L., Hamilton, G., Attar, M. J., Bell, J. D. & Conway, G. S. (2005). Excess visceral and hepatic adipose tissue in Turner syndrome determined by magnetic resonance imaging: estrogen deficiency associated with hepatic adipose content. *J Clin Endocrinol Metab*, *90*, 2631-2635.

[177] Lonardo, A., Carani, C., Carulli, N. & Loria, P. (2006). 'Endocrine NAFLD' a hormonocentric perspective of nonalcoholic fatty liver disease pathogenesis. *J Hepatol*, *44*, 1196-1207.

[178] Maffei, L., Murata, Y., Rochira, V., Tubert, G., Aranda, C., Vazquez, M., Clyne, C. D., Davis, S., Simpson, E. R. & Carani, C. (2004). Dysmetabolic syndrome in a man with a novel mutation of the aromatase gene: effects of testosterone, alendronate, and estradiol treatment. *J Clin Endocrinol Metab*, *89*, 61-70.

[179] Cerda, C., Perez-Ayuso, R. M., Riquelme, A., Soza, A., Villaseca, P., Sir-Petermann, T., Espinoza, M., Pizarro, M., Solis, N., Miquel, J. F. & Arrese, M. (2007). Nonalcoholic fatty liver disease in women with polycystic ovary syndrome. *J Hepatol*, *47*, 412-417.

[180] (2004). Revised 2003 consensus on diagnostic criteria and long-term health risks related to polycystic ovary syndrome. *Fertil Steril*, *81*, 19-25.

[181] Azziz, R., Carmina, E., Dewailly, D., amanti-Kandarakis, E., Escobar-Morreale, H. F., Futterweit, W., Janssen, O. E., Legro, R. S., Norman, R. J., Taylor, A. E. & Witchel, S. F. (2006). Positions statement: criteria for defining polycystic ovary syndrome as a predominantly hyperandrogenic syndrome: an Androgen Excess Society guideline. *J Clin Endocrinol Metab*, *91*, 4237-4245.

[182] Ameen, C. & Oscarsson, J. (2003). Sex difference in hepatic microsomal triglyceride transfer protein expression is determined by the growth hormone secretory pattern in the rat. *Endocrinology*, *144*, 3914-3921. ·

[183] Shapiro, B. H., Agrawal, A. K. & Pampori, N. A. (1995). Gender differences in drug metabolism regulated by growth hormone. *Int J Biochem Cell Biol*, *27*, 9-20.

[184] Clasey, J. L., Weltman, A., Patrie, J., Weltman, J. Y., Pezzoli, S., Bouchard, C., Thorner, M. O. & Hartman, M. L. (2001). Abdominal visceral fat and fasting insulin are important predictors of 24-hour GH release independent of age, gender, and other physiological factors. *J Clin Endocrinol Metab*, *86*, 3845-3852.

[185] Friend, K. E., Hartman, M. L., Pezzoli, S. S., Clasey, J. L. & Thorner, M. O. (1996). Both oral and transdermal estrogen increase growth hormone release in postmenopausal women--a clinical research center study. *J Clin Endocrinol Metab*, *81*, 2250-2256.

[186] Nemoto, Y., Toda, K., Ono, M., Fujikawa-Adachi, K., Saibara, T., Onishi, S., Enzan, H., Okada, T. & Shizuta, Y. (2000). Altered expression of fatty acid-metabolizing enzymes in aromatase- deficient mice. *J Clin Invest*, *105*, 1819-1825.

[187] Van, H. M., Rahier, J. & Horsmans, Y. (1996). Tamoxifen-induced steatohepatitis. *Ann Intern Med*, *124*, 855-856.

[188] Oien, K. A., Moffat, D., Curry, G. W., Dickson, J., Habeshaw, T., Mills, P. R. & MacSween, R. N. (1999). Cirrhosis with steatohepatitis after adjuvant tamoxifen. *Lancet*, *353*, 36-37.

[189] Saibara, T., Onishi, S., Ogawa, Y., Yoshida, S. & Enzan, H. (1999). Non-alcoholic steatohepatitis. *Lancet*, *354*, 1299-1300.

[190] Zimmet, P., Alberti, K. G. & Shaw, J. (2001). Global and societal implications of the diabetes epidemic. *Nature*, *414*, 782-787.

[191] Farrell, G. C. (2002). Hepatitis C, other liver disorders, and liver health: a practical guide. Sydney: MacLennan & Petty Pty.

[192] Ratziu, V., Giral, P., Charlotte, F., Bruckert, E., Thibault, V., Theodorou, I., Khalil, L., Turpin, G., Opolon, P. & Poynard, T. (2000). Liver fibrosis in overweight patients. *Gastroenterology, 118,* 1117-1123.

[193] Calle, E. E., Rodriguez, C., Walker-Thurmond, K. & Thun, M. J. (2003). Overweight, obesity, and mortality from cancer in a prospectively studied cohort of U.S. adults. *N Engl J Med, 348,* 1625-1638.

[194] Yalniz, M., Bahcecioglu, I. H., Ataseven, H., Ustundag, B., Ilhan, F., Poyrazoglu, O. K. & Erensoy, A. (2006). Serum adipokine and ghrelin levels in nonalcoholic steatohepatitis. *Mediators Inflamm,* 2006, 34295.

[195] Wolk, A., Gridley, G., Svensson, M., Nyren, O., McLaughlin, J. K., Fraumeni, J. F. & Adam, H. O. (2001). A prospective study of obesity and cancer risk (Sweden). *Cancer Causes Control, 12,* 13-21.

[196] Farrell, G. C. & Larter, C. Z. (2006). Nonalcoholic fatty liver disease: from steatosis to cirrhosis. *Hepatology, 43,* S99-S112.

[197] Bugianesi, E., Leone, N., Vanni, E., Marchesini, G., Brunello, F., Carucci, P., Musso, A., De, P. P., Capussotti, L., Salizzoni, M. & Rizzetto, M. (2002). Expanding the natural history of nonalcoholic steatohepatitis: from cryptogenic cirrhosis to hepatocellular carcinoma. *Gastroenterology, 123,* 134-140.

[198] Becker, U., Deis, A., Sorensen, T. I., Gronbaek, M., Borch-Johnsen, K., Muller, C. F., Schnohr, P. & Jensen, G. (1996). Prediction of risk of liver disease by alcohol intake, sex, and age: a prospective population study. *Hepatology, 23,* 1025-1029.

[199] Tanaka, F., Shiratori, Y., Yokosuka, O., Imazeki, F., Tsukada, Y. & Omata, M. (1996). High incidence of ADH2*1/ALDH2*1 genes among Japanese alcohol dependents and patients with alcoholic liver disease. *Hepatology, 23,* 234-239.

[200] Eriksson, C. J., Fukunaga, T., Sarkola, T., Lindholm, H. & Ahola, L. (1996). Estrogen-related acetaldehyde elevation in women during alcohol intoxication. *Alcohol Clin Exp Res, 20,* 1192-1195.

[201] Sherlock, S. & Dooley, J. (2002). Diseases of the liver and biliary system, Eleventh Edition ed. Oxford: *Blackwell Science.*

[202] Lieber, C. S. (2004). Alcoholic fatty liver: its pathogenesis and mechanism of progression to inflammation and fibrosis. *Alcohol, 34,* 9-19.

[203] Mathurin, P., Deng, Q. G., Keshavarzian, A., Choudhary, S., Holmes, E. W. & Tsukamoto, H. (2000). Exacerbation of alcoholic liver injury by enteral endotoxin in rats. *Hepatology, 32,* 1008-1017.

[204] Tamai, H., Kato, S., Horie, Y., Ohki, E., Yokoyama, H. & Ishii, H. (2000). Effect of acute ethanol administration on the intestinal absorption of endotoxin in rats. *Alcohol Clin Exp Res, 24,* 390-394.

[205] Bode, C. & Bode, J. C. (2005). Activation of the innate immune system and alcoholic liver disease: effects of ethanol per se or enhanced intestinal translocation of bacterial toxins induced by ethanol? *Alcohol Clin Exp Res, 29,* 166S-171S.

[206] Potter, J. J., Yang, V. W. & Mezey, E. (1993). Regulation of the rat class I alcohol dehydrogenase gene by growth hormone. *Biochem Biophys Res Commun, 191,* 1040-1045.

[207] Mezey, E. (2000). Influence of sex hormones on alcohol metabolism. *Alcohol Clin Exp Res*, *24,* 421.

[208] Ikejima, K., Enomoto, N., Iimuro, Y., Ikejima, A., Fang, D., Xu, J., Forman, D. T., Brenner, D. A. & Thurman, R. G. (1998). Estrogen increases sensitivity of hepatic Kupffer cells to endotoxin. *Am J Physiol*, *274,* G669-G676.

[209] Schultze, R. L., Gangopadhyay, A., Cay, O., Lazure, D. & Thomas, P. (1999). Tyrosine kinase activation in LPS stimulated rat Kupffer cells. *Cell Biochem Biophys*, *30,* 287-301.

[210] Yin, M., Ikejima, K., Wheeler, M. D., Bradford, B. U., Seabra, V., Forman, D. T., Sato, N. & Thurman, R. G. (2000). Estrogen is involved in early alcohol-induced liver injury in a rat enteral feeding model. *Hepatology*, *31,* 117-123.

[211] Jarvelainen, H. A., Lukkari, T. A., Heinaro, S., Sippel, H. & Lindros, K. O. (2001). The antiestrogen toremifene protects against alcoholic liver injury in female rats. *J Hepatol*, *35,* 46-52.

[212] Agrawal, A. K. & Shapiro, B. H. (2001). Intrinsic signals in the sexually dimorphic circulating growth hormone profiles of the rat. *Mol Cell Endocrinol*, *173,* 167-181.

[213] Chen, Z. M., Liu, B. Q., Boreham, J., Wu, Y. P., Chen, J. S. & Peto, R. (2003). Smoking and liver cancer in China: case-control comparison of 36,000 liver cancer deaths vs. 17,000 cirrhosis deaths. *Int J Cancer*, *107,* 106-112.

[214] (2004). Smoking and infertility. *Fertil Steril*, *81,* 1181-1186.

[215] Arase, Y., Ikeda, K., Suzuki, F., Suzuki, Y., Saitoh, S., Kobayashi, M., Akuta, N., Someya, T., Koyama, R., Hosaka, T., Sezaki, H., Kobayashi, M. & Kumada, H. (2007). Long-term outcome after interferon therapy in elderly patients with chronic hepatitis C. *Intervirology*, *50,* 16-23.

[216] Chitturi, S. & Farrell, G. C. (2001). Etiopathogenesis of nonalcoholic steatohepatitis. *Semin Liver Dis*, *21,* 27-41.

[217] Oelkers, W. (2004). Drospirenone, a progestogen with antimineralocorticoid properties: a short review. *Mol Cell Endocrinol*, *217,* 255-261.

[218] Chang, M. H., Chen, C. J., Lai, M. S., Hsu, H. M., Wu, T. C., Kong, M. S., Liang, D. C., Shau, W. Y. & Chen, D. S. (1997). Universal hepatitis B vaccination in Taiwan and the incidence of hepatocellular carcinoma in children. Taiwan Childhood Hepatoma Study Group. *N Engl J Med*, *336,* 1855-1859.

[219] Hickman, I. J., Clouston, A. D., MacDonald, G. A., Purdie, D. M., Prins, J. B., Ash, S., Jonsson, J. R. & Powell, E. E. (2002). Effect of weight reduction on liver histology and biochemistry in patients with chronic hepatitis C. *Gut*, *51,* 89-94.

In: Menopause: Vasomotor Symptoms, Systematic...
Editors: J. Michalski, I. Nowak, pp. 55-95

ISBN: 978-1-60876-930-8
© 2010 Nova Science Publishers, Inc.

Chapter II

An Overview of Post-Menopausal Care: Cardiovascular Aspects

Saeid Golbidi[1], Fung Ping Leung[2], Suk Ying Tsang[3], Yu Huang[4,] and Ismail Laher[1,]*

[1]Department of Pharmacology and Therapeutics, Faculty of Medicine University of British Colombia Vancouver, BC CANADA V6T 1Z3
[2]School of Biomedical Sciences Chinese, University of Hong Kong, Hong Kong, China
[3]Department of Biochemistry (Science), Chinese University of Hong Kong, Hong Kong, China
[4]School of Biomedical Sciences and Institute of Vascular Medicine Chinese University of Hong Kong, Hong Kong, China

Findings in Human Pathophysiology and Treatment Strategies

Epidemiology

By 2030, an estimated 47 million women will be undergoing menopause each year (1). The loss of circulating hormones (estrogens) that occur during the menopausal transition manifests itself through a variety of symptoms, including those related to changes in the cardiovascular system. Cardiovascular disease is often regarded as a problem that only men face, since most women do not consider cardiovascular disease as a serious health problem and in fact report that they are not well informed about their risks (2). This is despite the fact that, over their life span, women are more likely to experience cardiovascular disease and disability than men and will require intervention to improve survival. The Framingham Heart

---
* Corresponding author: Department of Pharmacology and Therapeutics. Faculty of Medicine. University of British Colombia, 2176 Health Sciences Mall, Vancouver, BC, CANADA V6T 1Z3, e-mail: ilaher@interchange.ubc.ca, Phone: (604) 822-5882, Fax: (604) 224-5142

Study revealed that there is a gradual increase in the incidence of cardiovascular morbidity and mortality between the ages of 40 and 55 years in premenopausal women, which were significantly elevated in postmenopausal women of all age groups. Furthermore, at any age, the incidence of cardiovascular disease was significantly higher in postmenopausal compared to premenopausal women, suggesting that cessation of ovarian function and the consequent ovarian hormone deficiency exacerbates the impact of cardiovascular risk factors (3, 4).

In Europe, 55% of women will die of cardiovascular causes as opposed to 43% of men. Coronary heart disease (CHD) accounts for 23% of deaths in women, while stroke accounts for a further 18% and other cardiovascular diseases for 15%. By comparison, in men, CHD is responsible for 21% of deaths, stroke for 11% and other cardiovascular diseases for 11%. Many women have a greater fear of cancer and identify breast cancer as a leading cause of death, although in reality breast cancer is responsible for only 3% of female deaths, but causes considerable morbidity (5).

Thus, coronary artery disease is a major cause of death in adult women, just as it is for men. Although breast cancer is responsible for 43,000 deaths annually and lung cancer for 51,000 deaths annually of women in the United States, coronary artery disease causes 236,000 annual deaths, and 87,000 strokes (3). Even though there was a 20% reduction in mortality resulting from coronary artery disease in women from 1979 to 1989, the absolute number of women dying due to this pathology continues to increase. With the progressive increase in life expectancy, the number of women older than 50, and consequently in menopause, is much higher today than in previous decades. In the United States, the average life expectancy for women is about eighty years (6), indicating not only a greater number of postmenopausal women but also that these women will live more than one third of their lives deprived of estrogen.

Gender Differences in Epidemiology of Cardiovascular Disease

The epidemiology, symptoms and progression of cardiovascular disease differs in women and men. Typically, women are about 10 years older than men when they develop cardiovascular disease (7). Although cardiovascular events are a rare occurrence in premenopausal women, their incidence increases most markedly after the age of 45–54 years (i.e. at the time of the menopause). Kayan et al. (8) determined that a 50-year old woman has 45% chance of aortic atherosclerosis and a 25% chance of coronary artery atherosclerosis, but the corresponding values in age matched males are 50% and 40%, respectively. By the time women are 75 years of age, these figures are 75% for aortic plaques and 55% for coronary artery atherosclerosis and the respective figures for men being 70% and 55%. This shows that there is a rapid progression in the development of coronary atherosclerotic disease in postmenopausal women, despite the rates being similar for aortic atherosclerosis in men and women of the same age.

There is an overall decline in the prevalence of cardiovascular diseases in developed countries, mainly attributable to the promotion of primary prevention (9). Despite an encouraging fall in age adjusted cardiovascular mortality in men, unfortunately this is not the same in women where there has been a gradual increase in the incidence of cardiovascular events (10). Furthermore, the prognosis of cardiovascular disease differs with regard to gender. For example, in-hospital and 1-year mortality after myocardial infarction are higher (two to three times) in women (11, 12), whereas in congestive heart failure the prognosis is better in women than in men (13). Some authors attribute this higher mortality to the prevalence of more risk factors for fatality, including the fact that most women outlive men (12, 14). Thus sexual biological factors could be considered independent variables in hospital mortality risks in patients with acute myocardial infarction.

Marked gender differences also exist in the pattern of stable angina, the most common manifestation of CHD. New cases of angina pectoris as an initial presentation are more common in women, with the incidence of uncomplicated angina in women equal to and, after the menopause, even exceeding that in men (15, 16). Men are more likely to present with an acute event, either myocardial infarction or sudden death, as the initial presentation of coronary disease in all age groups. After the menopause, the incidence of myocardial infarction in women also increases, although the absolute rates remain lower than in men until the eighth decade. Angina is often regarded as benign in women, but, despite presentations of normal or non-obstructive coronary disease, the morbidity rates are higher (17).

Gender Differences in Cardiovascular Risk Factors

Menopause negative impacts many traditional risk factors for cardiovascular disease (CVD), including increases in body weight, changes in fat distribution from a gynoid to an android pattern, detrimental lipid profiles, reduced glucose tolerance, increased blood pressure, increased sympathetic tone, endothelial dysfunction and vascular inflammation. These factors often have different impacts on the risks of CVD in women compared with men.

a- Lipid Changes Associated with the Menopause

Whilst abnormal plasma lipids are well recognized as a risk factor for CVD in men, high blood cholesterol is less important in postmenopausal women, as suggested from the analysis of data obtained during the Framingham Heart Study. The impact of high levels of triglycerides on the relative risk of CVD is more important in women compared with men (18). The total CVD risk in women may best be defined by high concentrations of triglycerides, a high level of lipoprotein (a) and low level of high density lipoprotein (HDL) cholesterol, with high levels of total cholesterol and low density lipoprotein (LDL) cholesterol having less impact (19). Some recent guidelines recommend treatment for those with HDL concentrations below 1 mmol/l. An increase of 1% in HDL is associated with a 3-5% decrease in risk of CVD in women but with only a 2% decrease for men (20). Menopausal induced changes in HDL may, however, be more complex than those indicated by measurement of plasma levels of total HDL alone. There is evidence for changes in the proportion of HDL subclasses during the transitional peri-menopausal period, in particular a decrease in levels of large, buoyant, cardioprotective HDL2 (by 25%) and a corresponding increase in HDL3. Additionally, the prevalence of atherogenic small dense LDL particles increases (by 30-49%) (21). These sex-dependent differences in CVD risk are underlined by the findings of interventional studies showing that a pharmacological reduction in cholesterol levels fails to reduce CVD events in both young and older women (22). It is recommended that all adults age 20 and older should be screened every 5 years using a fasting lipid profile consisting of total cholesterol, LDL, HDL, and TG. The frequency of measurement changes once an abnormality is found or other risk factors are identified (23).

In developing screening and treatment recommendations, the National Cholesterol Education Program (NCEP), Adult Treatment Panel III (ATP III) has incorporated risk factors into its recommendations *(Table 1)*. These risk factors include cigarette smoking, hypertension (blood pressure ≥140/90 mm Hg or treatment with antihypertensive medication), low HDL (<40mg/dL), family history of premature coronary artery disease (first degree relative, male <55 years old and female < 65 years old), and age (male ≥ 45 years old and female ≥ 55 years old) (24).

b- Obesity

Obesity continues to be a leading public health concern in the United States. Between 1980 and 2002, the prevalence of obesity has doubled in adults aged 20 years or older and overweight prevalence tripled in children and adolescents aged 6 to 19 years. In 2003-2004, 33.2% of women were obese and 6.9% were considered as extremely obese (25). Current clinical definitions of obesity in women are based on body mass index (BMI, body weight [in kg] divided by height [in m] squared), where a BMI ≥ 25 kg/m^2 is defined as overweight, and ≥ 30 kg/m^2 as obese and ≥ 40 is considered extreme obese.

Ageing alone has been associated with a decrease in lean body mass, a concomitant increase in body fat and a shifting of fat from peripheral subcutaneous depots to intra abdominal depots (26). Waist circumference and waist hip ratio, as indicators of abdominal adiposity, have been shown to be better than BMI as an indicator of total adiposity, for identifying individuals at higher risk of developing atherosclerotic diseases (27). A case controlled study involving populations worldwide reported that waist hip ratio was associated with acute myocardial infarction independently of, and more strongly than, BMI (28). Abdominal fat is located in two major compartments, subcutaneous and intraperitoneal (visceral). The subcutaneous adipose tissue is a much larger compartment than the intraperitoneal fat, and it is composed of truncal and gluteofemoral adipose tissues. The intraperitoneal adipose tissue consists of omental and mesenteric fat. The regional accumulation of fat in the visceral abdominal region (android or male pattern body fat distribution) causes greater increases the risk for hypertension, diabetes, cardiovascular disease, etc, culminating in the metabolic syndrome compared with abdominal fat stored in subcutaneous regions (gynoid or female pattern) (29, 30). Surgical removal of intra-abdominal adipose tissue in human results in decreased insulin and glucose levels (31), whereas removal of subcutaneous adipose tissue does not improve any aspect of the metabolic syndrome (32). The underlying reasons for why males and females store excess calories in different depots are presumably due to differential evolutionary and sexual selection pressures (33). Visceral fat can be mobilized rapidly to respond to shorter-term energetic challenges. Consequently, one reason to store fat in the visceral depot is to make it more accessible for specific intermittent activities. If males are more responsible for hunting, gathering, or immediate protection, then it would make sense to store calories in a fat depot with greater lipolytic activity, which would facilitate rapid mobilization. In contrast, the lower lipolytic rates in subcutaneous adipose tissue allows this fat depot to respond to chronic metabolic challenges such as those that occur during gestation and lactation in females. Therefore, there is a disproportionate weight gain in subcutaneous adipose tissue during pregnancy, thereby facilitating the female's ability to counteract the metabolic challenge associated with gestation and lactation. These findings support the concept that subcutaneous, but not visceral, adipose tissue is the preferred energy source utilized during late gestation in female rats. Additionally, in women, subcutaneous fat depots are more lipolytically active during lactation than are visceral fat depots; thus subcutaneous adipose tissue is utilized as an important source of energy supply during lactation.

Even though there is some controversy about menopause related changes in body fat distribution, the use of dual energy X-ray absorptiometry shows that a postmenopausal status is associated with a preferential increase in intra-abdominal fat. A study of 53 women shows that postmenopausal women have 36% more trunk fat, 49% greater intra-abdominal fat area, and 22% increased subcutaneous abdominal fat area than premenopausal women (34).

It is possible that the decrease in sex steroid hormones associated with menopause may facilitate age-related increases in body fat. Food intake and body weight regulation is potently influenced by estradiol in adult females of many species. Ovariectomy increases daily food intake and promotes weight gain in rodents. However, food intake and energy homeostasis following oophorectomy has not been extensively studied in humans. Changes in food intake directly related to the cycling of estrogen in women have been difficult to characterize due to the small differences in consumption over the days of the menstrual cycle. In women who displayed intermittent anovulatory cycles, food diaries reflected changes in intake present during cycles in which ovulation occurred, but not during cycles when ovulation did not occur. The most direct evidence that estradiol controls feeding is that a cyclic regimen of estradiol treatment in ovariectomized rats, designed to mimic the changes in plasma estradiol levels across the estrus cycle, normalizes meal size, food intake, and body weight gain to the levels observed in rats with intact gonads (35).

The majority of obese persons who develop CVD have a clustering of risk factors described as the metabolic syndrome. This syndrome is a combination of risk factors including abdominal obesity, dyslipidaemia (elevated triglycerides, decreased high density lipoprotein (HDL)), glucose intolerance and hypertension. The metabolic syndrome is an increasingly common disorder whose prevalence varies substantially with age and ethnicity in both men and women. It has been estimated that 24% of men and 23% of women in the United States meet the NCEP/ATP III diagnostic criteria *(Table 2)*. Its prevalence increases markedly with age, occurring in <10% of individuals ages 20 to 29 years, 20% of individuals ages 40 to 49 years, and 45% in individuals ages 60 to 69 years (36).

Table 1. ATP III recommendations for LDL, total, and HDL cholesterol and triglycerides levels (mg/dl)

	LDL cholesterol	Total cholesterol	Triglycerides	HDL cholesterol	
Desirable (optimal)	< 100	< 200	< 150		
Near (above) optimal	100-129			low	< 40
Borderline high	130-159	200-239	150-199	high	≥ 60
High	160-189	≥ 240	200-499		
Very high	≥ 190		≥ 500		

Table 2. Diagnostic criteria of metabolic syndrome, which requires any three of five risk factors shown. (24).

Risk factor	Levels	
Abdominal obesity (waist circumference in inches)	Males > 102 cm or > 40	Females > 88 cm or > 35
HDL cholesterol (mg/dL)	Males < 40	Females < 50
Triglycerides (mg/dL)	≥ 150	
Blood pressure (mm Hg)	≥ 130/85	
Fasting blood glucose (mg/dL)	≥ 110	

It can be concluded that following menopause, women tend to increasingly display features of the metabolic syndrome, which may partially explain their heightened cardiovascular risk. The metabolic syndrome is also a precursor of type II diabetes, which increases cardiovascular risks (37). Once diabetes develops, the cardiovascular risk is greater in women than in men: among men, the presence of diabetes doubles the risk of cardiovascular disease, whereas in women the risk is increased three-fold (38).

c- Hyperglycemia

According to the criteria of the American Diabetes Association, abnormal glucose metabolism can be classified into three groups, diabetes mellitus, impaired glucose tolerance, and impaired fasting glucose (39, 40). Impaired glucose tolerance and impaired fasting glucose are referred to as prediabetic states with a relatively high risk for development of diabetes mellitus as well as cardiovascular disease (41). Abnormal glucose metabolism or elevated fasting plasma glucose (FPG) levels are also important constituents of the criteria for metabolic syndrome as defined by the National Cholesterol Education Program (24); higher FPG levels within the normoglycemic range constitute an independent risk factor for the development of type II diabetes mellitus among young men (42). As a result, elevated FPG levels--even when they are below the range of diabetes mellitus--are considered important clinical indexes for human health care.

Diabetes induced cardiovascular disease is greater in women than in men, especially when associated with increased blood pressure, as shown in the DECODE study (72).

Diabetes eliminates the protective effects enjoyed by females; premenopausal women with diabetes have approximately the same risk as diabetic men of the same age (73). After menopause, women gain approximately 0.55 kg/year with an increase in abdominal obesity. At the same time, lean body mass is reduced. These changes are associated with detrimental changes in insulin resistance, plasma lipids, blood pressure, and sympathetic drive. In particular, increased body weight and obesity are associated with reduced insulin sensitivity and increased blood pressure. Menopause is likely associated with significant changes in insulin metabolism (43), with decreases in insulin sensitivity occurring especially after 60 years of age (44).

Prospective studies show that hypertension develops more often in subjects with insulin resistance than in patients with normal insulin sensitivity, suggesting that insulin resistance is a key factor in the development of hypertension. Furthermore, it has been reported that decreased insulin sensitivity (by euglycemic clamp) is inversely associated with blood pressure (74). The link between insulin resistance and hypertension is supported by the observation that the worsening of insulin resistance that occurs with weight gain is associated with a greater incidence of hypertension; meanwhile, an improvement in insulin sensitivity, occurring with weight loss or with drugs that improve insulin sensitivity, is associated with decreases in blood pressure.

Early animal studies suggested that estrogens had a protective effect on experimental diabetes. Experiments in dogs (45) and monkeys (46) reported that estrogen administration improved diabetes after a 95% pancreatectomy. Moreover, subtotal pancreatectomy followed by implantation of an estrogen pellet in the remaining pancreatic tissue resulted in localized islet regeneration, suggesting a direct effect of estrogens on the pancreas (47). Estradiol has powerful antidiabetic properties in many spontaneous rodent models of type II diabetes mellitus, such as Zucker diabetic fatty rats (48) or db/db mice (49), in which male rodents develop hyperglycemia but female rodents are protected. In these models, although both sexes develop early obesity and insulin resistance, only male mice develop hyperglycemia. Moreover, in mice with experimental diabetes induced by streptozotocin (STZ), only male mice are susceptible to STZ-induced diabetes, whereas female mice are resistant unless they are ovariectomized. In addition, exogenous estradiol protects against the diabetogenic effect of STZ in male mice and in ovariectomized female mice (50, 51).

The effects of estradiol and conjugated equine estrogen (CEE) on glucose homeostasis have been studied in both healthy and diabetic post menopausal women (lacking endogenous estradiol secretion). These effects can be summarized as follows: a) Treatment of healthy women with unopposed estradiol (without progestin) or CEE usually improves insulin sensitivity and lowers blood glucose (52-54) and b) In women with type 2 diabetes mellitus, both unopposed estradiol and CEE improve insulin sensitivity and glycaemic control (55-57), an effect that is maintained when combined (with progestin) hormone replacement therapy (HRT) is given (58).

Of course, treatment with estradiol does not have a strong hypoglycemic effect on healthy women and does not reverse type II diabetes mellitus. Rather, it appears that estradiol has a more powerful antidiabetic effect in individuals predisposed to oxidative stress. A double-blind, placebo-controlled trial demonstrated that HRT in postmenopausal women with coronary heart disease (who are thus at high risk of developing type II diabetes mellitus) results in a 35% reduction in the incidence of diabetes at 4 years (59). In the Diabetes Prevention Program, metformin treatment in prediabetic individuals reduced the incidence of diabetes by 31% at 3 years (60), strongly suggesting that the antidiabetic effect of estrogen in women with high oxidative stress may be a useful therapeutic strategy.

d- Hypertension

Hypertension, another important cardiovascular risk factor, increases with age in both men and women (61). However, here again, there are clear gender differences; women develop high blood pressure, particularly systolic hypertension, at an increased rate as they grow older. This age-related increase in blood pressure is exaggerated by menopause, with the prevalence increasing three-fold in women aged 65–74 years compared with those between the ages of 45 and 54 years (62). By the age of 60 years, over 80% of women are hypertensive (61). Blood pressure, if measured carefully, is still one of the most powerful and accurate determinants of cardiovascular status and risk (63). The development of high blood pressure and diabetes are important risk factors for CVD, especially in postmenopausal women. Women with diabetes are at greater relative risk for CVD mortality than men with diabetes, and this risk extends across the full spectrum of CVD (64). Women with hypertension similarly have an increased CVD risk compared with men. Following adjustment for age, body mass index, smoking, and cholesterol, women with high blood pressure are at greater risk of CVD mortality compared with men (65). The combination of the two risk factors (hypertension and diabetes) doubles the risk of CVD for women compared with men. When diabetes and hypertension coexist, women have a relative risk of CVD mortality of 4.57 compared with 2.32 for men. However, it may be that hypertension rather than diabetes is the more important risk factor and therefore has a greater treatment priority. In patients with diabetes and hypertension, tight control of blood pressure (mean 144/82 mmHg) was more effective than tight control of blood glucose (goal <6.0 mmol/l or 108 mg/dl) for reducing a range of CVD risks (66). This is important because the prevalence of hypertension increases more sharply with age in women. After menopause, there is a doubling of the proportion of women with hypertension within 10 years (67). European guidelines for the management of hypertension indicate that, in the presence of one or two additional risk factors for CVD, even patients with normal (120–129 mmHg systolic or 80–84 mmHg diastolic) or high-normal (130–139 mmHg systolic or 85–89 mmHg diastolic) blood pressure should receive antihypertensive treatment following several months of lifestyle change (19).

Aggressive control of blood pressure is well recognized as being beneficial in terms of reducing the incidence of cardiovascular events. Rigorous control of blood pressure is particularly beneficial in women, especially in those with the metabolic syndrome (68). Reducing systolic blood pressure to 130 mmHg, as proposed by the Joint National Committee on Prevention, Detection Evaluation, and Treatment of High Blood Pressure Guidelines (69), reduces the incidence of coronary heart disease by 28.1% in men and by 12.5% in women. Additional control of systolic blood pressure to 120 mmHg resulted in no further advantage for men, in whom the decrease in incidence was 28%, whereas the incidence was reduced by

45% in women (68). A reduction in blood pressure also has a positive impact on the stroke mortality rate. The Prospective Studies Collaboration, using data from 61 observational studies of 12.7 million person-years at risk, demonstrated a strong, direct relationship between stroke mortality and usual systolic and diastolic blood pressures (70). Even a small reduction in blood pressure can improve prognosis, where a 2 mmHg reduction in usual systolic blood pressure was calculated to result in a 10% lower mortality from stroke. As suggested by the study authors, this seemingly minor reduction in blood pressure should avoid large absolute numbers of premature deaths and disabling stroke. Conversely, gaining 11–20 kg in adulthood increases the risk of ischemic stroke by 1.69–2.52 times (71). Hence, avoidance of obesity is also important in cerebrovascular disease prevention.

e- Smoking

Cigarette smoking is the single most important preventable risk factor for CVD in women. Nearly 30% of adult women in developed countries and about 22% adult women in the United States smoke. In recent years, smoking has also increased among middle and high school children as well as college students (75). The prevalence of smoking among women is higher in parts of Europe (76). Unfortunately, adult women have not quit smoking at the same rate as men have done, probably because they fear gaining weight. Therefore, the number of women who start to smoke in their teenage years and continue to smoke throughout adult life is increasing. Almost 50% of adults who do not smoke are exposed to smoke at home or in the workplace and so are many children and adolescents (77). In women, smoking is directly responsible for 21% of all mortality from CVD and for 50% of all acute coronary events before the age of 55 (78).

The effect of cigarette smoking on the risk of fatal coronary artery heart disease is dose related and its effect is synergistic with those of other coronary risk factors (79). Cigarette smoking exerts its adverse coronary effects via several known mechanisms. Nicotinic alkaloids stimulate the sympathetic nervous system and cause increases in plasma levels of free fatty acids and LDL-C (80). Nicotine increases platelet aggregability (80) and fibrinogen plasma levels (81). Cigarette smokers have a higher incidence of insulin resistance compared to non-smokers, and their plasma lipids demonstrate an unfavorable profile (82). Premenopausal women who smoke cigarettes are usually deficient in estrogen, and cigarette smoking eliminates the protective effects of estrogen on cardiovascular disease (83). Premenopausal cigarette smokers have a higher incidence of central (abdominal) adipose tissue distribution (84) which as discussed earlier, is associated with an increased risk of coronary artery heart disease. Post menopausal women on estrogen replacement therapy and who also smoke cigarettes have lower estrogen levels than do non smokers (85). Cigarette smoking is also positively correlated with the risk of early natural menopause, greater prevalence of hirsutism, oligomenorrhoeas and infertility in premenopausal women (86). These observations suggest that cigarette smoking in women can provoke a low estrogenic, high androgenic condition. This assumption is supported by several observations: pre and post menopausal smokers have a lower incidence of estrogen dependent cancers, such as endometrial cancer (87), and smoking eliminates the protective effect of oral estrogens on hip fracture in post menopausal women (83). Nicotinic alkaloids inhibit directly human granulose cell aromatase activity and the conversion of androgens to estrogens (88). Cigarette smoking induces hepatic microsomal mixed function oxidase systems that metabolize sex hormones; it enhances 2-hydroxylation, resulting in the synthesis of non agonistic estrogen metabolites (83, 89).

Cessation of smoking is associated with an estimated reduction of 50-70% in the risk of coronary artery heart disease. Women who are ex-smokers have decreased their risk after 2-3 years of cessation of smoking, resulting in a comparable risk with non smokers (90).

f- Lifestyle changes

- *Physical activity:* As in younger age groups, physical activity is considered one of the most important health promotion strategies for older women, with benefits outweighing the associated risks. The most studied area in this respect is, of course, the association between exercise, physical fitness and cardiovascular morbidity and mortality (91). The pathophysiological basis for the reduction in cardiovascular risk lies in the diversity of metabolic effects attributable to exercise. Exercise lowers body mass index (BMI), decreases total body fat as well as subcutaneous and visceral fat, diminishes waist circumference, improves maximal oxygen consumption, carbohydrate handling and the lipid profile, lowers blood pressure, and is associated with better endothelial function and thinner intima-media dimensions (92). These changes may also account for the neuropsychological benefits of physical activity, expressed in lessening of the symptoms of anxiety and depression (93). A large prospective cohort study over 12.5 years demonstrated that women who increased physical activity between initial assessment and follow-up had lower mortality from all causes, independent of age, smoking, comorbid conditions, BMI, and baseline activity level (94). The other two major observational studies on postmenopausal women, the Nurses' Health Study (NHS) and the Women's Health Initiative (WHI), presented quantitative data on exercise and primary prevention of coronary artery disease (95-97). A recent publication from the National Health Service (NHS) (95), summarizing 20 years of follow-up, revealed that women who exercised less than 1 h/week had 58% increased risk for coronary heart disease as compared to women exercising more than 3.5 h/week. Exercise was defined as moderate to vigorous activity, requiring three or more metabolic equivalent tasks METs per hour (one MET is the amount of energy spent at rest). Although the relative risks were attenuated after adjustments for other risk factors for coronary heart disease (BMI, smoking, lipids, etc.), they still remained highly significant. An earlier publication from the NHS examined the influence of exercise on mortality during 16 years of follow up (96). The reference group consisted of women who were active for less than 1 h/week. Devoted exercisers (47 h/week) had 31%, 77%, 13% and 44% lower risk for cardiovascular death, respiratory death, cancer death, and all other causes of death, respectively. Reduction in risk also occurred in the group with more moderate grades of physical activity. While the NHS recruited women in the age range 34–59 years, the WHI trial (observational study) included women aged 50–79 years (97). During a mean follow-up period of 3.2 years, the same pattern of a graded, inverse relation between increasing physical activity score and risk of cardiovascular events was evident. Compared to sedentary women, those who were either walking (energy expenditure of more than 10 METs per h/week) or engaged in vigorous exercise (more than 150 min of exercise/week), had a 40% decrease in age-adjusted relative risk for cardiovascular events. The type of exercise recommended for weight loss is aerobic, such as walking, jogging, swimming, cycling and aerobic dancing.

- *Diet:* Proper nutrition is an essential part of a healthy lifestyle. The dietary regimen is generally similar for the general population as is the case for weight loss, diabetics, cancer patients and prevention, and in many other health conditions. The nutritional plan for weight loss aims for a decreased energy intake (the amount of reduction varies on an individual basis), while providing enough bulk of food. Hence, it is rich in grains, fruits and vegetables, which bring additional benefits such as decreased incidence of CVD (98) or cancer (99). The American Heart Association has recently published updated diet recommendations to reduce cardiovascular disease risk (100), which is also suitable for postmenopausal women and their families. The first issue is to balance calorie intake with physical activity, in order to maintain a healthy body weight. On the diet part, this means being aware of the calorie content of foods and beverages per portion consumed, remembering to eat less if you are less active. Regarding meal and diet composition, the long-standing recommendation of consuming a diet rich in vegetables, fruits, whole-grains, fiber and fish is reinforced with updated studies. Fat should be limited so that 25–35% of total energy is fat, where <7% of energy is saturated fat, <1% is trans fat, and cholesterol is consumed at <300 mg/day. Saturated fat intake is associated with an increased risk of CVD, while fats derived from fish oils have been shown to be cardioprotective. Monounsaturated fats, present in olive oil, improve biomarkers of cardiovascular health (101). Although current recommendations are specific for the reduction in total and saturated fat intakes to decrease risk of disease, specific recommendations on changes in monounsaturated and polyunsaturated fatty acid intakes have been more difficult to define because of the inconsistent and insufficient evidence about the potential effects on health. Optimal intakes of mono and polyunsaturated fats in the diet are still unclear (102). Omega-3 fatty acids may reduce the risk of heart disease by preventing cardiac arrhythmia, lowering serum triglyceride levels, decreasing thrombotic tendency and improving endothelial function. A review of published epidemiological studies supports the protective effects of omega-3 fatty consumption in a range of different populations (101). In particular, studies show that consuming two or more servings of fish per week is associated with a 30 per cent lower risk of CHD in women (103). Plant sources of an omega-3 fatty acid, alpha linolenic acid, present in high levels in linseed and soybean oils may also reduce the risk of heart disease (104). An inverse association between alpha linolenic acid intake and risk of fatal CHD has been observed in several large prospective studies. In one study of women, frequent consumption of salad dressing (one of the main sources of alpha linolenic acid in the US diet) was associated with a reduced risk of CHD (101). The effect of omega-3 fatty acids on secondary prevention of heart disease has also been investigated and the available data suggest a reduced risk of recurrence of the disease with increased intake of omega-3 fatty acids from plant or fish sources (101).

Beverages and foods with added sugars should also be limited, while salt reduction may be achieved by preparing foods with little or no salt. Sodium intake should be limited to 2.3 g/day (100 mmol/day). Alcohol should be consumed in moderation and with meals, no more than one drink per day for women (up to 20 g alcohol/day) and two drinks per day for men (less than 30 g alcohol/day). When eating food that is prepared outside of home, these principles should be kept in mind, due to the ready availability of ever-increasing portion sizes with high energy density, saturated fat, trans fat, cholesterol, sugars and sodium, while low in fiber and micronutrients (so-called empty calories). Research findings suggest that older women are not adhering to appropriate dietary guidelines, indicating a need for more careful assessment of women's understanding of healthful diets, barriers to obtaining and preparing nutritious meals, and adequacy and timing of health education practices (105).

- *Phytoestrogens.* Although utilized for centuries in various cultures, phytoestrogens have recently gained popularity in the United States. Derived from plant sterols, phytoestrogens can be classified into three groups: isoflavones, lignans, and coumestans. The two forms of isoflavones found in soy, genistein and daidzein, contain the greatest concentration of phytoestrogens with structural and functional properties similar to estrogen (106). The mechanism of action relates to the sterol's ability to bind with estrogen receptor sites (107). When high amounts of circulating endogenous estrogen levels are available, receptor site binding is minimal, as the levels of endogenous estrogen decreases, the binding capacity of phytoestrogens increases to supplement the body's deficiencies (108).

The potential health benefits of phytoestrogens on endogenous hormone levels may profoundly impact the prevention of cardiovascular disease (109). For example, a 26% improvement in arterial compliance has been noted in peri and postmenopausal women who consume 80 mg isoflavones per day (110). Such findings, typically noted only in athletic women or those using hormone replacement therapy, represent improved arterial pliability and relaxation of the endothelium lining of the artery (110). In contrast, reduced arterial pliability and impaired vascular relaxation correlates with coronary artery disease. Another aspect related to the health benefits of phytoestrogens involves the improvement of plasma lipid levels. Studies of premenopausal women indicate a substantial reduction in cardiovascular risk with long term soy consumption (111), where intake of soy isoflavones significantly changed levels of total cholesterol, HDL-C and LDL-C across the menstrual cycle. Overall, a diet rich in isoflavones lowered LDL concentrations by 7.6-10%, total cholesterol to HDL ratio 10.2% and LDL to HDL ratio by 13.8%. In other studies, decreases in cholesterol concentrations by 6-9.6% have been observed in pre- and postmenopausal women receiving soy supplementation (112,113).

g- Changes in Hematologic Factors

Changes in the coagulation properties of blood are associated with an increased risk of CHD. Blood viscosity and fibrinogen levels are higher in patients compared to controls following acute cardiovascular events such as stroke, myocardial infarction or sudden cardiac death (114, 115). Increased blood viscosity can be caused by changes in red blood cell count or increased red cell deformity, or due to elevated levels of fibrinogen and other high molecular weight proteins, such as the coagulation factors, and dehydration. The risk of CHD correlates with increases in the level of thrombogenic factors such as fibrinogen, procoagulants and coagulation factors VII and VIII, and with reduced activity of thrombolytic and fibrinolytic factors such as antithrombin III and plasminogen activator (115). Factors that increase platelet aggregation and adherence also correlate with CHD risk.

h- Stress and Autonomic Imbalance

In women, menopause marks the onset of the change in autonomic control of the cardiovascular system where there is an increased sympathetic tone (117). Disordered autonomic regulation of the cardiovascular system is implicated in CAD (116). Importantly, menopause affects cardiovascular reactivity to psychological stressors. Postmenopausal women are more reactive to laboratory stress than their age matched premenopausal counterparts (118). Evidence that menopause can be associated with an altered stress response and with increased sympathetic activity originates from studies that looked into the effects of menopause and estrogen replacement on heart rate variability and beat to beat blood pressure dynamics. Post menopausal women had increased sympathetic tone, which was improved following estrogen replacement therapy (119). Estrogen replacement therapy also attenuated the low frequency vasomotor responses to posture changes and meal digestion, compared to non treated post menopausal women (120). These data suggest that hypo-estrogenism after menopause may increase sympathetic tone and increase the risk of coronary artery heart disease.

There is a complex interaction between physiological changes related to menopause and psychosocial factors. Stress can affect sympathetic neuroendocrine activity and the responses of the coronary vasculature to stimuli (121). In addition to the effect on vasotonus, sympathetic hormones and glucocorticoids can also promote arteriosclerosis (114). In females, stress can have some relation to estrogen production, and in animals there is an association between stress and hypo-estrogenism. In women, psychosocial stress may exacerbate natural falls in estrogen during the menstrual cycle and reduce peak levels of estrogens, causing menstrual and fertility problems. Stressful life events have been found to be significant predictors of the pre-menstrual syndrome and menstrual irregularity, possibly as a result of defective folliculogenesis and relative hypo-estrogenism (122).

Another phenomenon that also shows the association of psychological stress, CVD, and hypo-estrogenic state is "takotsubo cardiomyopathy". It is a unique form of an acute cardiac attack, which is characterized by elevation of the ST segment in electrocardiography and left ventricular apical ballooning in left ventriculography without coronary stenosis and spasm, and occurs predominantly in postmenopausal women in association with emotional or physical stress (123). Although the etiology of this syndrome is yet to be clarified, increases of serum norepinephrine, epinephrine, and neuropeptide Y levels at the onset of cardiomyopathy compared with acute myocardial infarction suggest that the exaggerated sympathoadrenal activation triggered by stress is the primary cause of this cardiomyopathy. Estrogen supplementation partially attenuates these cardiac changes (123, 124).

i- Depression

Depression is common, especially among older people, and strongly relates to cardiovascular events and mortality among men and women. In the NHANES I study that enrolled adults 30 years and older, 17.5% of the 5007 women and 9.7% of the 2886 men were depressed. Depressed men and women had a 1.7 fold increased risk of non-fatal CHD after adjustment for other risk factors; men, but not women, also had a statistically significant increased risk of CHD mortality and all-cause mortality (125). In the study of Osteoporotic Fractures, seven year mortality in 7518 women age 67 or older was strongly related to the number of depressive symptoms at study entry. The relationship between depression and mortality was also seen in the less-well selected cohorts enrolled in the Established Populations for the Epidemiological Studies of the Elderly Project and in the Cardiovascular Health Study (126,127). The strength of this relationship is evident from the detailed analyses performed in the latter study: depression remained an independent risk factor even after adjustment for socio-demographic factors, prevalent clinical disease, sub-clinical disease indicators, and biological and behavioral risk factors (127). In the Systolic Hypertension in the Elderly Program, baseline depression did not relate to subsequent events, but increases in depressive symptoms over time was highly prognostic, suggesting that change in depressive symptoms may be a marker for subsequent major disease events and could serve to alert practicing clinicians (128).

Depressed patients may be less compliant with their medications and less likely to follow recommendations by their physicians, thus leading to increased risk of cardiac events (143). Other explanations for this correlation include cardiac arrhythmia due to tricyclic antidepressant toxicity and abnormalities in serotonin in the platelets, leading to increased platelet aggregation (144). This hypothesis is supported by the reduced cardiovascular mortality in patients receiving selective serotonin reuptake inhibitors (145,146). Moreover, CRP, which is a strong predictor of cardiovascular events, is found to be increased in patients with depression. Increased CRP down regulates endothelial nitric oxide production and platelet endothelial nitric oxide synthase production (147). Another strong link is the possibility of diffuse atherosclerosis causing central nervous system abnormalities including depression.

Pathophysiology of Atherosclerosis

Atherosclerotic lesions (atheromata) are asymmetric focal thickenings of the innermost layer of the artery, the intima. The lesions consist of cells, connective-tissue elements, lipids, and debris (129). Blood-borne inflammatory and immune cells constitute an important part of an atheroma, the remainder being vascular endothelial and smooth-muscle cells. The atheroma is preceded by a fatty streak, an accumulation of lipid-laden cells beneath the endothelium (130). Most of these cells in the fatty streak are macrophages, together with some T cells. Fatty streaks are prevalent in young people, rarely (if ever) cause symptoms, and may progress to atheromata or eventually disappear. In the center of an atheroma, foam cells and extracellular lipid droplets form a core region, which is surrounded by a cap of smooth-muscle cells and a collagen-rich matrix. T cells, macrophages, and mast cells infiltrate the lesion and are particularly abundant in the shoulder region where the atheroma grows (129, 131, 132). Many of the immune cells exhibit signs of activation and produce inflammatory cytokines (132, 133). Myocardial infarction occurs when the atheromatous process prevents blood flow through the coronary artery. It was previously thought that progressive luminal narrowing from continued growth of smooth-muscle cells in the plaque was the main cause of infarction. Angiographic studies have, however, identified culprit lesions that do not cause marked stenosis, and it is now evident that the activation of plaque rather than stenosis precipitates ischemia and infarction (134). Coronary spasm may be involved to some extent, but most cases of infarction are due to the formation of an occluding thrombus on the surface of the plaque (135). Plaque rupture is the most common cause for coronary thrombosis. It is detectable in 60 to 70 percent of cases (136) and is dangerous because it exposes the highly thrombogenic macrophage tissue factor, von Willebrand factor, and subendothelial collagen within the plaque core to circulating blood which triggers the coagulation cascade and platelet aggregation, leading rapidly to arterial thrombosis that characterizes acute coronary syndromes (137).

Although plaque rupture remains the most common type of plaque complication, it is now recognized that thrombotic coronary death and acute coronary syndromes may also be associated with nonruptured and nonstenotic plaques. In cases involving nonruptured plaques, plaque erosion or nodular calcification usually accompanies the luminal thrombus (138). Despite a higher absolute risk of shear stress on the surface of plaques with severe stenosis, nonstenotic lesions outnumber stenotic plaques and account for a significant proportion of culprit lesions. The initial triggers for the inflammatory cascade leading to initiation and progression of atherosclerosis are not entirely clear. However, current evidence supports the role of the traditional cardiovascular risk factors and, to a lesser degree, novel risk factors such as infectious agents. Oxidized LDL and angiotensin II, a vasoconstrictor associated with hypertension, have been shown to increase the expression of vascular cell adhesion molecule-1 and MCP-1 (138, 139, 140). The metabolic abnormalities that characterize diabetes, particularly hyperglycemia, liberation of free fatty acids, and insulin resistance may provoke vascular dysfunction and inflammation via multiple mechanisms including increased oxidative stress, disturbances of intracellular signal transduction, and activation of receptor for advanced glycation end products (141). The current worldwide obesity epidemic resulting from changes in lifestyle patterns may lead to increased incidence of type II diabetes and atherosclerotic vascular complications (142). Genetic variables may also modify individual susceptibility and response to these proatherogenic mediators.

Evaluation of Cardiovascular Risk

Recent advances in our understanding of the pathophysiology of CHD have led to the discovery of several novel cardiovascular risk factors that may potentially enhance our ability to identify and manage patients most likely to have a future cardiovascular event. In epidemiologic studies, elevated levels of C-reactive protein (CRP), homocysteine, and lipoprotein (a) have been associated with an increased risk of CHD. However, the role of these biomarkers as CVD risk factors has not yet been borne out in randomized controlled trials and therefore routine screening in all adults is not recommended at this time.

C-reactive protein (CRP), a serum marker of systemic inflammation, has been shown to predict cardiovascular events in both healthy patients as well as those with a history of CHD (148-150). Nested case control and prospective studies have shown that high sensitivity (hs) CRP adds predictive value above that obtained from currently established risk factors, but additional prospective studies are needed to define risk stratification criteria and possible differences in risk between genders and races. Therefore, it is not recommended to screen the entire population, but it is optional to measure hs-CRP as an adjunct to major risk factors to guide therapy in patients judged to be at intermediate risk for CHD (10%-20% risk of CHD per 10 years) (151).

Elevated homocysteine levels have been associated with an increased risk of CHD in some epidemiologic studies, but not all (152). In addition, levels of homocysteine have been shown to be lower in women than men, and in premenopausal compared to postmenopausal women (153). The precise relationship between hyperhomocysteinemia and atherosclerosis remains to be elucidated but in vitro studies suggest homocysteine incites vascular inflammation via increased oxidative stress, smooth muscle cell proliferation, and decreased levels of nitric oxide (NO) (154). Because homocysteine may be an acute-phase reactant that is a marker of atherogenesis or an independent risk factor more closely linked to the development of cardiovascular disease, further prospective trials are needed to determine the effects of homocysteine-lowering therapy on CVD development and progression.

Lipoprotein (a) [Lp(a)] is considered an independent risk factor for CAD (155). Lp(a) is an atherogenic lipoprotein that resembles LDL cholesterol and may be prothrombotic owing to competitive inhibition of plasminogen binding and plasmin generation. Lp(a) is determined by a single gene, and its levels are not modified by dietary intervention. A number of studies suggest that it can not be a CAD predictor in the presence of low LDL. Howerer, its role is augmented in the presence of increased total cholesterol/ HDL ratio. In women with Lp(a) concentrations of >30 mg/dL combined with a total cholerserol/HDL ratio > 5.5 or other risk factors, therapy to lower LDL should start earlier and should be more aggressive (156, 157).

Hormone Replacement Therapy for Cardiovascular Dysfunction

Several observational studies were performed in the 1980s with the aim of evaluating the association of exogenous estrogens and the occurrence of cardiovascular events. A meta-analysis of these studies published in 1991 demonstrated a significant reduction in the relative risk for coronary heart disease associated with hormone replacement therapy (HRT) (158). Based on these observational studies, in 1992 the American College of Physicians recommended HRT for all postmenopausal women to prevent coronary heart disease (159). As a result, use of HRT substantially increased in the 1990s. However, observational studies have limitations, especially because of the lack of randomization. Subsequently, several controlled randomized trials have been accomplished with the purpose of evaluating the effects of HRT on cardiovascular diseases.

The HERS (Heart and Estrogen/Progestin Replacement Study) study was one of the first randomized clinical trial of HRT and cardiovascular diseases. The HERS study included 2763 postmenopausal women, with the mean age of 67 and established coronary heart disease and randomized them to receive 0.625 mg of conjugated equine estrogen and 2.5 mg of medroxyprogesterone acetate or placebo (160). Interestingly, there was an increased rate of cardiovascular events in the first year after randomization in spite of lower LDL and higher HDL cholesterol, which decreased in the subsequent years. There was no significant difference between the groups using the end point of non fatal myocardial infarction or cardiac death, after 4 years of follow up. In the placebo group, the event rate was lower than expected in the first year, and was higher in the subsequent years of follow up.

In 1991, the Womend Health Initiative (WHI) was started by the National Institutes of Health with the purposes of determining the most common causes of death, disability, and decreased quality of life (such as cardiovascular diseases, cancer, and osteoporosis) in postmenopausal women (161). It had two observational and randomized controlled clinical trial components. The clinical trial included postmenopausal women, 50-79 years of age, without previous cardiovascular events. Those with an intact uterus (16608 participants) received 0.625 mg/day of conjugated equine estrogen and 2.5 mg/day of medroxyprogesterone or placebo. Women with a prior history of hysterectomy (10739 women) were randomized to receive 0.625 mg/day of conjugated equine estrogen alone or placebo. The primary end point was the occurrence of coronary heart disease (non fatal myocardial infarction and cardiac death). The trial in women with intact uterus was stopped after 5.2 years of follow up, due to increased cases of breast cancer (26%), increased coronary heart diseases mainly non-fatal myocardial infarction (29%), and 41% increase in stroke. A 23% reduction in osteoporotic fractures and a 37% reduction in colorectal cancers were also observed. Much as in the HERS trail, there was a significant increase in coronary heart disease events in the first year which showed a decrease in the subsequent years of follow up.

The estrogen alone arm of the study in hysterectomized women was also stopped prematurely after 6.8 years of follow up because of a 39% increase in the occurrence of stokes and a 33% increase in venous thromboemboli. There was a 39% reduction in hip fractures and a 23 % reduction in breast cancers, while coronary heart disease and colorectal cancers did not change.

In both of these trials (HERS and WHI) the lack of a cardioprotective effect of HRT was observed in spite of a favorable action on lipid profile (significant reduction in LDL and increase in HDL cholesterol). Based on these results, the scientific guidelines for HRT have been changed and it is now not recommended for the prevention of cardiovascular diseases (162-164). As a consequence, there was a 66% reduction in combined estrogen progestin and 33% in unopposed estrogen prescriptions in the United States during 2002-2003 (165,166).

A recent meta-analysis of 31 randomized controlled trials which includes 44113 subjects shows that HRT is associated with an increased risk of stroke (odds ratio(OR) 1.32, confidence intervals (CI) 1.14-1.53), stroke severity and venous thromboembolism (OR 2.05, CI 1.44-2.92) but not of CHD events. Combined HRT increases the risk of venous thromboembolism compared with estrogen monotherapy (167).

Hormone Replacement Therapy with Regard to Age and Time Interval from Menopause

Discordance between observational studies and randomized control trials (RCTs) is best exemplified within the WHI that evaluated HRT in both an observational and RCT. The WHI observational part showed a 50% reduction in CHD in women who used estrogen plus progestin compared to placebo users. In contract, the risk of CHD was increased in those who randomized for combined estrogen, medroxyprogeşterone acetate relative to nonusers. This discrepancy in outcome might be partly explained by confounding factors or selection biases. Women who used HRT in the observational studies were relatively young at the time of HT initiation (30 to 55 years old), recently postmenopausal, were relatively lean (approximate BMI was 25 kg/m^2), were predominantly symptomatic mainly with flushing and other menopausal symptoms as these symptoms were the primary reason for using HRT, and continued hormone therapy for decades. Meanwhile, the randomized trials consisted of relatively older women (90% older 55 years) who initiated HRT even 10 to 20 years after the beginning of menopause and excluded those with significant menopausal symptoms (flushing). Mean duration of therapy in RCTs was also considerably less than that of the observational studies. Furthermore, subjects in RCTs were overweight (approximate BMI 29 kg/m^2).

In order to verify the relationship between hormone therapy and cardiovascular risks with age and years since menopause, a secondary analysis of the combined randomized trials of the WHI in both the postmenopausal women who had undergone a hysterectomy and those with intact uterus has been performed (168). For women with less than 10 years since menopause began, the hazard ratio for coronary heart disease was 0.76 (95% CI 0.50–1.16); 10–19 years, 1.10 (95% CI 0.84– 1.45); and 20 or more years, 1.28 (95% CI 1.03–1.58). For the age group of 50–59 years, the hazard ratio for coronary heart disease was 0.93 (95% CI 0.65–1.33); 60–69 years, 0.98 (95% CI 0.79–1.21); and 70– 79 years, 1.26 (95% CI 1.00– 1.59). The risk of stroke was increased but did not vary significantly by age or time since menopause. Thus, women who initiated hormone therapy closer to menopause tended to have a reduced risk for coronary heart disease compared with women more distant from menopause, who showed an increased risk. The risk of stroke was increased regardless of age or of years since menopause.

Similar to the effect of HT on CHD, the WHI data indicates that the effect of HT on total mortality is related to the age at which HT is initiated. Relative to placebo, women who were 50 to 59 years old when randomized to estrogen plus medroxyprogesterone had a 31% reduction in total mortality whereas women 60 to 69 years old when randomized had a 9% increased risk of total mortality and women 70 to 79 years old when randomized had a 6% increased risk of total mortality (168). Women who were randomized to conjugated estrogen therapy between the ages of 50 to 59 years had a 29% reduction in total mortality, those randomized between the ages of 60 to 69 years had a 2% increased risk of total mortality, and those randomized between the ages of 70 to 79 years had a 20% increased risk of total mortality, all relative to placebo-treated women. With the combination of both arms (estrogen alone and estrogen plus medroxyprogesterone) total mortality was significantly reduced 30% in women 50 to 59 years old when randomized, whereas women 60 to 69 years old when randomized had a 5% increased risk of total mortality and women 70 to 79 years old when randomized had a 14% increased risk of total mortality, all relative to placebo-treated women. The subgroup of younger women randomized to WHI is more representative of the women in observational studies, data from which also indicate that women who use HT relative to those who do not have a reduction in total mortality (169).

The beneficial effect of HT on total mortality according to age has also been demonstrated in another large meta-analysis (170). The effect of HT on total mortality according to age was examined using 30 RCTs (more than 6 months duration) comparing HT with placebo. In this study, the effect of HT on total mortality was null over all ages. However, when the data were examined by the age of subjects, a statistically significant reduction in total mortality was found for subjects <60 years old at randomization. The magnitude of the reduction in total mortality of 39% for the women younger than 60 years old was similar to that of observational studies, notably comparable with that of the Nurses' Health Study (171), the largest observational study. The age at initiation of HT among the women in the observational studies and the age of the younger women randomized to RCTs examined in the meta-analysis is similar. On the other hand, in this meta-analysis, the effect of HT on total mortality in women >60 years old was similar to that reported over all ages in RCTs. In this analysis, the totality of data from RCTs indicates that young postmenopausal women who initiate HT in close proximity to menopause have reduced total mortality and CHD. These results parallel the consistency of a reduction in total mortality and CHD seen in observational studies where almost all the women initiated HT in close proximity to menopause, typically within 6 years.

An interesting ancillary substudy of the WHI trial suggests a possible explanation of these findings. Manson et al. (172) reported a relationship between estrogen replacement (alone) and coronary artery calcium among the 50-59 year age group. Calcified atheroma detected by CT scan of the heart reflects the chronic inflammatory process associated with atherosclerosis and may be used as a measure of cardiovascular risk factor. They performed computed tomography of the heart in 1064 women after a mean of 7.4 years of treatment and 1.3 years after the trial was completed (8.7 years after randomization). The findings reveal that those women receiving conjugated estrogen were 42% less likely to have severe coronary artery calcium than women receiving placebo. And among those who were particularly compliant (>80% adherence for at least 5 years), women receiving conjugated estrogen had a 61% lower risk of severe coronary calcium. These data also provide some reassurance that estrogen is not harmful for younger women, who are the group that may benefit from estrogen's effects on menopausal symptoms.

Collectively, these findings proposes a "timing hypothesis" which suggests that estrogen hinders earlier stages of atherosclerosis through beneficial effects on endothelial function and lipids, but triggers events in the presence of advanced atherogenic lesions (173). This hypothesis provides a scientific framework within which to understand much of the clinical data on the relation between hormone treatment and the occurrence of cardiovascular disease from the past two decades, including data from observational studies, the HERS study and the WHI reports.

Longevity of hormone therapy and cardiovascular protection: RCTs such as WHI and HERS which have the longest randomized follow up can provide evidence for long term beneficial effect on HT on CHD. There was a significant trend toward reduction in CHD after 4-5 years of combined estrogen medroxyprogesterone therapy in comparison to the placebo group in HERS (160). Compatible results were observed in the WHI trail after 6 years of estrogen progestin therapy (174). Consistency between the WHI RCTs and the WHI observational study also supports the beneficial effects of long term HT on CHD. In both of the WHI trial and observational study (estrogen plus progestin) the relative risk for CHD decreased after 5 years of HT compared to controls (nonusers). This matter was also supported in WHI trial and observational study of estrogen (alone) therapy (173).

Cardiovascular Risks after Discontinuation of HRT

As stated before, the WHI trail stopped prematurely because the risks exceeded the benefits; nevertheless, follow up continued for three additional years. Analysis was made to evaluate health outcomes in women who did not undergo hysterectomy (estrogen plus medroxyprogesterone) at 3 years after stopping the intervention (175). The primary end points were coronary heart disease and invasive breast cancer; in addition a global index summarizing the balance of risks and benefits included the two primary end points plus stroke, pulmonary embolism, endometrial cancer, colorectal cancer, hip fracture and death due to other causes. The risk of cardiovascular events after the intervention was comparable by initial randomized assignments, 1.97% (annualized rate) in the treated and 1.91% in the placebo group. Therefore, the increased cardiovascular risks in women assigned to HRT observed during the intervention period did not persist during the follow up period. A greater risk of fatal and non-fatal malignancies occurred in the HRT than in the placebo group (1.56% vs 1.26%; hazard ratio [HR], 1.24; 95% CI, 1.04-1.48), which indicates that, the increased risk of malignancies was also present after the intervention was stopped.

Conclusion of Data Related to Human Menopause and HRT

Menopause-related estrogen deficiency increases the risk of cardiovascular disease. The presence of abdominal obesity, dyslipidemia, hypertension, fasting hyperglycemia or impaired glucose tolerance further aggravates the CVD risk imposed by menopause. The consistency of observational data demonstrating a reduction of coronary heart disease with exogenous postmenopausal hormone therapy has not been confirmed by randomized clinical trials. Indeed, those who were assigned to receive estrogen plus progesterone showed increased risk of CHD and stroke, and in those who randomized to get estrogen alone (hysterectomized women), the risk of CHD was not affected and an increased incidence of stroke was observed too. The differences in age at initiation and the duration of HRT are key points to be considered as well. HRT appears to decrease coronary disease in younger women, near menopause; yet, in older women, HRT increases risk of a coronary event. Although HRT is a recognized method in the prevention and treatment of osteoporosis (and decreases the incidence of colorectal cancer), it is not licensed as a first line of treatment; meanwhile, increased risk of breast cancer has been shown in women with intact uterus. The increased risk of CVD associated with HRT did not persist after the intervention was stopped, while the risk of breast cancer was present despite the interruption of therapy.

The American Association of Clinical Endocrinologists issued a position statement in 2008 concluding that for symptomatic menopausal women under the age of 60, the benefits of HT exceed the risks (176). Nevertheless, the bottom line remains that the cardioprotective hypothesis of HRT has to be elucidated further, since randomized trials have not been conducted in the same population of women from which the hypothesis was initially derived. However, this hypothesis will be directly evaluated in the ongoing Early versus Late Intervention Trial with Estradiol (ELITE) (177). This randomized trial, funded by the National Institute on Aging, is designed to clarify the effects of 17β-estradiol on the progression of atherosclerosis, cognition and other postmenopausal health issues in recently menopausal (<6 years) and remotely menopausal (>10 years) women with no history of cardiovascular disease or diabetes. Until data from trials like ELITE comes up, guidelines such as those from the North American Menopause Society are reasonable for clinical practice (178).

Animal Models of Menopause

Menopause, a normal biological phenomenon in middle-aged women, is related to loss of fertility and augmented risk for cardiovascular diseases and bone loss. Thus, suitable animal models should be employed to allow comprehensive investigation of the detailed biological mechanisms underlying the increased risk for adverse health incidence in menopausal women. It is known that some species of older female non-human primates also experience a menopause-like condition, with termination of reproductive cycles, reduced bone density and an increased threat for atherosclerotic events. However, many issues should be taken into account to determine their usefulness for scientific studies, for example, the expense of purchase and care, small numbers of animals available and risk for disease transmission to humans.

In 1998, Bellino reported that a workshop was held at the National Institutes of Health to investigate the non-primate animal species as potential models for pathophysiological changes associated with loss of reproductive function (179). The main theme of the workshop was on middle-aged, ovariectomized females of various laboratory animals and the capacity of exogenous estrogen to reverse pathophysiolgical changes in the bone, thermoregulatory control and cardiovascular system in these different animals. The conclusions they reached can be summarized as: (1) the animals considered (mice, rats, pigs, rabbits, dogs and sheep/ewe, mice (because of transgenic technology) have the potential to be good models to study the effects of ovariectomy and estrogen replacement on associated bone and cardiovascular changes; (2) rats are an excellent model for bone studies but a poor model for the cardiovascular system changes associated with loss of reproductive function (however, rats are frequently used to vascular reactivity, as addressed later); (3) pigs are considered to be a good model for the human cardiovascular system, but there is limited information on ovariectomized mature pigs in cardiovascular and bone studies, sensitivity of bone density to dietary calcium—and it is difficult to easily manage regular pigs, while there is a relatively high cost attached to using miniature pigs; (4) rabbits have a good potential as a cardiovascular model despite the limited numbers of studies and their differences from primates in terms of coronary artery structure. Although rabbits are the smallest species known to have Haversian bone remodeling processes, the small number of bone studies in ovariectomized rabbits are confounded by effects of dietary calcium. (5) Although there are basically no studies on the cardiovascular system of ovariectomized dogs, bone studies that have been performed suggest that it is a poor model for the menopausal human. Additionally, the role of estrogen in bone and the cardiovascular system is hard to understand because of the limitation of two estrus cycles per year in the dog. (6) The sheep/ewe seems to be a promising large animal model for the bone and cardiovascular systems, but more research is needed; (7) Of the animals studied for estrogen effects on vasomotor symptoms (guinea pig, mouse, rat, and monkey), only rats and monkeys show symptoms of hot flashes associated with loss of reproductive function.

From 1998 onwards, additional studies showed greater opinions using different species. In 1998, another reported by Thornidike and Turner discussed the use of aged ovariectomized ewes as a cost-effective large animal model to study coronary artery disease, oral bone loss, osteoporosis, osteoarthritis – conditions seen after menopause (180). Their studies of the effects of estrogen deficiency and estrogen therapy on the terminal aortas of the aged ovariectomized (OVX) ewes demonstrated that there is subintimal thickening in the distal aorta of animals that were estrogen deficient compared to the controls. This model may an opportunity to study postmenopausal conditions and the safety and efficacy of new therapeutic agents.

In 2002, Dalsgaard et al. evaluated the effect of estrogen replacement therapy on the functional characteristics of coronary and cerebral arteries using the OVX Watanabe heritable hyperlipidemic (WHHL) rabbit fed a diet free of phytoestrogens. They demonstrated that treatment 17-estradiol decreased the electromechanical tonus of atherosclerotic coronary arteries proximally, where the atherosclerosis was most formed. This could be one of the mechanisms behind the putative protective effect of hormone replacement therapy during ischemic heart disease. They suggested that this animal model as being useful for the investigation of postmenopausal coronary and cerebral artery function. (181).

In 2004, Appe *et al.* suggested that some of the important health issues for postmenopausal women include cardiovascular disease, osteoporosis, breast cancer, and relief of menopausal symptoms. Ovariectomized cynomolgus monkeys (Macaca fascicularis) have many advantages as research animals including a close phylogenetic relationship to humans, resemblance in lipid/lipoprotein metabolism and coronary artery anatomy, comparable skeletal anatomical and morphological characteristics, mammary glands with similar pathophysiological characteristics, and a 28-day menstrual cycle with similar hormonal cycles. Monkeys (macaques) also experience declining ovarian function and irregular menstrual cycles (natural menopause) when they reach 24 to 29 yrs of age. However, because of their very short life span after natural menopause, ovariectomized macaques are used to model postmenopausal women. The cynomolgus monkey model has been valuable in evaluating the potential cardiovascular benefits of soy foods and soy supplements. It remains largely unclear whether the observations are generalizable to all women or only to those who, like cynomolgus monkeys, convert the soy isoflavone daidzein to the metabolite equol. (182).

In 2006, *Wong et al.* reported that the lack of a sutiable animal model has delayed our understanding of mechanisms related to higher cardiovascular risk in women after menopause. The aging female rat may share some menopausal changes observed in women. However, most studies have attempted to mimic menopause by ovariectomizing young (6-12 weeks old) animals without considering the influence of aging and of declining ovarian function. They examined changes in vascular reactivity in the aging (15 months old) female rat after ovariectomy and the effects of chronic raloxifene therapy on vascular reactivity and eNOS protein expression. (183).

After menopause, high blood pressure develops in women. Hypertension is one of the major risk factors for cardiovascular disease. However, the mechanisms responsible for the postmenopausal increase in blood pressure are yet to be elucidated. For instance, changes in estrogen/androgen ratios, an elevation in endothelin level and oxidative stress, activation of the renin-angiotensin system (RAS), obesity, type II diabetes, and activation of the sympathetic nervous system may also play important roles in postmenopausal hypertension. Nonetheless, progress in elucidating the mechanisms responsible for postmenopausal hypertension has been hindered by the lack of a suitable animal model. The aging female spontaneously hypertensive rat (SHR) exhibits many of the characteristics found in postmenopausal women. Reckelhoff *et al.* (2004) reported that some of the possible mechanisms that could play a role in postmenopausal hypertension as well as the characteristics of the aged could be studied in female spontaneously hypertensive rats (SHR) (184). They showed that female SHR stop cycling at age 10 to 12 months and have low estradiol levels comparable to postmenopausal women. However, by age 16 to 18 months, the blood pressure increases by 25 to 35 mm Hg, compared with young females, and 15 mm Hg when compared with 8-month-old females. Moreover, sex related differences in blood pressure no longer exist because of the increase in blood pressure in old females, whereas blood pressure in male SHR remains fairly stable after age 8 months.

Another hypertensive rat strain that also shows increases in blood pressure with aging is the Dahl salt-sensitive rat. Even when fed a low-salt diet, blood pressure increases with time in both males and females. If young female Dahl rats are ovariectomized and fed a high-salt diet, the blood pressure elevated to higher levels than in normal females. At what age these animals cease cycling and what happens to their blood pressure after cessation of cycling is not presently understood (185).

In addition to the rat models of postmenopausal hypertension, the follicular-stimulating hormone receptor knockout mouse has been developed and also exhibits similar characteristics of postmenopausal women. These animals have low plasma estradiol levels, hypertension when compared with their wild-type controls, hypercholesterolemia, and weight gain. However, when studied at age 14 to 16 weeks, these animals did not exhibit increased oxidative stress or endothelial dysfunction, factors common to postmenopausal women (186).

Little information has been reported on cardiac apoptosis in menopausal women or in those after bilateral oophorectomy. Lee *et al.* (2008) evaluated whether cardiac Fas-dependent (type I) and mitochondria-dependent (type II) apoptotic pathways are activated in ovariectomized rats. They concluded that the absence of female ovaries might activate the cardiac Fas-dependent and mitochondria-dependent apoptotic pathways, representing a possible mechanism for developing heart failure in post-menopause women (187). Recently, Ricchiuti *et al.* (2009) tested the hypothesis that 17beta-estradiol (E_2) has dual effects on the heart, increasing levels of proteins thought to have beneficial cardiovascular effects (e.g. endothelial nitric oxide (NO) synthase (eNOS)) as well as those thought to have detrimental cardiovascular effects (e.g. type 1 angiotensin II (AngII) receptor (AT_1R)). Ovariectomized Wistar rats consuming a high-sodium diet were used as an animal model to study the cardiac physiology (188).

HRT – Functional, Biochemical, Molecular Aspects

Using resistance-sized arteries pressurized in vitro, myogenic tone of rat or mouse cerebral arteries does not differ in males and females animals (189-192). These differences appear to fully or partially result from estrogen enhancement of endothelial nitric oxide (NO) production. In the rat study, using middle cerebral artery segments pressurized *in vitro*, the luminal diameter was similar to the maximal passive diameters (in 0mM Ca^{2+} and 1mM EDTA) as in arteries from control, ovariectomized (Ovx) or Ovx treated with estrogen (Ovx+E2) rats. In response to a series of 10-mmHg step increases in transmural pressure (20-80 mmHg), myogenic tone was greater and a diminished vascular distensibility occured in arteries from Ovx females compared with arteries from either control or Ovx+E2 females. Addition of a NO synthase inhibitor increased myogenic tone in all arteries, while at the same time abolishing the differences in arterial diameter in the various groups; on the other hand the addition of L-arginine restored the differences in myogenic tone. This suggests that estrogen decreases myogenic tone by increasing cerebrovascular NO production and/or action. Similarly, in mouse cerebral arteries, chronic estrogen treatment was found to modulate myogenic reactivity through NO (191). But in this mouse study, there was a greater role for endothelium-derived cyclooxygenase-dependent mechanisms (in addition to NO-dependent mechanisms) in the beneficial effects of estrogen on vasculature (191). These effects of estrogen on mouse cerebral arteries were mediated through the α-isoform of estrogen receptors (ERα) (192)

Although NO is a well-studied endothelium-derived vasodilator that is modulated by estrogen, it is clear that in the absence of NO, estrogen will exert its effects on other vasodilators (193). While estrogen does not regulate prostacycline activity in cerebral blood vessels of control mice, when NO production was dysfunctional such as in endothelial NO synthase (eNOS) knockout mice or in arteries treated with an eNOS inhibitor, the estrogen increased the activity of a cyclooxygenase (COX)-sensitive vasodilator (193). Results from another study reported that estrogen decreased cerebrovascular tone by shifting the primary end product of the endothelial cyclooxygenase-1 pathway from the vasoconstrictor prostaglandin prostaglandin H2 (PGH2) to the vasodilator prostacyclin-dependent pathway (194). Taken together, these observed effects of estrogen may in part explain the enhanced thrombo-resistance and cerebral blood flow in postmenopausal women.

On the other hand, endothelium-intact rings of carotid arteries from sham-operated control, Ovx, and Ovx+E2 rats respond similarly to constrictors such as U46619 or phenylephrine (195). Removal of the endothelium unmasks enhanced contractions in Ovx rats, which was prevented by estrogen treatment. Contractions to high K^+, which are mediated by vascular smooth muscle cell depolarization, were higher in both endothelium-intact and endothelium-denuded arteries from Ovx rats, while estrogen treatment normalized this high K^+-induced contraction. Therefore, this study showed that estrogen can decrease the contractility of vascular smooth muscle cells. In addition, this study also showed that, in cases of estrogen deficiency, there could be an enhanced endothelial function to compensate for the increased vascular smooth muscle reactivity. Taken together, estrogen appears to have multiple endothelial targets.

Interleukin-1β (IL-1β) induces cerebrovascular endothelial COX-2 expression, increases PGE2 production and decreases vascular tone in isolated cerebral arteries from estrogen-deficient rats (196). In contrast, in animals treated with estrogen, IL-1β had no significant effect on COX-2 protein levels, PGE2 production, or vascular tone. The effect of estrogen was mediated through a reduction of nuclear factor-kappaB activity. When lipopolysaccharide (LPS) was used to induce inflammation, inflammatory enzymes inducible NO synthase (iNOS) and COX-2 were found to be increased in Ovx females, an effect that was reversed by estrogen treatment (197). Consistent with these observations are the findings that in intact females, LPS induction of iNOS and COX-2 in cerebral vessels varied with the stage of the estrous cycle, with LPS having the greatest effect during estrus, when circulating estrogen is low and progesterone is high. Since inflammation of the cerebral vasculature is a key process in ischemic brain injury, the anti-inflammatory effects of estrogen may have important implications for the incidence and severity of cerebrovascular disease during ischemia.

Cerebrovascular contractions to agents such as endothelin-1 or Ca^{2+} are augmented in arteries from Ovx rats, an effect that was reversed by estrogen treatment (198), while constrictor responses to melatonin are smaller in tail arteries from female rats in proestrus compared with other stages of the estrous cycle and after Ovx (199). Estrogen administration to Ovx female rats decreased the constriction to melatonin. It is likely that estrogen mediates its action by enhancing MT2 melatonin-receptor function, resulting in increased vasodilatation in response to melatonin. Taken together, these studies clearly showed that estrogen is able to attenuate agonist-induced vascular tone.

Apart from the modulatory effect on vasocontrictors, estrogen also modulates vasodilator-mediated vasorelaxation. In rat cerebral arteries, Ovx enhances the relaxing potency of nicardipine, which was reversed by estrogen treatment (195). At a molecular level, chronic estrogen treatment increases the expression of eNOS, COX-1 protein and prostacyclin-synthase protein in cerebral microvessels (200-202). Indeed, these molecular changes agree with previous findings indicating that estrogen exposure increases NO and prostacyclin production in cerebrovascular reactivity in both male and female animals. Its is likely that this increase in eNOS expression is mediated through ER (203). All forms of ER-α in cerebral vessels are decreased after Ovx but significantly increased after chronic estrogen exposure *in vivo* (204). On the other hand, apart from mediating its effect through the classical pathway (i.e. through nuclear ER), estrogen can also mediate its action through membrane-initiated signaling pathways. For instant, estrogen rapidly activates eNOS via the phosphorylation by a phosphoinositide-3 (PI-3) kinase-dependent pathway which is mediated by ERα located at the plasma membrane of endothelial cells lining cerebral arteries (205). Long-term estrogen exposure increases the levels of cerebrovascular p-Akt and p-eNOS as well as basal NO production (205).

Ovariectomy decreases the mRNA expression of subtype 1.5 of delayed rectifier potassium channel ($K_V1.5$) in vascular cells--while increasing the mRNA expression of α_{1C} subunit of L-type voltage-gated calcium channels (VGCCs) in endothelium-denuded aortas from female rats (206). These effects were reversed by estrogen replacement in Ovx rats. In contrast, the expression levels of genes encoding both α- and β-subunits of the large-conductance calcium-activated potassium channel (BK_{Ca}) remained the same with or without chronic estrogen. This study may help explain the decrease in vascular tone caused by estrogen in animal studies.

Apart from affecting expression of genes in the cytoplasm, estrogen also modulates mitochondrial function in the vasculature (207). Chronic estrogen treatment *in vivo* increases the levels of cytochrome c, subunit I and IV of complex IV, manganese superoxide dismutase, and nuclear respiratory factor-1 protein in the mitochrondria. Functionally, estrogen treatment increases the activities of mitochondrial citrate synthase and complex IV. Consistent with the increase in antioxidant expression such as superoxide dismutase, mitochondrial production of hydrogen peroxide was decreased in vessels from estrogen-treated animals (207-209); these effects were mediate through ERα receptors (209). These results of greater mitochondrial capacity for oxidative phosphorylation (and thereby greater energy-producing capacity) and decreased reactive oxygen species production by estrogen on mitochondria may help partially explain the effectiveness of estrogen against age-related cardiovascular disorders such as stroke. However, this protective, anti-inflammatory effect of estrogen on cerebral blood vessels was later found to be observed only in young adults but was attenuated in aged animals (210).

Although much has been learned regarding estrogen's effects on blood vessels, many of these studies used young, healthy animals. However, hormonal effects may be modified by aging or disease states such as diabetes. Therefore, more thorough investigations using aged animals, perhaps also some with diseased states are deemed necessary. Clearly, a better understanding of estrogen's actions on vascular function would not only provide information on the apparently contrasting results seen in previous animal studies and clinical trials, but it would also provide insights into the development of new therapeutic entities (e.g. selective estrogen receptor modulators) that could be useful in preventing or treating a wide variety of vascular diseases.

References

[1]   Hill, K. The demography of menopause. *Maturitas.*, 1996, 23, 113-27.

[2]   Mosca, L; Jones, WK; King, KB; Ouyang, P; Redberg, RF; Hill, MN. Awareness, perception, and knowledge of heart disease risk and prevention among women in the United States. American Heart Association Women's Heart Disease and Stroke Campaign Task Force. *Arch Fam Med.*, 2000, 9, 506-15.

[3]   Grodstein, F; Stampfer, M. The epidemiology of coronary heart disease and estrogen replacement in postmenopausal women. *Prog Cardiovasc Dis.*, 1995, 38, 199-210.

[4]   Rosano, GM; Vitale, C; Silvestri, A; Fini, M. Hormone replacement therapy and cardioprotection: the end of the tale? *Ann N Y Acad Sci.*, 2003, 997, 351-7.

[5]   Collins, P; Rosano, G; Casey, C; Daly, C; Gambacciani, M; Hadji, P; Kaaja, R; Mikkola, T; Palacios, S; Preston, R; Simon, T; Stevenson, J; Stramba-Badiale, M. Management of cardiovascular risk in the perimenopausal women: a consensus statement of European cardiologists and gynecologists. *Climacteric.*, 2007, 10(6), 508-26.

[6]   Kung HC; Hoyert DL; Xu J; Murphy SL. *National vital statistics reports.* CDC 2008, 56(10), 1-121.

[7]   Ouyang, P; Michos, ED; Karas, RH. Hormone replacement therapy and the cardiovascular system: lessons learned and unanswered questions. *J Am Coll Cardiol.*, 2006, 47, 1741-53.

[8]   Kagan, AR; Uemura, K. Atherosclerosis of the aorta and coronary arteries in five towns. *Bull Who.*, 1976, 53, 485-91.

[9]   Unal, B; Critchley, JA; Capewell, S. Explaining the decline in coronary heart disease mortality in England and Wales between 1981 and 2000. *Circulation.*, 2004, 109, 1101-7.

[10]   Tunstall-Pedoe, H; Kuulasmaa, K; Mahonen, M; Tolonen, H; Ruokokoski, E; Amouyel, P. Contribution of trends in survival and coronary-event rates to changes in coronary heart disease mortality: 10-year results from 37 WHO MONICA project populations. Monitoring trends and determinants in cardiovascular disease. *Lancet.*, 1999, 353, 1547-57.

[11]   Simon, T; Mary-Krause, M; Cambou, JP; Hanania, G; Guéret, P; Lablanche, JM; Blanchard, D; Genès, N; Danchin, N. USIC Investigators. Impact of age and gender on in-hospital and late mortality after acute myocardial infarction: increased early risk in younger women: results from the French nation-wide USIC registries. *Eur Heart J.*, 2006, 27, 1282-8.

[12] Greenland, P; Reicher-Reiss, H; Goldbourt, U; Behar, S. In-hospital and 1-year mortality in 1,524 women after myocardial infarction: comparison with 4,315 men. *Circulation.*, 1991, 83, 484-91.

[13] Simon, T; Mary-Krause, M; Funck-Brentano, C; Jaillon, P. Sex differences in the prognosis of congestive heart failure: results from the Cardiac Insufficiency Bisoprolol Study (CIBIS II). *Circulation.*, 2001, 103, 375-80.

[14] Pimenta, L; Bassan, R; Potsch, A; Soares, JF; Albanesi Filho, FM. Is female gender an independent risk factor for hospital mortality in acute myocardial infarction? *J Am Coll Cardiol.*, 1998, 31(suppl C): 403C.

[15] Reunanen, A; Suhonen, O; Aromaa, A; Knekt, P; Pyorala, K. Incidence of different manifestations of coronary heart disease in middle-aged Finnish men and women. *Acta Med Scand.*, 1985, 218, 19-26.

[16] Lerner, DJ; Kannel, WB. Patterns of coronary heart disease morbidity and mortality in the sexes: a 26-year follow-up of the Framingham population. *Am Heart J.*, 1986, 111, 383-90.

[17] Bugiardini, R; Bairey Merz, CN. Angina with "normal" coronary arteries: a changing philosophy. *JAMA.*, 2005, 293, 477-84.

[18] Castelli, WP. Cholesterol and lipids in the risk of coronary artery disease - the Framingham Heart Study. *Can J Cardiol.*, 1988, 4(Suppl A), 5-10A.

[19] European Society of Hypertension-European Society of Cardiology Guidelines Committee. European Society of Hypertension-European Society of Cardiology guidelines for the management of arterial hypertension. *J Hypertens.*, 2003, 21, 1011-53.

[20] Taggu, W; Lloyd, G. Treating cardiovascular disease in women. *Menopause Int.*, 2007, 13(4), 159-64.

[21] Collins, P. HDL-C in post-menopausal women: An important therapeutic target. *Int J Cardiol.*, 2008, 124(3), 275-82.

[22] Shepherd, J; Blauw, GJ; Murphy, MB; Bollen, EL; Buckley, BM; Cobbe, SM; Ford, I; Gaw, A; Hyland, M; Jukema, JW; Kamper, AM; Macfarlane, PW; Meinders, AE; Norrie, J; Packard, CJ; Perry, IJ; Stott, DJ; Sweeney, BJ; Twomey, C; Westendorp, RG; PROSPER study group. PROspective Study of Pravastatin in the Elderly at Risk. Pravastatin in elderly individuals at risk of vascular disease (PROSPER): a randomized controlled trial. *Lancet.*, 2002, 360, 1623-30.

[23] Schnatz, PF; Schnatz JD. Dyslipidemia in menopause: mechanisms and management. *Obstet Gynecol Surv.*, 2006, 61(9), 608-13.

[24] Third Report of the National Cholesterol Education Program (NCEP) Expert Panel on Detection, Evaluation, and Treatment of High Blood Cholesterol in Adults (Adult Treatment Panel III) final report. *Circulation.*, 2002, 106,, 3143-3421.

[25] Ogden, CL; Carroll, MD; Curtin, LR; McDowell, MA; Tabak, CJ; Flegal, KM. Prevalence of overweight and obesity in the United States, 1999-2004. *JAMA.*, 2006, 295(13), 1549-55.

[26] Kanaley, JA; Sames, C; Swisher, L; Swick, AG; Ploutz-Snyder, LL; Steppan, CM; Sagendorf, KS; Feiglin, D; Jaynes, EB; Meyer, RA; Weinstock, RS. Abdominal fat

distribution in pre- and postmenopausal women: The impact of physical activity, age, and menopausal status. *Metabolism.*, 2001, 50(8), 976-82.

[27]   Han, TS; van Leer, EM; Seidell, JC; Lean, ME. Waist circumference action levels in the identification of cardiovascular risk factors: prevalence study in a random sample. *BMJ.*, 1995, 311, 1401-5.

[28]   Yusuf, S; Hawken, S; Ounpuu, S; Bautista, L; Franzosi, MG; Commerford, P; Lang, CC; Rumboldt, Z; Onen, CL; Lisheng, L; Tanomsup, S; Wangai, P; Jr; Razak, F; Sharma, AM; Anand, SS. Obesity and the risk of myocardial infarction in 27,000 participants from 52 countries: a case-control study. *Lancet.*, 2005, 366, 1640-9.

[29]   Despres, JP. Abdominal obesity as important component of insulin resistance syndrome. *Nutrition.*, 1993, 9, 452-9.

[30]   Hunter, GR; Kekes-Szabo, T; Treuth, MS; Williams, MJ; Goran, M; Pichon, C. Intra-abdominal adipose tissue, physical activity and cardiovascular risk in pre- and post-menopausal women. *Int J Obes.*, 1996, 20, 860-5.

[31]   Thorne, A; Lonnqvist, F; Apelman, J; Hellers, G; Arner, P. A pilot study of long-term effects of a novel obesity treatment: omentectomy in connection with adjustable gastric banding. *Int J Obes Relat Metab Disord.*, 2002, 26, 193-9.

[32]   Klein, S; Fontana, L; Young, VL; Coggan, AR; Kilo, C; Patterson, BW; Mohammed, BS. Absence of an effect of liposuction on insulin action and risk factors for coronary heart disease. *N Engl J Med.*, 2004, 350, 2549-57.

[33]   Hoyenga, KB; Hoyenga, KT. Gender and energy balance: sex differences in adaptations for feast and famine. *Physiol Behav.*, 1982, 28, 545-63.

[34]   Toth, MJ; Tchernof, A; Sites, CK; Poehlman, ET. Menopause-related changes in body fat distribution. *Ann N Y Acad Sci.*, 2000, 904, 502-6.

[35]   Shi, H; Clegg, DJ. Sex differences in the regulation of body weight. *Physiol Behav.*, 2009, 97(2), 199-204.

[36]   Schneider, JG; Tompkins, C; Blumenthal, RS; Mora, S. The metabolic syndrome in women. *Cardiol Rev.*, 2006, 14(6), 286-91.

[37]   Eckel, RH; Grundy, SM; Zimmet, PZ. The metabolic syndrome. *Lancet.*, 2005, 365, 1415-28.

[38]   Kannel, WB; McGee, DL. Diabetes and cardiovascular risk factor: the Framingham Heart Study. *Circulation.*, 1979, 59, 8-13.

[39]   Expert Committee on the Diagnosis and Classification of Diabetes Mellitus. Report of the Expert Committee on the Diagnosis and Classification of Diabetes Mellitus. *Diabetes Care.*, 1997, 20, 1183-97.

[40]   Expert Committee on the Diagnosis and Classification of Diabetes Mellitus. Follow-up report on the diagnosis of diabetes mellitus. *Diabetes Care.*, 2003, 26, 3160-7.

[41]   Unwin, N; Shaw, J; Zimmet, P; Alberti, KG. Impaired glucose tolerance and impaired fasting glycaemia: the current status on definition and intervention. *Diabet Med.*, 2002, 19, 708-723.

[42]   Tirosh, A; Shai, I; Tekes-Manova, D; Israeli, E; Pereg, D; Shochat, T; Kochba, I; Rudich, A. Israeli Diabetes Research Group. Normal fasting plasma glucose levels and type 2 diabetes in young men. *N Engl J Med.*, 2005, 353, 1454-62.

[43] Walton, C; Godsland, IF; Proudler, AJ; Wynn, V; Stevenson, JC. The effect of the menopause on insulin sensitivity, secretion and elimination in non-obese healthy women. *Eur J Clin Invest.*, 1993, 23, 466-73.

[44] DeNino, WF; Tchernof, A; Dionne, IJ; Toth, MJ; Ades, PA; Sites, CK; Poehlman, ET. Contribution of abdominal adiposity to age-related differences in insulin sensitivity and plasma lipids in healthy nonobese women. *Diabetes Care.*, 2001, 24, 925-32.

[45] Barnes, BO; Regan, JF; Nelson, WO. Improvement in experimental diabetes following the administration of ammniotin. *JAMA.*, 1933, 101, 926-7.

[46] Nelson, WO; Overholser, M. The effect of estrogenic hormones on experimental pancreatic diabetes in the monkey. *Endocrinology.*, 1936, 20, 473-80.

[47] Houssay, BA; Foglia, VG; Rodriguez, RR. Production and prevention of some types of experimental diabetes by estrogens or corticosteroids. *Acta Endocrinol.*, 1954, 17, 146-164.

[48] Clark, JB; Palmer, CJ; Shaw, WN. The diabetic Zucker fatty rat. *Proc Soc Exp Biol Med.*, 1983, 173, 68-75.

[49] Leiter, EH; Chapman, HD. Obesity-induced diabetes (diabesity) in C57BL/KsJ mice produces aberrant trans-regulation of sex steroid sulfotransferase genes. *J Clin Invest.*, 1994, 93(5), 2007-13.

[50] Paik, SG; Michelis, MA; Kim, YT; Shin, S. Induction of insulin dependent diabetes by streptozotocin. Inhibition by estrogens and potentiation by androgens. *Diabetes.*, 1982, 31, 724-9.

[51] Puah, JA; Bailey, CJ. Insulinotropic effect of ovarian steroid hormones in streptozotocin diabetic female mice. *Horm Metab Res.*, 1985, 17, 216-8.

[52] Espeland, MA; Hogan, PE; Fineberg, SE; Howard, G; Schrott, H; Waclawiw, MA; Bush, TL. Effect of postmenopausal hormone therapy on glucose and insulin concentrations. PEPI Investigators. Post menopausal Estrogen/Progestin Interventions. *Diabetes Care.*, 1998, 21, 1589-95.

[53] Crespo, CJ; Smit, E; Snelling, A; Sempos, CT; Andersen, RE; Nhanes, III. Hormone replacement therapy and its relationship to lipid and glucose metabolism in diabetic and nondiabetic postmenopausal women: results from the Third National Health and Nutrition Examination Survey (NHANES III). *Diabetes Care.*, 2002, 25, 1675-80.

[54] Saglam, K; Polat, Z; Yilmaz, MI; Gulec, M; Akinci, SB. Effects of postmenopausal hormone replacement therapy on insulin resistance. *Endocrine.*, 2002, 18, 211-4.

[55] Andersson, B; Mattsson, LA; Hahn, L; Mårin, P; Lapidus, L; Holm, G; Bengtsson, BA; Björntorp, P. Estrogen replacement therapy decreases hyperandrogenicity and improves glucose homeostasis and plasma lipids in postmenopausal women with noninsulin-dependent diabetes mellitus. *J Clin Endocrinol Metab.*, 1997, 82, 638-43.

[56] Brussaard, HE; Gevers Leuven, JA; Frölich, M; Kluft, C; Krans, HM. Short-term oestrogen replacement therapy improves insulin resistance, lipids and fibrinolysis in postmenopausal women with NIDDM. *Diabetologia.*, 1997, 40, 843-9.

[57] Friday, KE; Dong, C; Fontenot, RU. Conjugated equine estrogen improves glycemic control and blood lipoproteins in postmenopausal women with type 2 diabetes. *J Clin Endocrinol Metab.*, 2001, 86, 48-52.

[58] Perera, M; Sattar, N; Petrie, JR; Hillier, C; Small, M; Connell, JM; Lowe, GD; Lumsden, MA. The effects of transdermal estradiol in combination with oral norethisterone on lipoproteins, coagulation, and endothelial markers in postmenopausal women with type 2 diabetes: a randomized, placebo- controlled study. *J Clin Endocrinol Metab.*, 2001, 86, 1140-3.

[59] Kanaya, AM; Herrington, D; Vittinghoff, E; Lin, F; Grady, D; Bittner, V; Cauley, JA; Barrett-Connor, E. Heart and Estrogen/progestin Replacement Study. Glycemic effects of postmenopausal hormone therapy: the Heart and Estrogen/ progestin Replacement Study. A randomized, double-blind, placebo-controlled trial. *Ann Intern Med.*, 2003, 138, 1-9.

[60] Knowler, WC; Barrett-Connor, E; Fowler, SE; Hamman, RF; Lachin, JM; Walker, EA; Nathan, DM. Diabetes Prevention Program Research Group. Reduction in the incidence of type 2 diabetes with lifestyle intervention or metformin. *N Engl J Med.*, 2002, 346, 393-403.

[61] Hajjar, I; Kotchen, TA. Trends in prevalence, awareness, treatment, and control of hypertension in the United States, 1988-2000. *JAMA.*, 2003, 290, 199-206.

[62] Rosenthal, T; Oparil, S. Hypertension in women. *J Hum Hypertens.*, 2000, 14, 691-704.

[63] Messerli, F; White, WB; Staessen, JA. If only cardiologists did properly measure blood pressure. Blood pressure recordings in daily practice and clinical trials. *J Am Coll Cardiol.*, 2002, 40, 2201-3.

[64] Hu, G. Gender difference in all-cause and cardiovascular mortality related to hyperglycaemia and newly-diagnosed diabetes. *Diabetologia.*, 2003, 46, 608-17.

[65] Balkau, B; Hu, G; Qiao, Q; Tuomilehto, J; Borch-Johnsen, K; Pyorala, K; DECODE Study Group. European Diabetes Epidemiology Group. Prediction of the risk of cardiovascular mortality using a score that includes glucose as a risk factor. The DECODE Study. *Diabetologia.*, 2004, 47, 2118-28.

[66] Bakris, GL; Williams, M; Dworkin, L; Elliott, WJ; Epstein, M; Toto, R; Tuttle, K; Douglas, J; Hsueh, W; Sowers, J. Preserving renal function in adults with hypertension and diabetes: a consensus approach. National Kidney Foundation Hypertension and Diabetes Executive Committees Working Group. *Am J Kidney Dis.*, 2000, 36, 646-61.

[67] Kannel, WB; Cupples, LA; D'Agostino, RB; Stokes, J. 3rd. Hypertension, antihypertensive treatment, and sudden coronary death. The Framingham Study. *Hypertension.*, 1988, 11, 1145-50.

[68] Wong, ND; Pio, JR; Franklin, SS; L'Italien, GJ; Kamath, TV; Williams, GR. Preventing coronary events by optimal control of blood pressure and lipids in patients with the metabolic syndrome. *Am J Cardiol.*, 2003, 91, 1421- 6.

[69] Chobanian, AV; Bakris, GL; Black, HR; et al. The Seventh Report of the Joint National Committee on Prevention, Detection, Evaluation, and Treatment of High Blood Pressure: the JNC 7 report. *JAMA.*, 2003, 289, 2560-72.

[70] Lewington, S; Clarke, R; Qizilbash, N; Peto, R; Collins, R; Prospective Studies Collaboration. Age-specific relevance of usual blood pressure to vascular mortality: a meta-analysis of individual data for one million adults in 61 prospective studies. Lancet 2002, 360, 1903-13.

[71] Kawachi, I. Physical and psychological consequences of weight gain. *J Clin Psychiatry.*, 1999, 60(Suppl 21), 5-9.

[72] Hu, G; Qiao, Q; Tuomilehto, J; Eliasson, M; Feskens, EJ; Pyorala, K. DECODE Insulin Study Group. Plasma insulin and cardiovascular mortality in non-diabetic European men and women: a meta-analysis of data from eleven prospective studies. *Diabetologia.*, 2004, 47, 1245-56.

[73] Lindheim, SR; Presser, SC; Ditkoff, EC; Vijod, MA; Stanczyk, FZ; Lobo, RA. A possible bimodal effect of estrogen on insulin sensitivity in postmenopausal women and the attenuating effect of added progestin. *Fertil Steril.*, 1993, 60, 664-7.

[74] Ferrannini, E; Natali, A; Capaldo, B; Lehtovirta, M; Jacob, S; Yki-Jarvinen, H. Insulin resistance, hyperinsulinemia, and blood pressure: role of age and obesity. European Group for the Study of Insulin Resistance (EGIR). *Hypertension.*, 1997, 30, 1144-9.

[75] Wechsler, H;Rigotti, NA; Gledhill-Hoyt, J; Lee, H. Increased levels of cigarette use among college students. A cause for national concern. *Jama.*, 1998, 280, 1673-1678.

[76] Kesteloot, H. Queen Margrethe II andmortality in Danish women. *Lancet.*, 2001, 357, 871-2.

[77] Thom, T; Haase, N; Rosamond, W; Howard, VJ; Rumsfeld, J; Manolio, T; Zheng, ZJ; Flegal, K; O'Donnell, C; Kittner, S; Lloyd-Jones, D; Goff, DC; Jr; Hong, Y; Adams, R; Friday, G; Furie, K; Gorelick, P; Kissela, B; Marler, J; Meigs, J; Roger, V; Sidney, S; Sorlie, P; Steinberger, J; Wasserthiel-Smoller, S; Wilson, M; Wolf, P. American Heart Association Statistics Committee and Stroke Statistics Subcommittee. Heart disease and stroke statistics-2006 update: a report from the American Heart Association Statistics Committee and Stroke Statistics Subcommittee. *Circulation.*, 2006, 113(6), e85-151.

[78] Willett, WC; Green, A; Stampfer, MJ; Speizer, FE; Colditz, GA; Rosner, B; Monson, RR; Stason, W; Hennekens, CH. Relative and absolute excess risks of coronary heart disease among women who smoke cigarettes. *N Engl J Med.*, 1987, 317, 1303-9.

[79] LaCroix, AZ; Lang, J; Scherr, P; Wallace, RB; Cornoni-Huntley, J; Berkman, L; Curb, JD; Evans, D; Hennekens, CH. Smoking and mortality among older men and women in three communities. *N Engl J.*, Med 1991, 324(23), 1619-25.

[80] Mjøs, OD. Lipid effects of smoking. *Am Heart J.*, 1988, 115, 272-5.

[81] Markowe, HL; Marmot, MG; Shipley, MJ; Bulpitt, CJ; Meade, TW; Stirling, Y; Vickers, MV; Semmence, A. Fibrinogen: a possible link between social class and coronary heart disease. *Br Med J (Clin Res Ed).*, 1985, 291, 1312-4.

[82] Facchini, FS; Hollenbeck, CB; Jeppesen, J; Chen, YD; Reaven, GM. Insulin resistance and cigarette smoking. *Lancet.*, 1992, 339, 1128-30.

[83] Kiel, DP; Baron, JA; Anderson, JJ; Hannan, MT; Felson, DT. Smoking eliminates the protective effect of oral estrogens on the risk for hip fracture among women. *Ann Intern Med.*, 1992, 116(9), 716-21.

[84] Daniel, M; Martin, AD; Faiman, C. Sex hormones and adipose tissue distribution in premenopausal cigarette smokers. *Int J Obes Relat Metab Disord.*, 1992, 16(4), 245-54.

[85] Jensen, J; Christiansen, C; Rødbro, P. Cigarette smoking, serum estrogens, and bone loss during hormone-replacement therapy early after menopause. *N Engl J Med.*, 1985, 313(16), 973-5.

[86] Hartz, AJ; Kelber, S; Borkowf, H; Wild, R; Gillis, BL; Rimm, AA. The association of smoking with clinical indicators of altered sex steroids--a study of 50,145 women. *Public Health Rep.*, 1987, 102, 254-9.

[87] Baron, JA; La Vecchia, C; Levi, F. The antiestrogenic effect of cigarette smoking in women. *Am J Obstet Gynecol.*, 1990, 162, 502-14.

[88] Barbieri, RL; McShane, PM; Ryan, KJ. Constituents of cigarette smoke inhibit human granulosa cell aromatase. *Fertil Steril.*, 1986, 46, 232-6.

[89] Michnovicz, JJ; Hershcopf, RJ; Naganuma, H; Bradlow, HL; Fishman, J. Increased 2-hydroxylation of estradiol as a possible mechanism for the anti-estrogenic effect of cigarette smoking. *N Engl J Med.*, 1986, 315, 1305-9.

[90] Rosenberg, L; Palmer, JR; Shapiro, S. Decline in the risk of myocardial infarction among women who stop smoking. *N Engl J Med.*, 1990, 322, 213-7.

[91] Wessel, TR; Arant, CB; Olson, MB; Johnson, BD; Reis, SE; Sharaf, BL; Shaw, LJ; Handberg, E; Sopko, G; Kelsey, SF; Pepine, CJ; Merz, NB. Relationship of physical fitness vs body mass index with coronary artery disease and cardiovascular events in women. *Jama.*, 2004, 292, 1179-87.

[92] Kuller, LH; Kinzel, LS; Pettee, KK; Kriska, AM; Simkin-Silverman, LR; Conroy, MB; Averbach, F; Pappert, WS; Johnson, BD. Lifestyle intervention and coronary heart disease risk factor changes over 18 months in postmenopausal women: The Women On the Move through Activity and Nutrition (WOMAN Study) clinical trial. *J Womens Health.*, 2006, 15, 962-74.

[93] LaFontaine, TP; DiLorenzo, TM; Frensch, PA; Stucky-Ropp, RC; Bargman, EP; McDonald, DG. Aerobic exercise and mood. A brief review, 1985-1990. *Sports Med.*, 1992, 13, 160-70.

[94] Gregg, EW; Cauley, JA; Stone, K; Thompson, TJ; Bauer, DC; Cummings, SR; Ensrud, KE; Study of Osteoporotic Fractures Research Group. Relationship of changes in physical activity and mortality among older women. *JAMA.*, 2003, 289(18), 2379-86.

[95] Li, TY; Rana, JS; Manson, JE; Willett, WC; Stampfer, MJ; Colditz, GA; Rexrode, KM; Hu, FB. Obesity as compared with physical activity in predicting risk of coronary heart disease in women. *Circulation.*, 2006, 113, 499-506.

[96] Rockhill, B; Willett, WC; Manson, JE; Leitzmann, MF; Stampfer, MJ; Hunter, DJ; Colditz, GA. Physical activity and mortality: a prospective study among women. *Am J Public Health.*, 2001, 91, 578-83.

[97] Manson, JE; Greenland, P; LaCroix, AZ; Stefanick, ML; Mouton, CP; Oberman, A; Perri, MG; Sheps, DS; Pettinger, MB; Siscovick, DS. Walking compared with vigorous exercise for the prevention of cardiovascular events in women. *N Engl J Med.*, 2002, 347, 716-25.

[98] Liu, S; Manson, JE; Lee, IM; Cole, SR; Hennekens, CH; Willett, WC; Buring, JE. Fruit and vegetable intake and risk of cardiovascular disease: the Women's Health Study. *Am J Clin Nutr.*, 2000, 4, 922-8.

[99] Danaei, G; Vander Hoorn, S; Lopez, AD; Murray, CJ; Ezzati, M. Comparative Risk Assessment collaborating group (Cancers). Causes of cancer in the world: comparative risk assessment of nine behavioural and environmental risk factors. *Lancet.*, 2005, 366, 1784-93.

[100] Diet and Lifestyle recommendations revision 2006, a scientific statement from the American Heart Association nutrition committee. *Circulation.*, 2006, 114, 82-96.

[101] Hu, FB; Willett, WC. Optimal diets for prevention of coronary heart disease. *JAMA.*, 2002, 288, 2569-78.

[102] Kris-Etherton, PM; Yu, S. Individual fatty acid effects on plasma lipids and lipoproteins: human studies. *Am J Clin Nutr.*, 1997, 1628S-44S.

[103] Hu, FB; Bronner, L; Willett, WC; Stampfer, MJ; Rexrode, KM; Albert, CM; Hunter, D; Manson, JE. Fish and omega-3 fatty acid intake and risk of coronary heart disease in women. *JAMA.*, 2002, 287, 1815-21.

[104] Hu, FB. Plant-based foods and prevention of cardiovascular disease: an overview. *Am J Clin Nutr.*, 2003, 78, 544S-51S.

[105] Hsia, J; Rodabough, R; Rosal, MC; Cochrane, B; Howard, BV; Snetselaar, L; Frishman, WH; Stefanick, ML. Compliance with National Cholesterol Education Program dietary and lifestyle guidelines among older women with self-reported hypercholesterolemia. The Women's Health Initiative. *Am J Med.*, 2002, 113, 384-92.

[106] Taffe, AM; Cauffield, J. "Natural" hormone replacement therapy and dietary supplements used in the treatment of menopausal symptoms. Lippincotts *Prim Care Pract.*, 1998, 2, 292-302.

[107] King, LA; Carr, BR. Phytoestrogens: fact and fiction. *Patient Care.*, 1999, 33, 127-8.

[108] Kass-Annese, B. Alternative therapies for menopause. *Clin Obstet Gynecol.*, 2000, 43, 162-83.

[109] Taylor, M. Alternatives to conventional HRT: Phytoestrogens and botanicals. *Contemporary OB/GYN.*, 1999, 44, 27-50.

[110] Nestel, PJ; Yamashita, T; Sasahara, T; Pomeroy, S; Dart, A; Komesaroff, P; Owen, A; Abbey, M. Soy isoflavones improve systemic arterial compliance but not plasma lipids in menopausal and perimenopausal women. *Arterioscler Thromb Vasc Biol.*, 1997, 17, 3392-8.

[111] Merz-Demlow, BE; Duncan, AM; Wangen, KE; Xu, X; Carr, TP; Phipps, WR; Kurzer, MS. Soy isoflavones improve plasma lipids in normocholesterolemic, premenopausal women. *Am J Clin Nutr.*, 2000, 71, 1462-9.

[112] Cassidy, A; Bingham, S; Setchell, K. Biological effects of a diet of soy protein rich in isoflavones on the menstrual cycle of premenopausal women. *Am J Clin Nutr.*, 1994, 60, 333-40.

[113] Potter, SM; Baum, JA; Teng, H; Stillman, RJ; Shay, NF; Erdman, JW; Jr. Soy protein and isoflavones: their effects on blood lipids and bone density in postmenopausal women. *Am J Clin Nutr.*, 1998, 68, 1375S-9S.

[114] Fuster, V; Badimon, L; Badimon, JJ; Chesebro, JH. The pathogenesis of coronary artery disease and the acute coronary syndromes (2). *N Engl J Med.*, 1992, 326, 310-8.

[115] Resch, KL; Ernst, E; Matrai, A; Paulsen, HF. Fibrinogen and viscosity as risk factors for subsequent cardiovascular events in stroke survivors. *Ann Intern Med.*, 1992, 117, 371-5.

[116] Kaplan, JR; Pettersson, K; Manuck, SB; Olsson, G. Role of sympathoadrenal medullary activation in the initiation and progression of atherosclerosis. *Circulation.*, 1991, 84, VI23-32.

[117] Rosano, GM; Patrizi, R; Leonardo, F; Ponikowski, P; Collins, P; Sarrel, PM; Chierchia, SL. Effect of estrogen replacement therapy on heart rate variability and heart rate in healthy postmenopausal women. *Am J Cardiol.*, 1997, 80(6), 815-7.

[118] Barrett-Connor, E. Estrogen and estrogen-progestogen replacement: therapy and cardiovascular diseases. *Am J Med.*, 1993, 95, 40S-43S.

[119] Yildirir, A; Kabakci, G; Yarali, H; Aybar, F; Akgul, E; Bukulmez, O; Tokgozoglu, L; Gurgan, T; Oto, A. Effects of hormone replacement therapy on heart rate variability in postmenopausal women. *Ann Noninvasive Electrocardiol.*, 2001, 6, 280-4.

[120] Lipsitz, LA; Connelly, CM; Kelley-Gagnon, M; Kiely, DK; Morin, RJ. Effects of chronic estrogen replacement therapy on beat-to-beat blood pressure dynamics in healthy postmenopausal women. *Hypertension.*, 1995, 26, 711-5.

[121] Herd, JA. Cardiovascular response to stress. *Physiol Rev.*, 1991, 71, 305-30.

[122] Ballinger, S. Stress as a factor in lowered estrogen levels in the early postmenopause. *Ann N Y Acad Sci.*, 1990, 95-113.

[123] Kurisu, S; Sato, H; Kawagoe, T; Ishihara, M; Shimatani, Y; Nishioka, K; Kono, Y; Umemura, T; Nakamura, S. Tako-tsubo-like left ventricular dysfunction with ST-segment elevation: a novel cardiac syndrome mimicking acute myocardial infarction. *Am Heart J.*, 2002, 143, 448-55.

[124] Wittstein, IS; Thiemann, DR; Lima, JA; Baughman, KL; Schulman, SP; Gerstenblith, G; Wu, KC; Rade, JJ; Bivalacqua, TJ; Champion, HC. Neurohumoral features of myocardial stunning due to sudden emotional stress. *N Engl J Med.*, 2005, 352, 539-48.

[125] Ferketich, AK; Schwartzbaum, JA; Frid, DJ; Moeschberger, ML. Depression as an antecedent to heart disease among women and men in the NHANES I study. *Arch Intern Med.*, 2000, 160, 1261-8.

[126] Mendes de Leon, CF; Krumholz, HM; Seeman, TS;Vaccarino, V; Williams, CS; Kasl, SV; et al. Depression and risk of coronary heart disease in elderly men and women. New Haven EPESE, 1982-1991. *Arch Intern Med*, 1998, 158, 2341-8.

[127] Schulz, R; Beach, SR; Ives, DG; Martire, LM; Ariyo, AA; Kop, WJ. Association between depression and mortality in older adults. The Cardiovascular Health Study. *Arch Intern Med.*, 2000, 160, 1761-8.

[128] Wassertheil-Smoller, S; Applegate, WB; Berge, K; Chang, CJ; Davis, BR; Grimm, R; Jr; Kostis, J; Pressel, S; Schron, E. Change in depression as a precursor of cardiovascular events. SHEP Cooperative Research Group (Systolic Hypertension in the elderly). *Arch Intern Med.*, 1996, 156, 553-61.

[129] Stary, HC; Chandler, AB; Dinsmore, RE; Fuster, V; Glagov, S; Insull, W; Jr; Rosenfeld, ME; Schwartz, CJ; Wagner, WD; Wissler, RW. A definition of advanced types of atherosclerotic lesions and a histological classification of atherosclerosis: a report from the Committee on Vascular Lesions of the Council on Arteriosclerosis, American Heart Association. *Circulation.*, 1995, 92, 1355-74.

[130] Stary, HC; Chandler, AB; Glagov, S; Guyton, JR; Insull, W; Jr; Rosenfeld, ME; Schaffer, SA; Schwartz, CJ; Wagner, WD; Wissler, RW. A definition of initial, fatty streak, and intermediate lesions of atherosclerosis: a report from the Committee on Vascular Lesions of the Council on Arteriosclerosis, American Heart Association. *Circulation.*, 1994, 89, 2462-78.

[131] Jonasson, L; Holm, J; Skalli, O; Bondjers, G; Hansson, GK. Regional accumulations of T cells, macrophages, and smooth muscle cells in the human atherosclerotic plaque. *Arteriosclerosis.*, 1986, 6, 131-8.

[132] Kovanen, PT; Kaartinen, M; Paavonen, T. Infiltrates of activated mast cells at the site of coronary atheromatous erosion or rupture in myocardial infarction. *Circulation.*, 1995, 92, 1084-8.

[133] Frostegård, J; Ulfgren, AK; Nyberg, P; Hedin, U; Swedenborg, J; Andersson, U; Hansson, GK. Cytokine expression in advanced human atherosclerotic plaques: dominance of proinflammatory (Th1) and macrophage-stimulating cytokines. *Atherosclerosis.*, 1999, 145, 33-43.

[134] Hackett, D; Davies, G; Maseri, A. Preexisting coronary stenosis in patients with first myocardial infarction are not necessarily severe. *Eur Heart J.*, 1988, 9, 1317-23.

[135] Davies, MJ. Stability and instability: two faces of coronary atherosclerosis: the Paul Dudley White Lecture 1995. *Circulation.*, 1996, 94, 2013-20.

[136] Falk, E; Shah, PK; Fuster, V. Coronary plaque disruption. *Circulation.*, 1995, 92, 657-71.

[137] Libby, P. Inflammation in atherosclerosis. *Nature.*, 2002, 420, 868-74.

[138] Ross, R. Mechanisms of disease: atherosclerosis, an inflammatory disease. *N Engl J Med.*, 1999, 340, 115-26.

[139] Libby, P; Ridker, P; Maseri, A. Inflammation and atherosclerosis. *Circulation.*, 2002, 105, 1135-43.

[140] Griendling, K; Ushio-Fukai, M; Lassegue, B; et al. Angiotensin II signaling in vascular smooth muscle cells: new concepts. *Hypertension.*, 1997, 29, 366-73.

[141] Creager, M; Luscher, T. Diabetes and vascular disease, pathophysiology, clinical consequences and medical therapy: part I. *Circulation.*, 2003, 108, 1527-32.

[142] Mokdad, A; Bowman, B; Ford, E. The continuing epidemics of obesity and diabetes in the United States. *JAMA.*, 2001, 286, 1195-2000.

[143] Somberg, TC; Arora, RR. Depression and heart disease: Therapeutic implications. *Cardiology.*, 2008, 111, 75-81.

[144] Glassman, AH; Roose, SP; Bigger, JT; Jr. The safety of tricyclic antidepressants in cardiac patients: Risk benefit reconsidered. *JAMA.*, 1993, 269, 2673-5.

[145] Shapiro, PA; Lespérance, F; Frasure-Smith, N; O'Connor, CM; Baker, B; Jiang, JW; Dorian, P; Harrison, W; Glassman, AH. An open-label preliminary trial of sertraline for treatment of major depression after acute myocardial infarction (the SADHAT Trial). Sertraline Anti-Depressant Heart Attack Trial. *Am Heart J.*, 1999, 137, 1100-6.

[146] Jaffe, AS; Krumholz, HM; Catellier, DJ; Freedland, KE; Bittner, V; Blumenthal, JA; Calvin, JE; Norman, J; Sequeira, R; O'Connor, C; Rich, MW; Sheps, D; Wu, C. Enhancing Recovery in Coronary Heart Disease Patients (ENRICHD) Trial Investigators. Prediction of medical morbidity and mortality after acute myocardial infarction in patients at increased psychosocial risk in the Enhancing Recovery in Coronary Heart Disease Patients (ENRICHD) study. *Am Heart J* 2006, 152, 126-35.

[147] Järvisalo, MJ; Harmoinen, A; Hakanen, M; Paakkunainen, U; Viikari, J; Hartiala, J; Lehtimäki, T; Simell, O; Raitakari, OT. Elevated serum C-reactive protein levels and

early arterial changes in healthy children. *Arterioscler Thromb Vasc Biol.*, 2002, 22, 1323-8.

[148] Ridker, PM; Hennekens, CH; Buring, JE; Rifai, N. C-reactive protein and other markers of inflammation in the prediction of cardiovascular disease in women. *N Engl J Med.*, 2000, 342, 836-43.

[149] Ridker, PM; Rifai, N; Rose, L; Buring, JE; Cook, NR. Comparison of C-reactive protein and low-density lipoprotein cholesterol levels in the prediction of first cardiovascular events. *N Engl J Med.*, 2002, 347, 1557-65.

[150] Pradhan, AD; Manson, JE; Rossouw, JE; Siscovick, DS; Mouton, CP; Rifai, N; Wallace, RB; Jackson, RD; Pettinger, MB; Ridker, PM. Inflammatory biomarkers, hormone replacement therapy, and incident coronary heart disease. *JAMA.*, 2002, 288, 980-7.

[151] Pearson, TA; Mensah, GA; Alexander, RW; Anderson, JL; Cannon, RO 3rd; Criqui, M; Fadl, YY; Fortmann, SP; Hong, Y; Myers, GL; Rifai, N; Smith, SC Jr; Taubert, K; Tracy, RP; Vinicor, F; Centers for Disease Control and Prevention; American Heart Association: Markers of inflammation and cardiovascular disease. *Circulation.*, 2003, 107, 499-511.

[152] Boushey, CJ; Beresford, SA; Omenn, GS; Motulsky, AG. A quantitative assessment of plasma homocysteine as a risk factor for vascular disease. Probable benefits of increasing folic acid intakes. *JAMA.*, 1995, 274, 1049-1057.

[153] Verhoef, P. Hyperhomocysteinemia and risk of vascular disease in women. *Semin Thromb Hemost.*, 2000, 26, 325-334.

[154] van Guldener, C; Stehouwer, CD. Hyperhomocysteinemia, vascular pathology, and endothelial dysfunction. Semin *Thromb Hemost.*, 2000, 26, 281-9.

[155] Nachman, RL. Lipoprotein(a): Molecular mischief in the microvasculature. *Circulation.*, 1997, 96, 2485-7.

[156] Danesh, J; Collins, R; Peto, R. Lipoprotein (a) and coronary heart disease. Meta-analysis of prospective studies. *Circulation.*, 2000, 102, 1082-5.

[157] Hopkins, PN; Wu, LL; Hunt, SC; James, BC; Vincent, GM; Williams, RR. Lipoprotein (a) interactions with lipid and non lipid risk factors in early familial coronary artery disease. *Arterioscler Thromb Vasc Biol.*, 1997, 17, 2783-92.

[158] Stampfer, MJ; Colditz, GA. Estrogen replacement therapy and coronary heart disease: a quantitative assessment of the epidemiologic evidence. *Prev Med.*, 1991, 20, 47-63.

[159] American College of Physicians. Guidelines for counseling postmenopausal women about preventive hormone therapy. *Ann Intern Med.*, 1992, 117, 1016-37.

[160] Hulley, S; Grady, D; Bush, T; Furberg, C; Herrington, D; Riggs, B; Vittinghoff, E. Randomized trial of estrogen plus progestin for secondary prevention of coronary heart disease in postmenopausal women. Heart and Estrogen/progestin Replacement Study (HERS) Research Group. *JAMA.*, 1998, 280, 605-13.

[161] Rossouw, JE; Anderson, GL; Prentice, RL; LaCroix, AZ; Kooperberg, C; Stefanick, ML; Jackson, RD; Beresford, SA; Howard, BV; Johnson, KC; Kotchen, JM; Ockene, J; Writing Group for the Women's Health Initiative Investigators. Risks and benefits of estrogen plus progestin in healthy postmenopausal women: principal results From the Women's Health Initiative randomized controlled trial. *JAMA.*, 2002, 288, 321-33.

[162] Mosca, L; Appel, LJ; Benjamin, EJ; Berra, K; Chandra-Strobos N; Fabunmi, RP; Grady, D; Haan, CK; Hayes, SN; Judelson, DR; Keenan, NL; McBride, P; Oparil, S; Ouyang, P; Oz, MC; Mendelsohn, ME; Pasternak, RC; Pinn, VW; Robertson, RM; Schenck-Gustafsson, K; Sila, CA; Smith, SC; Jr; Sopko, G; Taylor, AL; Walsh, BW; Wenger, NK; Williams, CL. American Heart Association. Evidence-based guidelines for cardiovascular disease prevention in women. *Circulation.*, 2004, 109, 672-93.

[163] Mosca, L; Banka, CL; Benjamin, EJ; Berra, K; Bushnell, C; Dolor, RJ; Ganiats, TG; Gomes, AS; Gornik, HL; Gracia, C; Gulati, M; Haan, CK; Judelson, DR; Keenan, N; Kelepouris, E; Michos, ED; Newby, LK; Oparil, S; Ouyang, P; Oz, MC; Petitti, D; Pinn, VW; Redberg, RF; Scott, R; Sherif, K; Smith, SC; Jr; Sopko, G; Steinhorn, RH; Stone, NJ; Taubert, KA; Todd, BA; Urbina, E; Wenger, NK. Expert Panel/Writing Group; American Heart Association; American Academy of Family Physicians; American College of Obstetricians and Gynecologists; American College of Cardiology Foundation; Society of Thoracic Surgeons; American Medical Women's Association; Centers for Disease Control and Prevention; Office of Research on Women's Health; Association of Black Cardiologists; American College of Physicians; World Heart Federation; National Heart, Lung, and Blood Institute; American College of Nurse Practitioners. Evidence-based guidelines for cardiovascular disease prevention in women. 2007 update. *Circulation.*, 2007, 115, 1481-1501.

[164] Naftolin, F; Schneider, HP; Sturdee, DW; Birkhäuser, M; Brincat, MP; Gambacciani, M; Genazzani, AR; Limpaphayom, KK; O'Neill, S; Palacios, S; Pines, A; Siseles, N; Tan, D; Burger, HG. Executive Committee of the International Menopause Society. Guidelines for hormone treatment of women in the menopausal transition and beyond. *Climacteric.*, 2004, 7, 333-7.

[165] Hersh, AL; Stefanick, ML; Stafford, RS. National use of postmenopausal hormone therapy: annual trends and response to recent evidence. *JAMA.*, 2004, 291, 47-53.

[166] Parente, L; Uyehara, C; Larsen, W; et al. Long-term impact of the women's health initiative on HRT. *Arch Gynecol Obstet.*, 2008, 277, 219-24.

[167] Sare, GM; Gray, LJ; Bath, PM. Association between hormone replacement therapy and subsequent arterial and venous vascular events: a meta-analysis. *Eur Heart J.*, 2008, 2031-41.

[168] Rossouw, JE; Prentice, RL; Manson, JE; Wu, L; Barad, D; Barnabei, VM; Ko, M; LaCroix, AZ; Margolis, KL; Stefanick, ML. Postmenopausal hormone therapy and risk of cardiovascular disease by age and years since menopause. *JAMA.*, 2007, 297, 1465-77.

[169] Prentice, RL; Langer, R; Stefanick, ML; Howard, BV; Pettinger, M; Anderson, G; Barad, D; Curb, JD; Kotchen, J; Kuller, L; Limacher, M; Wactawski-Wende, J; Women's Health Initiative Investigators. Combined postmenopausal hormone therapy and cardiovascular disease: toward resolving the discrepancy between observational studies and the Women's Health Initiative clinical trial. *Am J Epidemiol.*, 2005, 162, 404-14.

[170] Salpeter, SR; Walsh, JM; Greyber, E; Ormiston, TM; Salpeter, EE. Mortality associated with hormone replacement therapy in younger and older women: a meta-analysis. *J Gen Intern Med.*, 2004, 19, 791-804.

[171] Grodstein, F; Manson, JE; Colditz, GA; Willett, WC; Speizer, FE; Stampfer, MJ. A prospective, observational study of postmenopausal hormone therapy and primary prevention of cardiovascular disease. *Ann Intern Med.*, 2000, 133, 933-941.

[172] Manson, JE; Allison, MA; Rossouw, JE; Carr, JJ; Langer, RD; Hsia, J; Kuller, LH; Cochrane, BB; Hunt, JR; Ludlam, SE; Pettinger, MB; Gass, M; Margolis, KL; Nathan, L; Ockene, JK; Prentice, RL; Robbins, J; Stefanick, ML. WHI and WHI-CACS Investigators. Estrogen therapy and coronary-artery calcification. *N Engl J Med.*, 2007, 356, 2591-602.

[173] Prentice, RL; Langer, RD; Stefanick, ML; Howard, BV; Pettinger, M; Anderson, GL; Barad, D; Curb, JD; Kotchen, J; Kuller, L; Limacher, M; Wactawski-Wende, J; Women's Health Initiative Investigators. Combined analysis of Women's health Initiative observational and clinical trial data on postmenopausal hormone therapy and cardiovascular disease. *Am J Epidemiol.*, 2006, 163, 589-99.

[174] Manson, JE; Hsia, J; Johnson, KC; Rossouw, JE; Assaf, AR; Lasser, NL; Trevisan, M; Black, HR; Heckbert, SR; Detrano, R; Strickland, OL; Wong, ND; Crouse, JR; Stein, E; Cushman, M; Women's Health Initiative Investigators. Estrogen plus progestin and the risk of coronary heart disease. *N Engl J Med.*, 2003, 349, 523-34.

[175] Heiss, G; Wallace, R; Anderson, GL; Aragaki, A; Beresford, SA; Brzyski, R; Chlebowski, RT; Gass, M; LaCroix, A; Manson, JE; Prentice, RL; Rossouw, J; Stefanick, ML; WHI Investigators. Health risks and benefits 3 years after stopping randomized treatment with estrogen and progestin. *JAMA.*, 2008, 299, 1036-45.

[176] American Association of Clinical Endocrinologists (AACE) position statement on hormone replacement therapy (HRT) and cardiovascular risk. American Association of Clinical Endocrinologists Web site www.aace.com/pub/pdf/guidelines/ HRTCVRISKposition_ statement.pdf. *Accessed March.*, 5, 2008.

[177] http://clinicaltrials.gov/ct2/show/NCT00114517

[178] North American Menopause Society. Estrogen and progestogen use in peri- and postmenopausal women: March 2007 position statement of The North American Menopause Society. *Menopause.*, 2007, 14, 168-82.

[179] Bellino, FL. Nonprimate animal models of menopause: workshop report. *Menopause.*, 2000, 7, 14-24.

[180] Thorndike, EA; Turner, AS. In search of an animal model for postmenopausal diseases. *Front Biosci.*, 1998, 3, c17-26.

[181] Dalsgaard, T1; Larsen, CR; Mortensen, A; Larsen, JJ; Ottesen, B. New animal model for the study of postmenopausal coronary and cerebral artery function: the Watanabe heritable hyperlipidemic rabbit fed on a diet avoiding phytoestrogens. *Climacteric.*, 2002 , 5, 178-89.

[182] Appt, SE. Usefulness of the monkey model to investigate the role soy in postmenopausal women's health. *ILAR J.*, 2004, 45(2), 200-11.

[183] Wong, CM; Yao, X; Au, CL; Tsang, SY; Fung, KP; Laher, I; Vanhoutte, PM; Huang, Y. Raloxifene prevents endothelial dysfunction in aging ovariectomized female rats. *Vascul Pharmacol.*, 2006, 44, 290-8.

[184] Reckelhoff, JF; Fortepiani, LA. Novel mechanisms responsible for postmenopausal hypertension. *Hypertension.*, 2004, 43, 918-23.

[185] Hinojosa-Laborde, C; Lange, DL; Haywood, JR. Role of female sex hormones in the development and reversal of Dahl hypertension. *Hypertension.*, 2000, 35, 484-9.

[186] Javeshghani, D; Touyz, R; Sairam, M; Virdis, A; Neves, M; Schiffrin, E. Attenuated responses to angiotensin II in follitropin receptor knockout mice, a model of menopause-associated hypertension. *Hypertension.*, 2003, 42, 761-76.

[187] Lee, SD; Kuo, WW; Ho, YJ; Lin, AC; Tsai, CH; Wang, HF; Kuo, CH; Yang, AL; Huang, CY; Hwang, JM. Cardiac Fas-dependent and mitochondria-dependent apoptosis in ovariectomized rats. *Maturitas.*, 2008, Nov 20, 61(3), 268-77.

[188] Reckelhoff, JF; Fortepiani, LA. Novel mechanisms responsible for postmenopausal hypertension. *Hypertension.*, 2004, 43, 918-23.

[189] Geary, GG; Krause, DN; Duckles, SP. Estrogen reduces myogenic tone through a nitric oxide-dependent mechanism in rat cerebral arteries. *Am J Physiol.*, 1998, 275, H292-H300.

[190] Geary, GG; Krause, DN; Duckles, SP. Gonadal hormones affect diameter of male rat cerebral arteries through endothelium-dependent mechanisms. *Am J Physiol Heart Circ Physiol.*, 2000, H610-8.

[191] Geary, GG; Krause, DN; Duckles, SP. Estrogen reduces mouse cerebral artery tone through endothelial NOS- and cyclooxygenase-dependent mechanisms. *Am J Physiol Heart Circ Physiol.*, 2000, 279, H511-9.

[192] Geary, GG; McNeill, AM; Ospina, JA; Krause, DN; Korach, KS; Duckles, SP. Selected contribution: cerebrovascular nos and cyclooxygenase are unaffected by estrogen in mice lacking estrogen receptor-alpha. *J Appl Physiol.*, 2001, 91, 2391-9.

[193] Li, X; Geary, GG; Gonzales, RJ; Krause, DN; Duckles, SP. Effect of estrogen on cerebrovascular prostaglandins is amplified in mice with dysfunctional NOS. *Am J Physiol Heart Circ Physiol.*, 2004, 287, H588-94.

[194] Ospina, JA; Duckles, SP; Krause, DN. 17beta-estradiol decreases vascular tone in cerebral arteries by shifting COX-dependent vasoconstriction to vasodilation. *Am J Physiol Heart Circ Physiol.*, 2003, 285, H241-50.

[195] Tsang, SY; Yao, X; Chan, HY; Chan, FL; Leung, CS; Yung, LM; Au, CL; Chen, ZY; Laher, I; Huang, Y. Tamoxifen and estrogen attenuate enhanced vascular reactivity induced by estrogen deficiency in rat carotid arteries. *Biochem Pharmacol.*, 2007, 73, 1330-9.

[196] Ospina, JA; Brevig, HN; Krause, DN; Duckles, SP. Estrogen suppresses IL-1beta-mediated induction of COX-2 pathway in rat cerebral blood vessels. *Am J Physiol Heart Circ Physiol.*, 2004, 286, H2010-9.

[197] Sunday, L; Tran, MM; Krause, DN; Duckles, SP. Estrogen and progestagens differentially modulate vascular proinflammatory factors. *Am J Physiol Endocrinol Metab.*, 2006, 291, E261-7.

[198] Tsang, SY; Yao, X; Chan, FL; Wong, CM; Chen, ZY; Laher, I; Huang, Y. Estrogen and tamoxifen modulate cerebrovascular tone in ovariectomized female rats. *Hypertension.*, 2004, 44, 78-82.

[199] Doolen, S; Krause, DN; Duckles, SP. Estradiol modulates vascular response to melatonin in rat caudal artery. *Am J Physiol.*, 1999, 276, H1281-8.

[200] McNeill, AM; Zhang, C; Stanczyk, FZ; Duckles, SP; Krause, DN. Estrogen increases endothelial nitric oxide synthase via estrogen receptors in rat cerebral blood vessels: effect preserved after concurrent treatment with medroxyprogesterone acetate or progesterone. *Stroke.*, 2002, 33, 1685-91.

[201] Stirone, C; Chu, Y; Sunday, L; Duckles, SP; Krause, DN. 17 Beta-estradiol increases endothelial nitric oxide synthase mRNA copy number in cerebral blood vessels: quantification by real-time polymerase chain reaction. *Eur J Pharmacol.*, 2003, 478, 35-8.

[202] Ospina, JA; Krause, DN; Duckles, SP. 17beta-estradiol increases rat cerebrovascular prostacyclin synthesis by elevating cyclooxygenase-1 and prostacyclin synthase. *Stroke.*, 2002, 33, 600-5.

[203] Stirone, C; Chu, Y; Sunday, L; Duckles, SP; Krause, DN. 17 Beta-estradiol increases endothelial nitric oxide synthase mRNA copy number in cerebral blood vessels: quantification by real-time polymerase chain reaction. *Eur J Pharmacol.*, 2003, 478, 35-8.

[204] Stirone, C; Duckles, SP; Krause, DN. Multiple forms of estrogen receptor-alpha in cerebral blood vessels: regulation by estrogen. *Am J Physiol Endocrinol Metab.*, 2003, 284, E184-92.

[205] Stirone, C; Boroujerdi, A; Duckles, SP; Krause, DN. Estrogen receptor activation of phosphoinositide-3 kinase, akt, and nitric oxide signaling in cerebral blood vessels: rapid and long-term effects. *Mol Pharmacol.*, 2005, 67, 105-13. ,

[206] Tsang, SY; Yao, X; Wong, CM; Chan, FL; Chen, ZY; Huang, Y. Differential regulation of K+ and Ca2+ channel gene expression by chronic treatment with estrogen and tamoxifen in rat aorta. *Eur J Pharmacol.*, 2004, 483, 155-62.

[207] Stirone, C; Duckles, SP; Krause, DN; Procaccio, V. Estrogen increases mitochondrial efficiency and reduces oxidative stress in cerebral blood vessels. *Mol Pharmacol.*, 2005, 68, 959-65.

[208] Razmara, A; Duckles, SP; Krause, DN; Procaccio, V. Estrogen suppresses brain mitochondrial oxidative stress in female and male rats. *Brain Res.*, 2007, 1176, 71-81.

[209] Razmara, A; Sunday, L; Stirone, C; Wang, XB; Krause, DN; Duckles, SP; Procaccio, V. Mitochondrial effects of estrogen are mediated by estrogen receptor alpha in brain endothelial cells. *J Pharmacol Exp Ther.*, 2008, 325, 782-90.

[210] Sunday, L; Osuna, C; Krause, DN; Duckles, SP. Age alters cerebrovascular inflammation and effects of estrogen. Am J Physiol Heart Circ Physiol, 2007, 292, H2333-40.

In: Menopause: Vasomotor Symptoms, Systematic…   ISBN: 978-1-60876-930-8
Editors: J. Michalski, I. Nowak, pp. 97-110   © 2010 Nova Science Publishers, Inc.

Chapter III

Menopause: Vasomotor Symptoms, Systemic Treatments and Self-Care Measures

Lucia Alves da Silva Lara (Lara, LAS) and Ana Carolina Japur de Sá Rosa e Silva (Rosa-e-Silva, ACJS)
Sexual Medicina Service, Human Reproduction Sector, Department of Obstetrics and Gynecology, Faculty of Medicine of Ribeirão Preto, São Paulo University, SP, Brazil

Abstract

Since women's life expectancy is increasing all over the world, most of them are expected to live a significant part of their life in menopausal status. This period marks the end of the reproductive status and, in addition to bringing about negative feelings about this, might be accompanied by many complaints due to the decline of circulating estrogen levels. The most common complaint during this period is related to vasomotor symptoms such as hot flashes and night sweats. Although not all women are bothered by them, vasomotor symptoms represent a very frequent and distressing occurrence. The mechanism by which vasomotor symptoms are triggered has not been fully clarified but the link with low estrogen concentrations has been well established. Low estrogen levels result in disturbance of the temperature regulating mechanism situated in the anterior-preoptic hypothalamus, where there is a thermoneutral zone that is reduced after menopause, becoming hypersensitive to hot stimuli and abnormally inducing hot flashes. In this way the sweating threshold seems to be *reduced to a greater level* and the shivering threshold is increased. Also, estrogen is known to influence serotonin, endorphin, noradrenalin and dopamine levels, and neurotransmitters that have been associated with regulatory mechanisms in body temperature control. Additionally, hypoestrogenism may interfere with vascular reactivity to the inputs from this altered thermoneutral zone. This culminates with symptoms including sudden feelings of warmth and skin redness that begin in the chest and spread to the neck and face, accompanied by sweating, palpitations, anxiety and sleeping disturbance that potentially impair the quality of life of women. The management of these symptoms includes hormonal replacement therapy (HRT) that constitutes the basis of the treatment of menopause symptoms especially regarding hot flashes. Some measures including lifestyle changes are useful to reduce vasomotor symptoms and should be considered in all cases. The efficacy of complementary alternative medicine therapies remains inconclusive due to the lack of evidence.

Introduction

Since the life expectancy of women is increasing all over the world, most of them are expected to live a significant portion of their life in menopausal status. This period that marks the end of the reproductive status, in addition to bringing about negative feelings about this, might be accompanied by many complaints due to the decline of circulating estrogen levels. The most common complaint during this period is related to the vasomotor symptoms represented by hot flashes and night sweats. The hot flashes are a rapid and exaggerated response causing an intense heat sensation and skin reddening secondary to an increased skin blood flow, followed by changes in heart rate and blood pressure (Charkoudian 2003). An elevation of core body temperature, in general, precedes hot flashes, that are triggered by small elevations in body temperature acting within a reduced thermoneutral zone (Freedman, Norton et al. 1995). The vasomotor symptoms seem to result from a dysfunction in the circuitry of temperature control, leading to an exaggerated activation of heat dissipation responses resulting from an exacerbated peripheral vasodilatation response that culminates with hot flashes and sweating (Deecher 2005). Although not all women are bothered by them, vasomotor symptoms represent a very frequent and distressing occurrence. Thus, these symptoms need to be controlled with special strategies in order to provide a better quality of life.

Prevalence of Vasomotor Symptoms

The prevalence of vasomotor symptoms varies widely according to region and may be influenced by a range of factors, including climate, diet, lifestyle, women's roles, and attitudes related to the end of the reproductive period and aging (Freeman and Sherif 2007). On average, approximately 75% of climacteric woman suffer from hot flashes and night sweats that begin in general one to two years before menopause and commonly persist for 6 months to 5 years after the last menstrual period (Freedman 2005; Utian 2005). Examining 436 women in the pre- an post-menopausal period, some authors found that 37% of the premenopausal group and 79% of the postmenopausal women reported hot flashes (Freeman, Sammel et al. 2005). The vasomotor symptoms can start as early as at 38 years of age and peak in late perimenopause or early menopause by 52-54 years (Rodstrom, Bengtsson et al. 2002; 2005). In a longitudinal study conducted in Scandinavia these vasomotor symptoms were common, with a maximal prevalence of 64% at 54 years of age (Rodstrom, Bengtsson et al. 2002). They usually occur daily in women whose menstrual flow demonstrates changes or cessation, and for 25% of them, hot flushes persist for five years or more (McKinlay and Jefferys 1974; Kronenberg 1990).

Pathophysiology of Vasomotor Symptoms and Associated Factors

Maintaining body homeostasis involves a small oscillatory zone of core body temperature situated between a lower and upper threshold that is called thermoneutral zone (Cabanac and Massonnet 1977). The thermoneutral zone responds to stimuli from thermoregulatory zones that are spread on the body surface and in the gastrointestinal tract and other internal organs, in intraabdominal veins, in the spinal cord and in the Central Nervous System (CNS) (Kakitsuba, Mekjavic et al. 2007; Rintamaki 2007). In the CNS, specifically in the preoptic-anterior hypothalamus, there are warming and cooling areas responsible for body thermobalance. The warming area promotes dissipation of heat through sweating and increased skin blood flow, and the cooling area produces heat and promotes heat retention within the body core. The heat production response includes shivering and nonshivering thermogenesis, and heat retention responses include cutaneous vasoconstriction (Boulant 1998). These sensors signal temperature oscillation to the thermoregulatory centers in the preoptic-anterior hypothalamus area where these messages are processed and signalized as a response to maintain homeostatic thermoregulation. The capacity of the body to maintain this mechanism intact depends on adequate conditions mainly linked to the hormonal status. In pre- and post-menopausal women, the reduction of estrogen levels results in rupture of this mechanism that culminates with vasomotor symptoms.

The pathophysiology of vasomotor symptoms is not entirely clear but three mechanisms such as alterations of the hypothalamic area that controls the core body temperature, the hypersensitivity of the peripheral thermoregulatory zone and neurochemical imbalances have been proposed to explain them. These mechanisms seem to be linked to changes in various substances such as hypothalamic β-endorphin levels, adrenergic and cholinergic receptor activity and noradrenalin and serotonin concentrations, that are under the control of estrogen action.

In normal conditions, the way that environmental temperature induces a body response to maintain adequate core body temperature includes both vasodilation to dissipate heat and vasoconstriction to conserve heat. Probably the hot flashes are a result of a thermoregulatory dysfunction which originates in the hypothalamus due to estrogen reduction. The thermoneutral zone is formed by a stable range within preset limits that vary over the circadian cycle (Hensel 1973) within witch the body temperature oscillates to maintain its homeostasis. After menopause, this thermoregulatory threshold is modified, permitting the occurrence of sudden peripheral vasodilatation that results in increased skin blood flow and excessive sweating with a rapid loss of body heat. This promotes a reduction of central temperature to levels below normal and the onset of tremors, a body artifice that tries to increase body temperature. Vasoconstriction occurs in parallel, preventing a greater loss of body heat (Miller and Li 2004). On this basis, when the core body temperature increases above or below threshold, vasodilatation occurs, resulting in hot flushes followed by sweating that leads to loss of heat and shivering (Freedman, Norton et al. 1995; Freedman and Krell 1999).

Some individual characteristics are responsible for the degree of activation of body thermal sensors, and hence these individual characteristics outline the neurochemical response that controls the dynamics of the peripheral vasculature (Deecher 2005). The vasomotor symptoms may appear even during the menopausal transition period due to neurochemical imbalances associated with sexual steroid changes in the brain resulting in thermoregulatory dysfunction (Shanafelt, Barton et al. 2002).

Estrogen controls the synthesis and action of many neurotransmitter molecules such as serotonin and noradrenalin that have been proposed to be involved in this mechanism, which in turn may affect thermoregulatory responses (McEwen and Alves 1999; Rybaczyk, Bashaw et al. 2005). Additionally, estrogen modulates the synthesis and action of neuropeptides such as nitric oxide and vasoactive intestinal peptides that are co-responsible for vascular reactivity (Przewlocka-Kosmala 2002). The changes in the levels of these substances may interfere with the ability of blood vessels to respond rapidly and to the appropriate extent, resulting in an exaggerated response (Charkoudian 2003).

Also, there is supportive evidence for the role of estrogen, opioids and neurotransmitters such as norepinephrine (NE) and serotonin (5-HT) in temperature regulation. It has been demonstrated that serotonin 2a receptors (5-HT(2A)) play a role in temperature regulation by promoting heat loss (Blum, Vered et al. 1996) and estrogen withdrawal is associated with decreased serotonin concentration in the blood and in the hypothalamus (Fink, Sumner et al. 1996). This condition is gradually worsened by age (Gonzales and Carrillo 1993; Blum, Vered et al. 1996). On the other hand, hypoestrogenism culminates with abnormal noradrenergic hyperactivity that leads to an increased hypothalamic release of norepinephrine and serotonin. These substances promote a lowering of the set point in the thermoregulatory nucleus, that culminates with subtle changes in core body temperature (Casper and Yen 1985). In summary, the hormonal mechanism linked to these symptoms has not been fully clarified, but the role of estrogen reduction in this condition is presumed to activate the cascade of events that culminates with hot flashes and sweating. In fact, it has been proposed that the rate of change of plasma estrogen concentrations other than the levels of estrogens itself influences the thermoregulatory system via the hypothalamus (Andrikoula and Prelevic 2009). This theory is based on the fact that young women with gonadal dysgenesia, a condition in which very low circulating levels of estrogen are present since birth without pubertal changes, rarely present hot flushes. Unless they receive estrogen replacement therapy followed by discontinuation, these complaints never appear.

Additionally, estrogen improves vasomotion by modulation of vasoconstrictor and vasodilator systems through endothelium-dependent and endothelium-independent mechanisms (Joswig, Hach-Wunderle et al. 1999). The changes in estrogen levels culminate with an increased peripheral blood flow provoked by a reduced response of the peripheral vasculature to the changes of body core temperature (Charkoudian 2003), and a compensatory increase of heart rate.

Another hypothesis raised to explain the triggering of hot flashes is the reduction of endogenous opioids that accompanies the dramatic reduction of estrogen concentrations after menopause. This theory is supported by experimental studies in rats in which endorphin injection in the preoptic-anterior hypothalamus resulted in an increase of body temperature (Thornhill and Wilfong 1982). In hypoestrogenic conditions the levels of endorphin decrease in the hypothalamus and hypothalamic norepinephrine and serotonin release increases, resulting in lowering of the thermoregulatory nucleus threshold, which in turn promotes heat loss that activates the cascade of events that culminates with changes in core body temperature.

Some conditions are associated with the vasomotor symptoms instead of being responsible for them. It has been shown that anxiety is significantly associated with the occurrence and with the severity and frequency of hot flashes (Freeman, Sammel et al. 2005). Also, alterations in the concentrations of other endogenous substances have been observed in patients with hot flashes and seem to be more an association rather than a causative factor (Kronenberg, Cote et al. 1984; Zhao, Wang et al. 2000). An example is the increase in luteinizing hormone (LH) levels after hot flashes. In addition to LH, other substances such as adrenaline, corticotropin, cortisol, androstenedione, dihydroepiandrostenedione, beta-endorphins and growth hormone are at highest levels during hot flushes. Estradiol levels and estrone, prolactin, TSH, and FSH do not change.

Similarly, progesterone appears to influence skin blood flow control (Brooks, Paulson et al. 1997) and the decrease of both estrogen and progesterone, in addition to reducing the elasticity of blood vessels, may affect vascular reactivity, resulting in delayed responses of the vessels. The proximity of the thermoregulatory center to the neurons that produce GnRH possibly activates the release of this hormone simultaneously to the alterations of body temperature.

Clinical Manifestations

The classic manifestations of vasomotor symptoms are hot flushes and night sweats that vary greatly in intensity among women (Rodstrom, Bengtsson et al. 2002). The symptoms include a sudden feeling of warmth and skin redness that begins in the chest and spreads to the neck and the face, accompanied by sweating, palpitations, anxiety and sleeping disturbances that potentially impair women's relationships and quality of life (McKinlay and Jefferys 1974). This process lasts 2 or 4 minutes and sometimes is followed by a cold sensation and tremors.

The vasomotor symptoms occur both during the day and at night. Complaints of sleep disturbances are frequently reported following these symptoms, and it has been also demonstrated to occur immediately before the hot flashes. On this basis, the increased frequency of sleep disturbances during menopause may be due to disorders that are screened out, such as sleep apnea and drug use (Freedman and Roehrs 2004). The Study of Women's Health Across the Nation pointed out important factors associated with bothersome hot flashes including mood, symptom sensitivity, symptom duration, sleep problems, age, frequency, and race. Thus, strategies to control hot flashes should include measures to control all of these factors (Thurston, Bromberger et al. 2008).

Studies have shown that the time of menopause is associated with the frequency of hot flashes and in general four or five years after this event there is a dramatic decrease in this complaint. Analyses of longitudinal and cross-sectional studies including 35,445 menopausal women showed that menopause symptoms increase in the two years before the final menstrual period and persist, but declining, for about eight years after the final menstrual period. In general, the first year after the final menstrual period corresponds to the higher level of complaints; 50% of the women report vasomotor symptoms up to four years after menopause and in 10% of them, these symptoms persist for more than 12 years (Politi, Schleinitz et al. 2008).

Body temperature increases in parallel to higher concentrations of progesterone and estrogen according to the ovulatory period and the control of the thermoregulatory reflex of cutaneous vasodilation is modified (Brooks, Morgan et al. 1997). In hypoestrogenic conditions this effect changes, resulting in enhancement of the vasodilator response to local warming. These data are consistent with reports of the influence of estrogen on the enhancement of nitric oxide-dependent vasodilator responses (Charkoudian, Stephens et al. 1999).

The use of estrogen antagonist drugs such as tamoxifen and raloxifene can also cause hot flashes. Some diseases such as thyroidopathies frequently associated with menopause can disrupt temperature homeostasis and can also lead to hot flashes.

Prevention and Treatment of Vasomotor Symptoms

Hormonal replacement therapy (HRT) has been the basis of treatment, especially for the relief of moderate-to-severe menopause-associated vasomotor symptoms (Umland 2008) and is currently the only FDA-approved treatment for hot flashes (Pinkerton, Stovall et al. 2009). The effectiveness treatment seems to be based on estrogen replacement that culminates with relief of symptoms in about 80% to 90% of cases. It is recommended that hormonal therapy use should be limited to the lowest effective dosage over the shortest period of time, and continued use should be reevaluated on a periodic basis (2008). Oral micronized 17 beta-estradiol at an initial dose of 1 mg is effective in reducing the daily number and severity of hot flushes and in reducing the number of night sweats (Notelovitz, Lenihan et al. 2000; Gambacciani, Spielmann et al. 2005). The risk and benefit must be controlled in this kind of treatment. A negative effect of HRT on secondary coronary heart disease was detected by The Heart and Estrogen/Progestin Replacement Study (HERS) and Women's Health Initiative (WHI). However, it has been recently demonstrated that women in early menopause who are in good cardiovascular health are at low risk of adverse cardiovascular effects with HRT (Welty 2003; 2008). It is important to point out that greater proven benefits of HRT are obtained when the therapy is applied during the first years post-menopause, in a so-called "window of opportunity", exactly when the hot flashes are more intense (Utian, Archer et al. 2008). Additionally, oral 17 beta-estradiol with or without cyclic progestin had no effect on the progression of atherosclerosis or reinfarction and transdermal 17 beta-estradiol plus cyclic progestin is associated with a non-significant increase in coronary heart disease events in women with coronary heart disease (Welty 2003).

The use of medroxyprogesterone acetate (MPA) is a suitable alternative to estrogen therapy for reducing vasomotor symptoms (Lobo, McCormick et al. 1984), being a possible choice for those women that are at risk of thromboembolism. A single MPA dose seems to be well tolerated and effective in these cases (Loprinzi, Levitt et al. 2006). Megestrol acetate is a synthetic progestogen used for the treatment of patients with breast cancer. When orally administered at doses of 20 to 80 mg/day, megestrol has proved to be effective in reducing by as much as 85% the frequency of heat waves (Warren 2008). A transitory increase in the occurrence of symptoms may be observed at the beginning of treatment that almost always disappears within one or two weeks. The side effects of megestrol acetate at high doses or during prolonged treatment include Cushing's syndrome, new-onset diabetes and suppression of plasma ACTH and cortisol levels. It is important to monitor adrenal function due to suppression of the pituitary-adrenal axis after treatment discontinuation since megestrol has a glucocorticoid-like activity (Gonzalez Villarroel, Fernandez Perez et al. 2008).

The potential risk for breast cancer after HRT has been demonstrated. The WHI, a randomized controlled trial that involved 16608 postmenopausal women, demonstrated an increase of invasive breast cancer after 5 years of follow-up (Rossouw, Anderson et al. 2002). The association of HRT and ovarian cancer remains controversial. A meta-analysis of data from 15 case-control studies of estrogen replacement therapy did not find a correlation between HRT and epithelial ovarian cancer incidence (Coughlin, Giustozzi et al. 2000). However, another recent meta-analysis demonstrated that HRT use is associated with an increased risk of ovarian cancer and it seems that the use estrogen replacement alone is more strongly associated with this event than the use of combined HRT (Lacey, Mink et al. 2002; Zhou, Sun et al. 2008). In conclusion, the results of the Women's Health Initiative in combination with other recent reports suggest that long-term estrogen therapy should not be recommended for most women at this time (Shanafelt, Barton et al. 2002).

Alternative therapy for vasomotor symptoms with the use of newer antidepressants and alternative medicine has been shown to have variable benefits. In special conditions when women are at risk of breast cancer, ovarian cancer, endometrial cancer, venous thromboembolism and cardiovascular risk, interventions other than hormones should be considered (Shanafelt, Barton et al. 2002) mainly when the symptoms do not interfere with daily function. In this case some measures considered to be reasonable as an initial approach are recommended (Rabin, Cipparrone et al. 1999; Shanafelt, Barton et al. 2002). Although a current tendency to an increased adoption of complementary and alternative medicine to control vasomotor symptoms has been observed (Kupferer, Dormire et al. 2009), its efficacy and the efficacy of herbal remedies such as soy isoflavones, red clover isoflavones, black cohosh, and vitamin E remain inconclusive, mainly due to the lack of well designed trials (Green, Denham et al. 2007; Welty, Lee et al. 2007). Additionally, modest effectiveness of these therapies has been reported and data about their long-term safety are lacking (Bordeleau, Pritchard et al. 2007). However, they appear to be safe when used for 6 months but they are less effective then HRT and may be appropriate to control only mild symptoms (Umland 2008).

Alternatively, the use of centrally active agents has been recommended, such as selective serotonin reuptake inhibitors, serotonin-norepinephrine reuptake inhibitors, mainly venlafaxine, paroxetine, and the anti seizure agent gabapentin, as well as the alpha-2 adrenergic agonist clonidine, all of them regarded as the most promising nonhormonal agents for the treatment for hot flashes. These agents affect the release and reuptake of a variety of neurotransmitters at multiple sites in the central nervous system, including the hypothalamus and other specific and nonspecific effects on neurotransmitter kinetics may contribute to their clinical effects (Loprinzi, Pisansky et al. 1998; Loprinzi, Stearns et al. 2005). They are effective in reducing hot flashes by 50%-60% (Stearns and Hayes 2002). However, there are controversies about this kind of treatment, which is supposed to be based on poor evidences of not well designed studies (Loprinzi, Barton et al. 2009). In addition, recent studies have shown important indications for this drugs that probably restore levels of 5-HT and norepinephrine that are believed to be altered by the loss of modulation by estrogens (Deecher, Alfinito et al. 2007; Nelson 2008). In this case, the benefit of noradrenaline and norepinephrine antagonists as nonhormonal therapies that comprises the selective 5-HT and 5-HT/NE reuptake inhibitors (SNRI) has been considered for the treatment of vasomotor symptoms (Deecher, Alfinito et al. 2007; Santoro 2008).

Venlafaxine, a 5-HT/NE reuptake inhibitor, is effective for the treatment of hot flashes. However, its efficacy must be balanced against the drug's side-effects that include hypertension, mouth dryness, decreased appetite, nausea, and constipation (Loprinzi, Kugler et al. 2000). Other selective 5-HT reuptake inhibitors such as fluoxetine at a dose of 20 mg/d are well tolerated and result in a modest improvement of hot flashes (Loprinzi, Sloan et al. 2002); paroxetine promoted a reduction of hot flash frequency (67%) and of severity score (75%), with significant improvement of depression, sleep, anxiety, and quality of life scores (Stearns, Isaacs et al. 2000). Hence, paroxetine may constitute an effective and acceptable alternative to hormone replacement and other therapies (Stearns, Beebe et al. 2003)..
Citalopram has little effect on hot flushes and cannot be recommended for the treatment of vasomotor symptoms (Suvanto-Luukkonen, Koivunen et al. 2005). Overall, other commonly reported side effects are decreased appetite, discontinuation syndrome, sexual dysfunction (Chen, Wang et al. 2008), and elevated blood pressure with venlaflaxine. Considering the effectiveness hierarchy of these drugs, paroxetine is the most potent inhibitor of serotonin re-uptake, being effective in controlling vasomotor symptoms in about 41% of women (Marks, Park et al. 2008), followed by venlafaxine, fluoxetine, and sertraline, which have shown scores of 33% and 13%, respectively (Loprinzi, Sloan et al. 2009). Schemes using small and medium doses lead to a similar improvement of symptoms when compared to schemes using high doses, in addition to involving a lower occurrenmce of side effects. Thus, the recommendation is to start treatment with low doses to be gradually increased until the desired effect is obtained. Thus, venlaflaxine and paroxetine are effective at a daily dose of 75 mg/d (Loprinzi, Kugler et al. 2000) and 20 mg, respectively (Stearns, Isaacs et al. 2000)

Another centrally active drug that has been considered to be effective in controlling vasomotor symptoms is gabapentin. Comparison of the efficacy of estrogen and gabapentin in the treatment of moderate-to-severe hot flushes demonstrated that gabapentin is effective and well-tolerated in the control of hot flashes at a dose of 900 mg/day (Butt, Lock et al. 2008) and appears to be as effective as estrogen (Reddy, Warner et al. 2006). This drug is considered to be an appropriate alternative for women who cannot or will not use HRT, such as breast cancer survivors (Pandya, Morrow et al. 2005; Bordeleau, Pritchard et al. 2007); its adverse effects, that comprise somnolence, dizziness, ataxia, headache, decrease or loss of libido, anemia, thrombocytopenia and others, must also be considered (Nelson 2008).

Anticholinergic drugs such as Oxybutynin seem to be promising in the management of hot flashes in refractory patients (Sexton, Younus et al. 2007) based on the notion that the cholinergic system is involved in the genesis of vasomotor symptoms. However, the scarcity of available data does not permit a formal recommendation of this drug for the control of vasomotor symptoms.

Clonidine is a central agonist of alpha-2 adrenergic receptors which acts by reducing vascular reactivity, but its effect on hot flashes relief is controversial. This medicine administered at a dose of 0.1 mg/day has a modest effect in reducing hot flash frequency. The most common side effects of clonidine are dry mouth, constipation, somnolence, and local irritation. The use of the antihypertensive drugs alpha-methyldopa and belladonna may be helpful for some women (Santoro 2008), although their modest efficacy and adverse effects should be considered (Shanafelt, Barton et al. 2002).

Veralipride, a synthetic benzamide derivative with an antidopaminergic action, is effective in reducing the frequency and severity of hot flushes. The adverse effects of this drug include acute dyskinesia, which may occur after many months of treatment (De Leo, Morgante et al. 2006). All trials that tested this drug were considered to be inadequate to support the use of this medicine due to their poor quality; hence, this drug should not be prescribed for the control of vasomotor symptoms.

A randomized controlled trial using acupuncture and auricular acupressure demonstrated that this therapy significantly relieves both the severity and frequency of hot flashes in menopausal ovariectomized women (Zhou, Qu et al. 2009), representing an alternative treatment for selected patients who feel comfortable with this kind of therapy.

Tibolone is a synthetic *hormone*-type drug with estrogenic, progestational and androgenic effects that has been used as an alternative to estrogen to treat menopausal symptoms for 30 years. Vasomotor symptoms improve significantly with tibolone (Kenemans, Bundred et al. 2009). However, the Million Women Study demonstrated an increase in the relative risk of breast cancer (Bundred and Morris 2003). Despite its beneficial effect on vasomotor symptoms, this treatment must be discouraged for breast cancer survivors due to the significantly increased risk of breast cancer recurrence (Goodwin 2009; Kenemans, Bundred et al. 2009). There was also an increased risk of cancer of the endometrium. The long-term effects regarding cardiovascular disease are not known.

The use of phytoestrogens is increasingly common, although there is no clinical evidence of their real benefits. Soy contains large amounts of phytoestrogens and is the food containing the highest levels of isoflavones available for consumption, representing one of the most popular treatments based on foods that have an estrogenic action. Since isoflavones are similar to endogenous estrogens, they compete with the latter for the same receptors, with alternately pro- and anti-estrogenic functions. The effects of soy consumption on menopausal symptoms seem to be mild, but more studies are needed in order to reach more definitive conclusions. A recent meta-analysis reported that isoflavone supplementation was associated with a 34% reduction in hot flashes and the dose of at least 15 mg of genistein, rather than total isoflavones, was responsible for a reduction in symptoms (Kurzer 2008). Another review including 11 randomized studies, only 3 of which evaluated soy or isoflavone supplementation with at least six weeks of follow-up, reported beneficial effects of these compounds. It is important to emphasize that this was a short-term follow-up for definitive conclusions. And one of the studies was unable to prove any benefit of isoflavone supplementation. In fact, some of the trials that found that phytoestrogen treatments alleviated the frequency and severity of vasomotor symptoms are considered of low quality and underpowered (Lethaby, Brown et al. 2007). Hence, the use of phytoestrogen treatment is not based on sufficient evidence to be indicated as a suitable alternative to conventional HRT because of the lack of evidence of its effectiveness in the alleviation of menopausal symptoms (Lethaby, Brown et al. 2007). In addition, there is no evidence that the same side effects observed for conventional HRT will not occur with soy or isoflavone supplementation.

One of the most popular botanicals is known as Black Cohosh (*Cimicifuga racemosa*), which is the most extensively studied phytoestrogen for the treatment of hot flashes. Although its real mechanism of action is still unknown, this phytoestrogen is believed to compete with estrogen for its receptors and to mimic its effects. Nevertheless, more recent data suggest that it may act as a selective estrogen receptor modulator depending on which specific kind of tissue it is acting. Also, it may play a role as an agonist for serotonin receptors. Normally it is not used for long-term treatment. The present results are controversial, varying from no action to an 84% reduction of symptoms (Maki, Rubin et al. 2009). The American College of Gynecology and Obstetrics recommends that this sort of phytoestrogen may be useful for short-term treatment of hot flashes (up to six months). Since it may have an estrogenic effect on the breast, it should not be indicated for patients with a past history of breast cancer or with a high risk for neoplasias (Davis, Jayo et al. 2008). Same neuroactive agents such as estrogen receptor-beta-targeted herbal therapy, MF-101 and bazedoxifene, a selective estrogen receptor modulator, are under investigation for the relief of vasomotor symptoms (Pinkerton, Stovall et al. 2009).

Self-Care Measures

General measures to be followed by both symptomatic and asymptomatic menopausal woman include lifestyle changes such as wearing light clothing, avoiding a fat diet, using relaxation techniques, regular physical activity, smoking cessation, avoiding high environmental temperatures, and avoiding stressful conditions (Gold, Block et al. 2004). In a recent analysis of 6 studies of physical exercise aiming to ameliorate hot flashes, the investigators did not find positive effects, possibly because exercise raises core body temperature, thereby triggering hot flashes (Freedman 2005). Other lifestyle measures such as avoiding alcohol, caffeine and spicy foods, keeping the core body temperature cool and paced respiration seem to have positive effect on hot flashes (2004). Thus, the preferential intake of fruit and vegetables is recommended.

References

(2004). "Treatment of menopause-associated vasomotor symptoms: position statement of The North American Menopause Society." *Menopause* **11**(1): 11-33.

(2005). "National Institutes of Health State-of-the-Science Conference statement: management of menopause-related symptoms." *Ann Intern Med* **142**(12 Pt 1): 1003-1013.

(2008). "ACOG Committee Opinion No. 420, November 2008: hormone therapy and heart disease." *Obstet Gynecol* **112**(5): 1189-1192.

Andrikoula, M. and G. Prelevic (2009). "Menopausal hot flushes revisited." *Climacteric* **12**(1): 3-15.

Blum, I., Y. Vered, et al. (1996). "The effect of estrogen replacement therapy on plasma serotonin and catecholamines of postmenopausal women." *Isr J Med Sci* **32**(12): 1158-1162.

Bordeleau, L., K. Pritchard, et al. (2007). "Therapeutic options for the management of hot flashes in breast cancer survivors: an evidence-based review." *Clin Ther* **29**(2): 230-241.

Boulant, J. A. (1998). "Hypothalamic neurons. Mechanisms of sensitivity to temperature." *Ann N Y Acad Sci* **856**: 108-115.

Brooks, B. P., H. L. Paulson, et al. (1997). "Characterization of an expanded glutamine repeat androgen receptor in a neuronal cell culture system." *Neurobiol Dis* **3**(4): 313-323.

Brooks, E. M., A. L. Morgan, et al. (1997). "Chronic hormone replacement therapy alters thermoregulatory and vasomotor function in postmenopausal women." *J Appl Physiol* **83**(2): 477-484.

Bundred, N. J. and J. Morris (2003). "Breast cancer and hormone-replacement therapy: the Million Women Study." *Lancet* **362**(9392): 1329; author reply 1330-1321.

Butt, D. A., M. Lock, et al. (2008). "Gabapentin for the treatment of menopausal hot flashes: a randomized controlled trial." *Menopause* **15**(2): 310-318.

Cabanac, M. and B. Massonnet (1977). "Thermoregulatory responses as a function of core temperature in humans." *J Physiol* **265**(3): 587-596.

Casper, R. F. and S. S. Yen (1985). "Neuroendocrinology of menopausal flushes: an hypothesis of flush mechanism." *Clin Endocrinol (Oxf)* **22**(3): 293-312.

Charkoudian, N. (2003). "How do female reproductive hormones influence vascular control in the hand?" *Clin Auton Res* **13**(3): 178-179.

Charkoudian, N., D. P. Stephens, et al. (1999). "Influence of female reproductive hormones on local thermal control of skin blood flow." *J Appl Physiol* **87**(5): 1719-1723.

Chen, Z. X., H. Q. Wang, et al. (2008). "[Selective serotomin reuptake inhibitor is more likely to induce sexual dysfunction than mirtazapine in treating depression]." *Zhonghua Nan Ke Xue* **14**(10): 896-899.

Coughlin, S. S., A. Giustozzi, et al. (2000). "A meta-analysis of estrogen replacement therapy and risk of epithelial ovarian cancer." *J Clin Epidemiol* **53**(4): 367-375.

Davis, V. L., M. J. Jayo, et al. (2008). "Black cohosh increases metastatic mammary cancer in transgenic mice expressing c-erbB2." *Cancer Res* **68**(20): 8377-8383.

De Leo, V., G. Morgante, et al. (2006). "The safety of veralipride." *Expert Opin Drug Saf* **5**(5): 695-701.

Deecher, D. C. (2005). "Physiology of thermoregulatory dysfunction and current approaches to the treatment of vasomotor symptoms." *Expert Opin Investig Drugs* **14**(4): 435-448.

Deecher, D. C., P. D. Alfinito, et al. (2007). "Alleviation of thermoregulatory dysfunction with the new serotonin and norepinephrine reuptake inhibitor desvenlafaxine succinate in ovariectomized rodent models." *Endocrinology* **148**(3): 1376-1383.

Fink, G., B. E. Sumner, et al. (1996). "Estrogen control of central neurotransmission: effect on mood, mental state, and memory." *Cell Mol Neurobiol* **16**(3): 325-344.

Freedman, R. R. (2005). "Hot flashes: behavioral treatments, mechanisms, and relation to sleep." *Am J Med* **118 Suppl 12B**: 124-130.

Freedman, R. R. and W. Krell (1999). "Reduced thermoregulatory null zone in postmenopausal women with hot flashes." *Am J Obstet Gynecol* **181**(1): 66-70.

Freedman, R. R., D. Norton, et al. (1995). "Core body temperature and circadian rhythm of hot flashes in menopausal women." *J Clin Endocrinol Metab* **80**(8): 2354-2358.

Freedman, R. R. and T. A. Roehrs (2004). "Lack of sleep disturbance from menopausal hot flashes." *Fertil Steril* **82**(1): 138-144.

Freeman, E. W., M. D. Sammel, et al. (2005). "The role of anxiety and hormonal changes in menopausal hot flashes." *Menopause* **12**(3): 258-266.

Freeman, E. W. and K. Sherif (2007). "Prevalence of hot flushes and night sweats around the world: a systematic review." *Climacteric* **10**(3): 197-214.

Gambacciani, M., D. Spielmann, et al. (2005). "Efficacy on climacteric symptoms of a continuous combined regimen of 1 mg 17beta-estradiol and trimegestone versus two regimens combining 1 or 2 mg 17beta-estradiol and norethisterone acetate." *Gynecol Endocrinol* **21**(2): 65-73.

Gold, E. B., G. Block, et al. (2004). "Lifestyle and demographic factors in relation to vasomotor symptoms: baseline results from the Study of Women's Health Across the Nation." *Am J Epidemiol* **159**(12): 1189-1199.

Gonzales, G. F. and C. Carrillo (1993). "Blood serotonin levels in postmenopausal women: effects of age and serum oestradiol levels." *Maturitas* **17**(1): 23-29.

Gonzalez Villarroel, P., I. Fernandez Perez, et al. (2008). "Megestrol acetate-induced adrenal insufficiency." *Clin Transl Oncol* **10**(4): 235-237.

Goodwin, P. J. (2009). "Tibolone: the risk is too high." *Lancet Oncol* **10**(2): 103-104.

Green, J., A. Denham, et al. (2007). "Treatment of menopausal symptoms by qualified herbal practitioners: a prospective, randomized controlled trial." *Fam Pract* **24**(5): 468-474.

Hensel, H. (1973). "Neural processes in thermoregulation." *Physiol Rev* **53**(4): 948-1017.

Joswig, M., V. Hach-Wunderle, et al. (1999). "Postmenopausal hormone replacement therapy and the vascular wall: mechanisms of 17 beta-estradiol's effects on vascular biology." *Exp Clin Endocrinol Diabetes* **107**(8): 477-487.

Kakitsuba, N., I. B. Mekjavic, et al. (2007). "Individual variability in the peripheral and core interthreshold zones." *J Physiol Anthropol* **26**(3): 403-408.

Kenemans, P., N. J. Bundred, et al. (2009). "Safety and efficacy of tibolone in breast-cancer patients with vasomotor symptoms: a double-blind, randomised, non-inferiority trial." *Lancet Oncol* **10**(2): 135-146.

Kronenberg, F. (1990). "Hot flashes: epidemiology and physiology." *Ann N Y Acad Sci* **592**: 52-86; discussion 123-133.

Kronenberg, F., L. J. Cote, et al. (1984). "Menopausal hot flashes: thermoregulatory, cardiovascular, and circulating catecholamine and LH changes." *Maturitas* **6**(1): 31-43.

Kupferer, E. M., S. L. Dormire, et al. (2009). "Complementary and alternative medicine use for vasomotor symptoms among women who have discontinued hormone therapy." *J Obstet Gynecol Neonatal Nurs* **38**(1): 50-59.

Kurzer, M. S. (2008). "Soy consumption for reduction of menopausal symptoms." *Inflammopharmacology* **16**(5): 227-229.

Lacey, J. V., Jr., P. J. Mink, et al. (2002). "Menopausal hormone replacement therapy and risk of ovarian cancer." *Jama* **288**(3): 334-341.

Lethaby, A. E., J. Brown, et al. (2007). "Phytoestrogens for vasomotor menopausal symptoms." *Cochrane Database Syst Rev*(4): CD001395.

Lobo, R. A., W. McCormick, et al. (1984). "Depo-medroxyprogesterone acetate compared with conjugated estrogens for the treatment of postmenopausal women." *Obstet Gynecol* **63**(1): 1-5.

Loprinzi, C. L., D. L. Barton, et al. (2009). "Newer antidepressants for hot flashes--should their efficacy still be up for debate?" *Menopause* **16**(1): 184-187.

Loprinzi, C. L., J. W. Kugler, et al. (2000). "Venlafaxine in management of hot flashes in survivors of breast cancer: a randomised controlled trial." *Lancet* **356**(9247): 2059-2063.

Loprinzi, C. L., R. Levitt, et al. (2006). "Phase III comparison of depomedroxyprogesterone acetate to venlafaxine for managing hot flashes: North Central Cancer Treatment Group Trial N99C7." *J Clin Oncol* **24**(9): 1409-1414.

Loprinzi, C. L., T. M. Pisansky, et al. (1998). "Pilot evaluation of venlafaxine hydrochloride for the therapy of hot flashes in cancer survivors." *J Clin Oncol* **16**(7): 2377-2381.

Loprinzi, C. L., J. Sloan, et al. (2009). "Newer Antidepressants and Gabapentin for Hot Flashes: An Individual Patient Pooled Analysis." *J Clin Oncol* **30**: 30.

Loprinzi, C. L., J. A. Sloan, et al. (2002). "Phase III evaluation of fluoxetine for treatment of hot flashes." *J Clin Oncol* **20**(6): 1578-1583.

Loprinzi, C. L., V. Stearns, et al. (2005). "Centrally active nonhormonal hot flash therapies." *Am J Med* **118 Suppl 12B**: 118-123.

Maki, P. M., L. H. Rubin, et al. (2009). "Effects of botanicals and combined hormone therapy on cognition in postmenopausal women." *Menopause* **8**: 8.

Marks, D. M., M. H. Park, et al. (2008). "Paroxetine: safety and tolerability issues." *Expert Opin Drug Saf* **7**(6): 783-794.

McEwen, B. S. and S. E. Alves (1999). "Estrogen actions in the central nervous system." *Endocr Rev* **20**(3): 279-307.

McKinlay, S. M. and M. Jefferys (1974). "The menopausal syndrome." *Br J Prev Soc Med* **28**(2): 108-115.

Miller, H. G. and R. M. Li (2004). "Measuring hot flashes: summary of a National Institutes of Health workshop." *Mayo Clin Proc* **79**(6): 777-781.

Nelson, H. D. (2008). "Menopause." *Lancet* **371**(9614): 760-770.

Notelovitz, M., J. P. Lenihan, et al. (2000). "Initial 17beta-estradiol dose for treating vasomotor symptoms." *Obstet Gynecol* **95**(5): 726-731.

Pandya, K. J., G. R. Morrow, et al. (2005). "Gabapentin for hot flashes in 420 women with breast cancer: a randomised double-blind placebo-controlled trial." *Lancet* **366**(9488): 818-824.

Pinkerton, J. V., D. W. Stovall, et al. (2009). "Advances in the treatment of menopausal symptoms." *Womens Health (Lond Engl)* **5**(4): 361-842; quiz 383-364.

Politi, M. C., M. D. Schleinitz, et al. (2008). "Revisiting the duration of vasomotor symptoms of menopause: a meta-analysis." *J Gen Intern Med* **23**(9): 1507-1513.

Przewlocka-Kosmala, M. (2002). "[Arterial hypertension in perimenopausal women]." *Pol Merkur Lekarski* **12**(72): 535-538.

Rabin, D. S., N. Cipparrone, et al. (1999). "Why menopausal women do not want to take hormone replacement therapy." *Menopause* **6**(1): 61-67.

Reddy, S. Y., H. Warner, et al. (2006). "Gabapentin, estrogen, and placebo for treating hot flushes: a randomized controlled trial." *Obstet Gynecol* **108**(1): 41-48.

Rintamaki, H. (2007). "Human responses to cold." *Alaska Med* **49**(2 Suppl): 29-31.

Rodstrom, K., C. Bengtsson, et al. (2002). "A longitudinal study of the treatment of hot flushes: the population study of women in Gothenburg during a quarter of a century." *Menopause* **9**(3): 156-161.

Rossouw, J. E., G. L. Anderson, et al. (2002). "Risks and benefits of estrogen plus progestin in healthy postmenopausal women: principal results From the Women's Health Initiative randomized controlled trial." *Jama* **288**(3): 321-333.

Rybaczyk, L. A., M. J. Bashaw, et al. (2005). "An overlooked connection: serotonergic mediation of estrogen-related physiology and pathology." *BMC Womens Health* **5**: 12.

Santoro, N. (2008). "Symptoms of menopause: hot flushes." *Clin Obstet Gynecol* **51**(3): 539-548.

Sexton, T., J. Younus, et al. (2007). "Oxybutynin for refractory hot flashes in cancer patients." *Menopause* **14**(3 Pt 1): 505-509.

Shanafelt, T. D., D. L. Barton, et al. (2002). "Pathophysiology and treatment of hot flashes." *Mayo Clin Proc* **77**(11): 1207-1218.

Stearns, V., K. L. Beebe, et al. (2003). "Paroxetine controlled release in the treatment of menopausal hot flashes: a randomized controlled trial." *Jama* **289**(21): 2827-2834.

Stearns, V. and D. F. Hayes (2002). "Approach to menopausal symptoms in women with breast cancer." *Curr Treat Options Oncol* **3**(2): 179-190.

Stearns, V., C. Isaacs, et al. (2000). "A pilot trial assessing the efficacy of paroxetine hydrochloride (Paxil) in controlling hot flashes in breast cancer survivors." *Ann Oncol* **11**(1): 17-22.

Suvanto-Luukkonen, E., R. Koivunen, et al. (2005). "Citalopram and fluoxetine in the treatment of postmenopausal symptoms: a prospective, randomized, 9-month, placebo-controlled, double-blind study." *Menopause* **12**(1): 18-26.

Thornhill, J. A. and A. Wilfong (1982). "Lateral cerebral ventricle and preoptic-anterior hypothalamic area infusion and perfusion of beta-endorphin and ACTH to unrestrained rats: core and surface temperature responses." *Can J Physiol Pharmacol* **60**(10): 1267-1274.

Thurston, R. C., J. T. Bromberger, et al. (2008). "Beyond frequency: who is most bothered by vasomotor symptoms?" *Menopause* **15**(5): 841-847.

Umland, E. M. (2008). "Treatment strategies for reducing the burden of menopause-associated vasomotor symptoms." *J Manag Care Pharm* **14**(3 Suppl): 14-19.

Utian, W. H. (2005). "Psychosocial and socioeconomic burden of vasomotor symptoms in menopause: a comprehensive review." *Health Qual Life Outcomes* **3**: 47.

Utian, W. H., D. F. Archer, et al. (2008). "Estrogen and progestogen use in postmenopausal women: July 2008 position statement of The North American Menopause Society." *Menopause* **15**(4 Pt 1): 584-602.

Warren, M. P. (2008). "Is megestrol acetate a suitable option for treatment of hot flashes in women with breast cancer?" *Nat Clin Pract Endocrinol Metab* **4**(12): 650-651.

Welty, F. K. (2003). "Alternative hormone replacement regimens: is there a need for further clinical trials?" *Curr Opin Lipidol* **14**(6): 585-591.

Welty, F. K., K. S. Lee, et al. (2007). "The association between soy nut consumption and decreased menopausal symptoms." *J Womens Health (Larchmt)* **16**(3): 361-369.

Zhao, G., L. Wang, et al. (2000). "Menopausal symptoms: experience of Chinese women." *Climacteric* **3**(2): 135-144.

Zhou, B., Q. Sun, et al. (2008). "Hormone replacement therapy and ovarian cancer risk: a meta-analysis." *Gynecol Oncol* **108**(3): 641-651.

Zhou, J., F. Qu, et al. (2009). "Acupuncture and Auricular Acupressure in Relieving Menopausal Hot Flashes of Bilaterally Ovariectomized Chinese Women: A Randomized Controlled Trial." *Evid Based Complement Alternat Med* **2**: 2.

In: Menopause: Vasomotor Symptoms, Systematic...   ISBN: 978-1-60876-930-8
Editors: J. Michalski, I. Nowak, pp. 111-123   © 2010 Nova Science Publishers, Inc.

Chapter IV

Follicle Stimulating Hormone and Estradiol Levels during Perimenopause in a Cohort of Japanese Women: The Radiation Effects Research Foundation Adult Health Study

Michiko Yamada[*]

Department of Clinical Studies, Radiation Effects Research Foundation,
Hiroshima, Japan.

Abstract

Background: Among Caucasian populations, it is reported that changes in hormone levels (decreased E2 and increased FSH) occur within one to two years on each side of the final menstrual period, and that variations of hormone levels between individuals are large.

Objective: To investigate the levels of the two important hormones, FSH and E2, during perimenopause in a Japanese cohort.

Method: The Adult Health Study (AHS) is a longitudinal population-based study. Non-menopausal women, aged 47-54 years, were measured in terms of FSH and E2 levels every six months. For 89 women whose FSH and E2 levels were measured within three months from their final menstrual period (FMP), the trends of FSH and E2 within 21 months of FMP were investigated at six-month intervals. For 17 women whose hormone levels were measured for a period of more than 50 months, the individual trends of FSH and E2 were observed.

---

[*] Corresponding author: Department of Clinical Studies, Radiation Effects Research Foundation, 5-2 Hijiyama Park, Minami-ku, Hiroshima 732–0815, Japan, Telephone: +81-82-261-3131, Fax: +81-82-263-7279, e-mail: yamada@rerf.or.jp

Results: The FSH and E2 levels within three months of FMP exhibited a wide range. Although FSH increased and E2 decreased during perimenopause, FSH and E2 levels at individual time points were found to not be a reliable marker of biological menopause, since the trends for the combination of FSH and E2 displayed such wide variations longitudinally. Temporal fluctuations in a single individual exhibited various patterns, and the trends of the hormone levels were not uni-directional during perimenopause, displaying remarkably increased E2 levels in some case. Longitudinal hormone changes within 21 months of FMP in this study are compatible with previous studies in which the length of perimenopausal transition was estimated to be approximately four years.

Conclusions: Among Japanese women who had natural menopause around the age of 50, hormone levels in and between individuals exhibited a wide variation throughout perimenopause, with a convergence of the biochemical menopausal pattern characterized by high FSH and low E2 by approximately two years after the FMP.

Keywords: estradiol, follicle stimulating hormone, perimenopause, final menstrual period

Introduction

It is well known that menopause carries a significant risk for heart disease and osteoporosis[1] and that vasomotor symptoms affect most women during the menopausal transition.[2] These are caused by endocrine changes which occur during the perimenopause. Cross-sectional studies have reported that major changes, characterized by significant increase of serum follicle stimulating hormone (FSH) and significant decrease of estradiol (E2), occur in the pituitary-gonadal axis in relation to the menopausal transition and the menopause.[3-5] However, cross-sectional studies also suggest that laboratory test results, including those of FSH and E2, do not reliably distinguish among women in the reproductive, menopause transition, and postmenopause, because there was considerable overlap of the hormone level ranges among women in different reproductive stages.[5, 6]

The cycle-by-cycle hormonal variability of individual woman can be observed by prospective observation. Observations of continuing menstrual cycles among a limited number of perimenopausal women showed marked fluctuation of individual hormone levels. [7-9] Additional information on changes in FSH and E2 during perimenopause has been obtained from longitudinal studies using relatively large samples. Mean FSH started to increase from aproximately 5 years before the final menstrual period (FMP) and followed a marked increase in a period of two years before to one year after the FMP.[10,11] The mean E2 started to decrease from approximately 2 years before the FMP.[12] It is concluded that substantial changes in reproductive hormone levels occur within one to two years on each side of the FMP,[12,13] and that the length of the perimenopausal transition is estimated to be nearly four years.[14]

Both cross-sectional and longitudinal studies have been conducted in Caucasian populations. The Study of Women's Health Across the Nation (SWAN) reported the effects of ethnicity and age on the menopausal transition.[15, 16] Although Japanese women living in the U.S. had lower E2 but similar FSH levels compared with Caucasian women,[15] the longitudinal changes in FSH and E2 during perimenopause among Japanese living in Japan remained unknown.

The Radiation Effects Research Foundation (RERF)'s Adult Health Study (AHS) is examining the potential effect of prior atomic-bomb radiation exposure in atomic-bomb survivors. The observation of serum FSH and E2 during perimenopause is important for an understanding of factors that influence the baseline parameters related to various diseases. The aim of this study was to observe the levels of the two important perimenopausal hormone, serum FSH and E2, among Japanese living in Japan in relation to FMP.

Materials and Methods

The study subjects were part of the AHS, which is described elsewhere.[17] In the AHS, biennial health examinations (comprising medical history, physical examination, and laboratory tests) have been conducted since 1958. In December 1993, 212 women (47-54 years old) who had menstruated within the preceding 12 months, who had not undergone hysterectomy or oophorectomy, and who were not undergoing hormone therapy were selected for the study. The study was approved by the RERF institutional ethics committee (the Human Investigation Committee), and written informed consent was obtained from the subjects. Serum FSH and E2 levels were measured by radioimmunoassay at SRL, Inc., Tokyo, at six-month intervals from December 1993 to October 2003. Blood samples were drawn in the morning between the second and fourth days of the menstrual cycle in subjects having regular menstrual cycles, or after a six-month interval for the others. Quality control for the reproducibility and consistency of the hormone assays was conducted on a regular basis. The lower detection limit of E2 was 10 pg/ml. At each examination, women were asked to make a calendar record of menstrual bleeding. Based on the calendar, the menstrual period that preceded 12 months of continued amenorrhea was designated the FMP. Nineteen women who had surgery or took exogenous hormones during the study period were excluded. Among the residual 193 subjects, FSH and E2 levels were measured within three months on each side of the FMP in 89 subjects. Scatter plot of FSH and E2 was shown in Figure 1. Using a t-test, we analyzed whether FSH or E2 levels within three months of the FMP differed for subjects on the bases of their age, weight, body mass index (weight/height^2), smoking, drinking, and three- months amenorrhea before testing. For those 89 subjects, all samples obtained within 21 months on each side of the FMP were grouped in six-month intervals (21 to 16 months before FMP, 15 to 10 months before FMP, nine to four months before FMP, within three months of FMP, four to nine months after FMP, 10 to 15 months after FMP, and 16 to 21 months after FMP). The FSH and E2 levels at the quartiles and the distribution of the combination of the individual FHS and E2 levels, using 30 mIU/ml of FSH and 20 pg/ml of E2 as the cutoff points, were calculated. For 17 women whose hormone levels were measured every six months for a period of more than 50 months, the individual trends of FSH and E2 were observed.

Fourteen volunteer women, in their twenties and having regular menstrual cycles, served as young controls. Among those young controls, blood samples were drawn in the morning between at the 6th - 8th days, 13th - 15th days, and 20th -22nd days of same cycle.

Results

Figure 1 shows the FSH and E2 levels of the 89 selected subjects with measurements performed within three months of FMP. The characteristics of the subjects are shown in Table 1. Age at FMP ranged from 48 to 55 years. The range of FSH within three months of FMP was 2 to 170 mIU/ml and that of E2 was < 10 to 385 pg/ml. Neither FSH nor E2 levels differed by age, weight, BMI, smoking, or alcohol consumption. (data not shown) Although the FSH levels appear to be lower and the E2 levels higher among subjects not having three months of amenorrhea, there is no significant statistical difference. The minimal, maximal and quartiles levels of FSH and E2, and the distribution of a combination of the individual FHS and E2 levels, are shown in Table 2. The median FSH level within three months of FMP was 57 mIU/ml and the median E2 was 17.4 pg/ml. Within three months of FMP, a pattern of low FSH (< 30 mIU/ml) and high E2 (≥ 20 pg/ml), high FSH and high E2, or high FSH and low E2 were found in 21.1%, 24.4%, and 54.4% of subjects, respectively. FSH at each quartile increased gradually until four to nine months after FMP, and then leveled off. Although the E2 of the lowest quartile and the second lowest quartile decreased gradually, the E2 of the highest quartile was highest within three months of FMP, and then dropped markedly at four to nine months after FMP. The maximal E2 level was greater than 200 pg/ml until 10 to 15 months after FMP, which was a remarkably higher E2 level than observed in young controls, as shown in Table 3. The fraction of subjects with low FSH and high E2, which is a biochemical pattern of a pre-menopausal condition, decreased gradually, and the fraction of subjects with high FSH and low E2, which is biochemically a post-menopausal condition, increased gradually during perimenopause. Approximately 30% of the subjects 21 to 16 months before FMP, and over 70% of subjects four months and later after FMP, exhibited a high FSH and low E2. For 62 of 89 subjects who provided both of the measurements at four to nine months before and after FMP, Figure 2 shows the distribution of FSH and E2 in three time categories. The fraction of subjects with low FSH and high E2 decreased and the fraction of subjects with high FSH and low E2 increased, at four to nine months after FMP. The distribution of individualized FSH and E2 levels within three months of FMP was not predictable by the distribution of hormone levels in the categories of before and after. For 17 women whose hormone levels were measured every six months for a period of more than 50 months, observed individual trends of FSH and E2 were not uni-directional and had a wide variation. (Figure 3)

Table 1. Characteristics of 89 selected subjects within three months of the final menstrual period.

Age	mean	51.4
	S.D.	1.9
Weight	mean	55.2
	S.D.	8.0
Body mass index (kg/m^2)	mean	23.1
	S.D.	3.1
Tobacco smoking	%	11.2
Alcohol	%	31.5

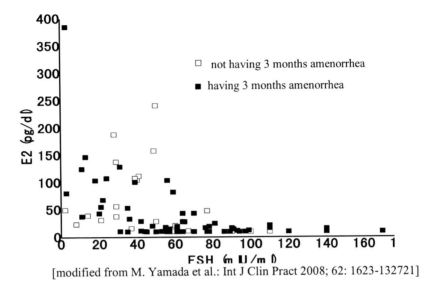

[modified from M. Yamada et al.: Int J Clin Pract 2008; 62: 1623-132721]

Figure 1. Follicle stimulating hormone and estradiol within three months (from) of final menstrual period

Discussion

Although a recent multi-ethnic study in the U.S. (SWAN) showed that Chinese and Japanese women had lower E2 but similar FSH levels compared to Caucasian women across the early phase of menopausal transition, no longitudinal hormone study has previously been conducted on Japanese women living in Japan. To observe serum FSH and E2 levels among Japanese living in Japan in relation to FMP, frequent hormone measurements among a relatively large number of subjects were required, since FMP was determined retrospectively after 12 months of amenorrhea. We measured FSH and E2 every six months in 212 pre- or perimenopausal women aged 47-54 years at baseline. There were shorter measurement intervals in this study than SWAN [15] or the Melbourne Women's Midlife Health Project , [12] where reproductive hormones were measured annually. That enabled the observation of hormone levels near FMP and the identification of precise trends during perimenopause among 89 women. It was possible to observe not only trends of a single hormone, but also trends of the combination of FSH and E2.

Table 2. FSH and E2 min, max, each quartile, and combination of FSH and E2 by six-month time categories relative to FMP

	No.	FSH					E2					FSH and W2 combination (%)			
		min.	max.	quarter	median	Three-quarter	min.	max.	quarter	median	Three-quarter	a	b	c	d
before FMP															
21 to 16 months	54	4.5	100	13	32	48	<10	641	15.2	32.7	88.7	40.7	5.6	24.1	29.6
15 to 10 months	61	7.3	140	31	44	73	<10	474	11.6	24.4	58.6	23.0	1.3	32.8	42.6
9 to 4 months	71	4.2	140	29	50	79	<10	207	<10	20.3	60.2	23.9	4.2	26.8	45.1
Within 3 months	89	2.2	170	35	57	94	<10	385	<10	17.4	105	21.1	0	24.4	54.4
after FMP															
4 to 9 months	75	8.3	190	51.5	80	95.5	<10	235	<10	11.3	16.4	6.7	1.3	16.0	76.0
10 to 15 months	67	7.5	140	43	73	95	<10	271	<10	11.4	20.3	7.5	3.0	19.4	70.1
16 to 21 months	42	35	150	60	71.5	94	<10	66.2	<10	<10	15.5	0	0	14.3	85.7

FSH: follicle stimulating hormone

E2: estradiol

FMP: final menstrual period

a: FSH < 30 mIU/ml and E2 ≥20pg/ml

b: FSH < 30 mIU/ml and E2 < 20pg/m

c: FSH ≥ 30 mIU/ml and E2 ≥ 20pg/ml

d: FSH ≥ 30 mIU/ml and E2 < 20pg/ml

[modified from M. Yamada et al.: Int J Clin Pract 2008; 62: 1623-1327[21]]

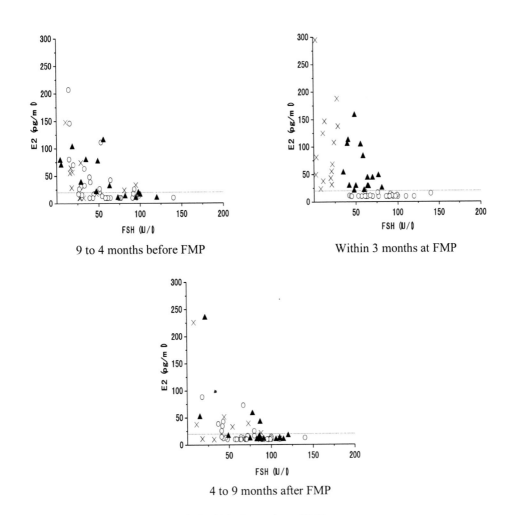

9 to 4 months before FMP

Within 3 months at FMP

4 to 9 months after FMP

×: FSH < 30 mIU/ml and E2 ≥20pg/ml within 3 months at FMP
▲: FSH ≥ 30 mIU/ml and E2 ≥ 20pg/ml within 3 months at FMP
○: FSH ≥ 30 mIU/ml and E2 < 20pg/ml within 3 months at FMP

Figure 2. Trends of the combination of the FSH and E2 levels before and after the final menstrual period (FMP)

Our study subjects, compared with the subjects in previous Caucasian studies, were characterized by a relatively older age at baseline, lower weight and BMI, and less of a proportion of smokers. Women in the AHS displayed low rates of hormone therapy (<5%) and study subjects were not undergoing hormone therapy. Although Chinese and Japanese women had lower E2 concentrations compared with Caucasian women in the cross-sectional[16] and the longitudinal the SWAN study,[15] we can not compare the hormone levels directly with previous results due to the difference in the methods employed.

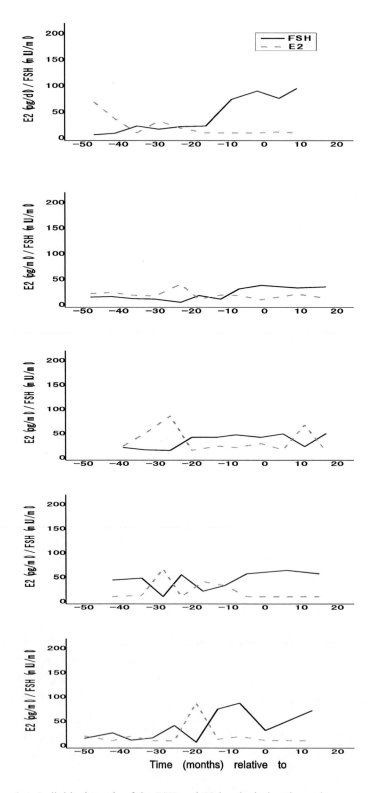

Figure 3-1. Individual trends of the FSH and E2 levels during the perimenopause

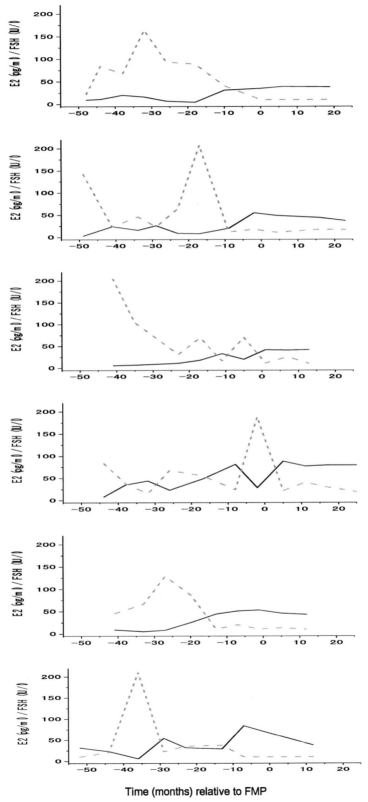

Time (months) relative to FMP

Figure 3-2. Individual trends of the FSH and E2 levels during the perimenopause

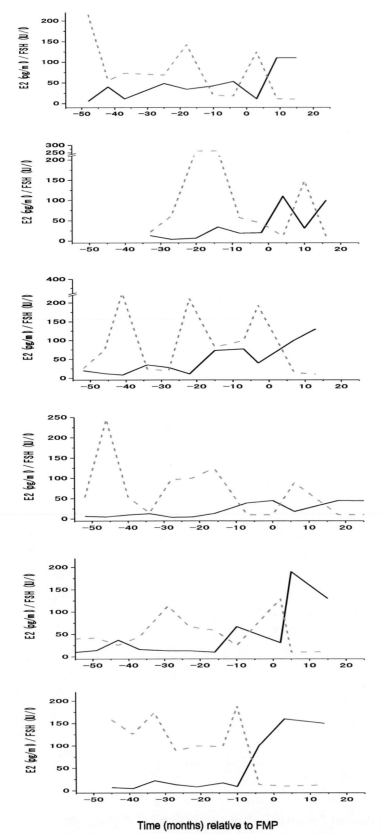

Time (months) relative to FMP

Figure 3-3. Individual trends of the FSH and E2 levels during the perimenopause

Table 3. FSH and E2 levels among young controls on three different menstrual days

Days in menstrual cycle		FSH	E2
6th - 8th day	mean	7.2	49.0
	S.D.	1.8	24.5
	min.	4.1	23.9
	max.	10	96.1
13th – 15th day	mean	5.7	103.4
	S.D.	1.5	78.0
	min.	3.2	32.2
	max.	8.2	318
20th – 22nd day	mean	4.5	148.3
	S.D.	3.2	48.8
	min.	2.2	81.4
	max.	8.9	253

FSH: follicle stimulating hormone
E2: estradiol

The wide-range of the distributions of FSH and E2 in the proximity of FMP in this study was compatible with previous reports.[3, 8, 12, 15, 18, 19] Increased FSH and decreased E2 with large variations in temporal patterns of the hormone level between and in individuals during perimenopause were observed in Japanese women, as was the case in Caucasian women. [3, 8, 12, 15, 18, 19] Some subjects showed a biochemically post-menopausal pattern (high FSH and low E2) at 21 to 16 months before FMP. Some subjects showed relatively high E2 at 10 months and longer after FMP. Evidence of a sporadically higher E2 level in which increased estrogen levels rose to exceed normal cycle concentrations by 2- or 3-fold,[20] and a relative preservation of E2 during perimenopause, [4, 9] were confirmed in this study. Longitudinal hormone changes within 21 months of FMP in this study are compatible with the results from the Melbourne study [12] and from the Massachusetts study, [14] in which the length of perimenopausal transition was estimated to be approximately four years.

Since temporal fluctuations in a single individual were broad and hormone level trends were not uni-directional in this study, neither FSH nor E2 was a reliable hormone marker of menopause by itself for individual women, as previously reported.[19] Six month measurement intervals during the approximate 10 years in this study allow us to demonstrate various patterns of temporal fluctuations, including remarkably increased E2 levels in some cases.

It is concluded that the longitudinal hormone measurements among Japanese women who had natural menopause around the age of 50 have a similar duration of perimenopause as well as similar trends of FSH and E2 levels as reported for Caucasian women. Although information regarding subjects who undergo menopause at younger ages is still required, the results of this study suggest applicability to other Japanese populations.

Acknowledgments

I wish to acknowledge the contributions of Dr. Midori Soda of the Radiation Effects Research Foundation, Nagasaki, Japan. The Radiation Effects Research Foundation, Hiroshima and Nagasaki, Japan, is a private nonprofit foundation funded by the Japanese Ministry of Health, Labour and Welfare (MHLW) and the U.S. Department of Energy (DOE), the latter in part through the National Academy of Sciences. This publication was based on RERF Research Protocol RP #5-93.

References

[1] Greendale, GA; Lee, NP; Arriola, ER. The menopause. *Lancet.*, 1999, 353, 571-80.
[2] Gold, EB; Colvin, A; Avis, N; et al. Longitudinal analysis of the association between vasomotor symptoms and race/ethnicity across the menopausal transition: study of women's health across the nation. *Am J Public Health.*, 2006, 96, 1226-35.
[3] Burger, HG; Dudley, EC; Hopper, JL; et al. The endocrinology of the menopausal transition: a cross-sectional study of a population-based sample. *J Clin Endocrinol Metab.*, 1995, 80, 3537-45.
[4] Prior, JC. Perimenopause: the complex endocrinology of the menopausal transition. *Endocr Rev.*, 1998, 19, 397-428.
[5] Henrich, JB; Hughes, JP; Kaufman, SC; Brody, DJ; Curtin, LR. Limitations of follicle-stimulating hormone in assessing menopause status: findings from the National Health and Nutrition Examination Survey (NHANES 1999-2000)*. *Menopause.*, 2006, 13, 171-7.
[6] Bastian, LA; Smith, CM; Nanda, K. Is this woman perimenopausal? *JAMA.*, 2003, 289, 895-902.
[7] Hee, J; MacNaughton, J; Bangah, M; Burger, HG. Perimenopausal patterns of gonadotrophins, immunoreactive inhibin, oestradiol and progesterone. *Maturitas.*, 1993, 18, 9-20.
[8] Metcalf, MG; Donald, RA. Fluctuating ovarian function in a perimenopausal women. *N Z Med J.*, 1979, 89, 45-7.
[9] Santoro, N; Brown, JR; Adel, T; Skurnick, JH. Characterization of reproductive hormonal dynamics in the perimenopause. *J Clin Endocrinol Metab.*, 1996, 81, 1495-501.
[10] Rannevik, G; Jeppsson, S; Johnell, O; Bjerre, B; Laurell-Borulf, Y; Svanberg, L. A longitudinal study of the perimenopausal transition: altered profiles of steroid and pituitary hormones, SHBG and bone mineral density. *Maturitas.*, 1995, 21, 103-13.
[11] Sowers, MR; Zheng, H; McConnell, D; Nan, B; Harlow, S; Randolph, JF; Jr. Follicle stimulating hormone and its rate of change in defining menopause transition stages. *J Clin Endocrinol Metab.*, 2008, 93, 3958-64.
[12] Burger, HG; Dudley, EC; Hopper, JL; et al. Prospectively measured levels of serum follicle-stimulating hormone, estradiol, and the dimeric inhibins during the menopausal

transition in a population-based cohort of women. *J Clin Endocrinol Metab.*, 1999, 84, 4025-30.

[13] Longcope, C; Franz, C; Morello, C; Baker, R; Johnston, CC. Jr. Steroid and gonadotropin levels in women during the peri-menopausal years. *Maturitas.*, 1986, 8, 189-96.

[14] McKinlay, SM; Brambilla, DJ; Posner, JG. The normal menopause transition. *Maturitas.*, 1992, 14, 103-15.

[15] Randolph, JF; Jr.; Sowers, M; Bondarenko, IV; Harlow, SD; Luborsky, JL; Little, RJ. Change in estradiol and follicle-stimulating hormone across the early menopausal transition: effects of ethnicity and age. *J Clin Endocrinol Metab.*, 2004, 89, 1555-61.

[16] Santoro, N; Lasley, B; McConnell, D; et al. Body size and ethnicity are associated with menstrual cycle alterations in women in the early menopausal transition: The Study of Women's Health across the Nation (SWAN) Daily Hormone Study. *J Clin Endocrinol Metab.*, 2004, 89:2622-31.

[17] Yamada, M; Wong, FL; Fujiwara, S; Akahoshi, M; Suzuki, G. Noncancer disease incidence in atomic bomb survivors, 1958-1998. *Radiat Res.*, 2004, 161, 622-32.

[18] Metcalf, MG; Donald, RA; Livesey, JH. Pituitary-ovarian function in normal women during the menopausal transition. *Clin Endocrinol (Oxf).*, 1981, 14, 245-55.

[19] Burger, HG; Dudley, EC; Robertson, DM; Dennerstein L. Hormonal changes in the menopause transition. *Recent Prog Horm Res.*, 2002, 57, 257-75.

[20] Shideler, SE; DeVane, GW; Kalra, PS; Benirschke, K; Lasley, BL. Ovarian-pituitary hormone interactions during the perimenopause. *Maturitas.*, 1989, 11, 331-9.

[21] Yamada, M; Soda, M; Fujiwara, S. Follicle-stimulating hormone and oestradiol levels during perimenopause in a cohort of Japanese women. *Int J Clin Pract.*, 2008, 62, 1623-7.

In: Menopause: Vasomotor Symptoms, Systematic…
Editors: J. Michalski, I. Nowak, pp. 125-131
ISBN: 978-1-60876-930-8
© 2010 Nova Science Publishers, Inc.

Chapter V

Thyrotropin Levels during the Perimenopause: The Radiation Effects Research Foundation Adult Health Study

Michiko Yamada [*], *Misa Imaizumi and Waka Ohishi*

Department of Clinical Studies, Radiation Effects Research Foundation,
Hiroshima, Japan

Abstract

Objective: Climacteric symptoms resemble those of thyroid dysfunction, raising the possibility of changes in thyrotropin (TSH) during the perimenopause. The objective of the study was to investigate TSH levels in association with reproductive hormone.

Methods: Non-menopausal women of the Adult Health Study of the Radiation Effects Research Foundation, aged 47-54 years, were followed between 1993 and 2003 for changes in reproductive hormonal levels during the perimenopause. The TSH levels of 35 perimenopausal women whose frozen sera had been preserved after the measurements of follicle stimulating hormone (FSH), and estradiol (E2), were measured in 2008.

Results: Although FSH increased and E2 decreased, there was no uniform pattern in individual trend of TSH. Two cases developed hyperthyroidism during the perimenopause without specific onset of symptoms or reproductive hormone changes.

[*] Corresponding author: Department of Clinical Studies, Radiation Effects Research Foundation 5-2 Hijiyama Park, Minami-ku, Hiroshima 732–0815, Japan, Telephone: +81-82-261-3131, Fax: +81-82-263-7279, e-mail: yamada@rerf.or.jp

Conclusions: Although there was no association between TSH and reproductive hormone found, it is suggested that caution is required in diagnosing thyroid dysfunction during the perimenopause.

Keywords: thyrotropin; thyroid dysfunction; follicle stimulating hormone; estradiol; menopause; longitudinal study

Introduction

The relationship between reproductive function and thyroid hormone activity has attracted considerable attention. There are reports of climacteric syndrome and thyroid dysfunction. Since climacteric symptoms, such as hot flashes, resemble those attributed to thyroid dysfunction, women with climacteric syndrome may include patients with thyroid dysfunction.[1] Overlie [2] reported that high levels of thyrotropin (TSH) during menopause were related to vasomotor complaints. Custro[3] reported transient mild hyperthyroidism cases with inappropriate TSH secretion in those afflicted with vasomotor symptoms. The increased TSH level among women with estrogen replacement therapy,[4] along with the increased serum inhibin B levels in postmenopausal women with thyroid dysfunction,[5] suggests a relationship between reproductive and thyroid function.

The major changes during the perimenopause are reported to be increased follicle stimulating hormone (FSH) and decreased estradiol (E2),[6] while the trend of these hormones in a given individual commonly exhibits large fluctuations.[7] Changes in TSH in association with reproductive function during perimenopause have been reported in recent years,[8, 9] but there is no data on Japanese living in Japan.

The Adult Health Study (AHS) of the Radiation Effects Research Foundation (RERF) is being conducted for the purpose of examining the potential effects of prior atomic-bomb exposure in atomic-bomb survivors.[10, 11] FSH and E2 levels were measured at six-month intervals among the perimenopausal women in this cohort between 1993 and 2003 to understand hormone changes during the perimenopause. The previous study reported that FSH increased and E2 decreased during the perimenopause, exhibiting wide variations longitudinally.[12] To investigate the changes in TSH in association with reproductive function, we examined the TSH level among 35 perimenopausal women whose frozen sera had been preserved at -80°C after the measurements of FSH and E2.

Materials and Methods

The study subjects took part in the AHS, in which biennial health examinations of atomic-bomb survivors have been conducted since 1958, the details of which are provided elsewhere.[11] In the AHS, in December 1993, 212 women (47-54 years old) who had menstruated within the preceding 12 months, who had not undergone hysterectomy or oophorectomy, and who were not undergoing hormone therapy, were selected for the study. The study was approved by the RERF institutional ethics committee (the Human Investigation Committee), and written informed consent was obtained from all subjects.

Serum FSH and E2 levels were measured by radioimmunoassay at SRL, Inc., Tokyo, at six-month intervals from December 1993 to October 2003. At each examination, women were asked to record menstrual bleeding on a calendar and symptoms and medication on a questionnaire. The final menstrual period (FMP) was designated by 12 months of continued amenorrhea. A detailed description of the study methods is available elsewhere.[12] In 2008, using the frozen serum samples preserved at -80˚C after the measurement of FSH and E2, the TSH levels for 35 women without either a history of thyroid disease or a history of treatment for thyroid disease before the menopause transition were measured at RERF by immunometric techniques based on chemiluminescence (Fujirebio Inc, Tokyo, Japan). In total, 141 frozen serum samples were measured for the TSH level (average, 4.0 per woman). The antithyroid peroxidase antibody (TPOAb) level in the early sample of each individual was measured by enzyme-linked immunosorbent assay (Medical & Biological Laboratories Co Ltd, Nagoya, Japan). We defined hyperthyroidism as TSH levels $<0.4\mu$IU/ml, and hypothyroidism as TSH levels $>5\mu$IU/ml. Women with hyperthyroidism were further investigated with free thyroxine (T4) (reference range: 0.71-1.52 ng/dl) and TSH receptor antibody.

Results

For 35 subjects, 93 samples (average, 2.7 per woman) obtained within a period of 21 months on each side of the FMP were grouped in six-month intervals (21 to 16 months before FMP, 15 to 10 months before FMP, nine to four months before FMP, within three months of FMP, four to nine months after FMP, 10 to 15 months after FMP, and 16 to 21 months after FMP). The median, minimal, and maximal levels of FSH, E2, and TSH in the six-month intervals are shown in Table 1. Although FSH in a single individual increased and E2 decreased with wide fluctuations, as in our previous report,[12] there is no uniform pattern in the individual trends of TSH (data not shown). Those results did not change after excluding five subjects with positive TPOAb (10 IU/ml or more). Among 35 women, 26 women (74%) complained of hot flashes, 8 women (23%) had more than 3kg weight loss, and 9 women (26%) had more than 3kg weight gain during the perimenopause.

Two hyperthyroidism cases were detected during the study period. The trends of the FSH, E2, and TSH levels for the two cases are shown in Figure 1. In case 1, TSH levels until 30 months before FMP were in the normal range, while TSH at 2 months after FMP was 0.01μIU/ml. The free-T4 in frozen serum at 2 months after FMP was 0.91 ng/dl and TSH receptor antibody was negative at this point. Hot flashes started nearly 30 months and weight loss started near 10 months before FMP. Although this patient was detected to have hyperthyroidism (free-T4: 1.76 ng/dl, TSH: 0.003μIU/ml) at 26 months after FMP at an AHS examination in 2002, reproductive hormones were not measured in 2002 and she did not receive any medication for thyroid disease, or climacteric syndrome, up until TSH was measured using the frozen sera in 2008. In case 2, TSH levels until 16 months before FMP were in the normal range. That case had complaints of body-weight loss, fatigue, and mood disturbance from 5 months after FMP, but no hot flash. The TSH level at 16 months after FMP was $<0.003\mu$IU/ml and the free T4 level was 1.45ng/dl. TSH receptor antibody was negative at this point. That case consulted an endocrinologist complaining of the above mentioned symptoms at 16 months after FMP and the TSH returned to the normal range after 9 months of medication.

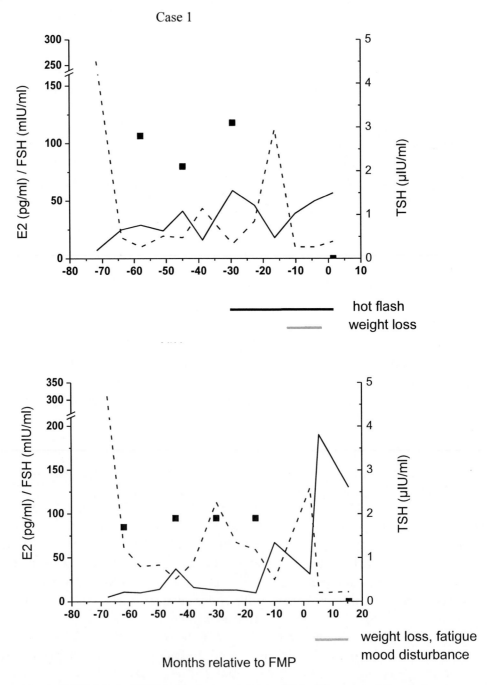

Figure 1. Trend of FSH, E2, and TSH for the two cases who exhibited hyperthyroidism during the perimenopause. The solid line displays FSH levels. The dotted line displays E2 levels. The points display TSH levels. FSH: follicle stimulating hormone E2: estradiol TSH: thyrotropin

Table 1. FSH, E2 and TSH levels by six-month time intervals relative to FMP

Time of measurement		before FMP			within	after FMP		
		21 to 16 M	15 to 10 M	9 to 4 M	-3 to 3 M	4 to 9 M	10 to 15 M	16 to 21 M
Number of subjects		17	19	12	17	12	11	5
FSH (mIU/ml)	median	26	33	58	47	65.5	85	80.5
	minimal	6.6	4	8.3	6	38	23	38
	maximal	69	96	120	160	110	140	89
E2 (pg/ml)	median	55.4	33.7	19.4	17.3	13	<10	10.9
	minimal	<10	<10	<10	<10	<10	<10	<10
	maximal	260	262	226	396	73.2	148	24.4
TSH (μIU/ml)	median	2.1	1.8	1.6	1.7	1.6	1.6	1.6
	minimal	1.1	0.9	0.7	1.0	0.9	0.7	0.7
	maximal	3.9	2.8	2.6	4.3	3.6	3.7	2.5

FSH: follicle stimulating hormone
E2: estradiol
TSH: thyrotropin
FMP: final menstrual period

Discussion

In this study, TSH did not exhibit an association with FSH or E2 during the perimenopause, as in previous studies.[8, 9] No uniform pattern in the individual trends of TSH in this study is also consistent with the reports that the prevalence of hyperthyroidism or hypothyroidism is basically stable near the menopause transition.[13, 14]

Despite the overall constancy of TSH, two cases of hyperthyroidism among 35 women were detected during the perimenopause. The pathogenesis of hyperthyroidism in this study differs from mild hyperthyroidism, which exhibits transient inappropriately-high TSH, as reported by Custro [3]. Regarding the association between TSH and climacteric symptoms, no association with self-reported hot flash and/or mood disturbance was found by Sowers et al.[9] Although most climacteric symptoms are reportedly less frequent in Japanese and Chinese than Caucasians in the Study of Women's Health Across the Nation (SWAN),[15] approximately three fourths of women in our study complained of hot flashes at some points during the perimenopause. Weight change, which is a common sign of thyroid dysfunction,[16] was observed in half of the subjects. The symptoms identified in our study are not indicators of thyroid dysfunction as the SWAN.[9] The limited previous studies reported no association between TSH and reproductive hormone based on the baseline cross-sectional data, not longitudinal data.[8,9] The two hyperthyroidism cases in this study exhibited in postmenopause with normal TSH during the menopausal transition, so TSH measurement at a single point could not have afforded the detection of hyperthyroidism. It is therefore suggested that caution is required in diagnosing thyroid dysfunction during the perimenopause.

Acknowledgments

The Radiation Effects Research Foundation (RERF), Hiroshima and Nagasaki, Japan, is a private, non-profit foundation funded by the Japanese Ministry of Health, Labour and Welfare (MHLW) and the U.S. Department of Energy (DOE), the latter in part through the National Academy of Sciences. This publication was supported by RERF Research Protocol RP #5-93 and in part by a grant from the Japan Arteriosclerosis Prevention Fund.

References

[1]   Badawy, A; State O; Sherief, S. Can thyroid dysfunction explicate severe menopausal symptoms? *J Obstet Gynaecol.*, 2007, 27, 503-5.

[2]   Overlie, I; Moen, MH; Holte, A; Finset, A. Androgens and estrogens in relation to hot flushes during the menopausal transition. *Maturitas.*, 2002, 41, 69-77.

[3]   Custro, N; Scafidi, V. Transient mild hyperthyroidism with inappropriate TSH secretion in postmenopause. Follow-up of 4 cases. *Minerva Endocrinol.*, 1988, 13, 111-4.

[4]   Abech, DD; Moratelli, HB; Leite, SC; Oliveira, MC. Effects of estrogen replacement therapy on pituitary size, prolactin and thyroid-stimulating hormone concentrations in menopausal women. *Gynecol Endocrinol.*, 2005, 21, 223-6.

[5]   Viceconti, N; Luisi, S; Nardo, S; et al. Increased serum inhibin B levels in postmenopausal women with altered thyroid function. *Horm Metab Res.*, 2003, 35, 498-501.

[6]   Randolph, JF; Jr; Sowers, M; Bondarenko, IV; Harlow, SD; Luborsky, JL; Little, RJ. Change in estradiol and follicle-stimulating hormone across the early menopausal transition: effects of ethnicity and age. *J Clin Endocrinol Metab.*, 2004, 89, 1555-61.

[7]   Santoro, N; Brown, JR; Adel, T; Skurnick, JH. Characterization of reproductive hormonal dynamics in the perimenopause. *J Clin Endocrinol Metab.*, 1996, 81, 1495-501.

[8]   Rojas, LV; Nieves, K; Suarez, E; Ortiz, AP; Rivera, A; Romaguera, J. Thyroid-stimulating hormone and follicle-stimulating hormone status in Hispanic women during the menopause transition. *Ethn Dis.*, 2008, 18, S2-230-4.

[9]   Sowers, M; Luborsky, J; Perdue, C; Araujo, KL; Goldman, MB; Harlow, SD. Thyroid stimulating hormone (TSH) concentrations and menopausal status in women at the mid-life: SWAN. *Clin Endocrinol (Oxf).*, 2003, 58, 340-7.

[10] Imaizumi, M; Usa, T; Tominaga, T; et al. Radiation dose-response relationships for thyroid nodules and autoimmune thyroid diseases in Hiroshima and Nagasaki atomic bomb survivors 55-58 years after radiation exposure. *Jama.*, 2006, 295, 1011-22.

[11] Yamada, M; Wong, FL; Fujiwara, S; Akahoshi, M; Suzuki, G. Noncancer disease incidence in atomic bomb survivors, 1958-1998. *Radiat Res.*, 2004, 161, 622-32.

[12] Yamada, M; Soda, M; Fujiwara, S. Follicle-stimulating hormone and oestradiol levels during perimenopause in a cohort of Japanese women. *Int J Clin Pract.*, 2008, 62, 1623-7.

[13] Steinmetz, J; Spyckerelle, Y; De Talance, N; et al. Factors of variation and reference values for TSH in 45-70 year old women. *Ann Endocrinol (Paris).*, 2000, 61, 501-7.

[14] Surks, MI; Hollowell, JG. Age-specific distribution of serum thyrotropin and antithyroid antibodies in the US population: implications for the prevalence of subclinical hypothyroidism. *J Clin Endocrinol Metab.*, 2007, 92, 4575-82.

[15] Gold, EB; Sternfeld, B; Kelsey, JL; et al. Relation of demographic and lifestyle factors to symptoms in a multi-racial/ethnic population of women 40-55 years of age. *Am J Epidemiol.*, 2000, 152, 463-73.

[16] Knudsen, N; Laurberg, P; Rasmussen, LB; et al. Small differences in thyroid function may be important for body mass index and the occurrence of obesity in the population. *J Clin Endocrinol Metab.*, 2005, 90, 4019-24.

In: Menopause: Vasomotor Symptoms, Systematic…   ISBN: 978-1-60876-930-8
Editors: J. Michalski, I. Nowak, pp. 133-164   © 2010 Nova Science Publishers, Inc.

Chapter VI

Menopause and Cancer*

Jennifer M. Blake†

Department of Obstetrics and Gynecology, University of Toronto, Toronto, Canada

Abstract

Objectives: To address the many symptoms of menopause experienced by women as a result of treatment for their cancer.

Discussion: There is a relationship of premature ovarian failure with atherosclerosis and osteoporosis. Options for treating vasomotor symptoms may include environmental factors, physical activity, paced respiration, herbal and botanical, phytoestrogens, non-hormonal and hormonal therapy. Management of sleep disturbances will be reviewed. Risk factors for a depressed mood and management including conventional modalities and estrogen will be discussed. Vulvo-vaginal symptoms, joint pain and stiffness and sexuality concerns will be reviewed.

Conclusion: With increasing numbers of cancer patients living longer, quality of survivorship becomes an important issue. Menopausal symptoms are important for women and treatment options need to be made available.

Introduction

Menopause poses unique challenges for women with cancer, some may have experienced premature ovarian failure and an early menopause as a result of their cancer or its treatment,

---

* A version of this chapter was also published in *Women and Cancer*, edited by Laurie Elit, published by Nova Science Publishers, Inc. It was submitted for appropriate modifications in an effort to encourage wider dissemination of research.
† Correspondence concerning this article should be addressed to Jennifer Blake MD MSc FRCSC, Email: Jennifer.Blake@sunnybrook.ca.

for others, with natural menopause, symptom relief that is available to other women, is not an option for them. The symptoms of menopause are not unique, and can be confused with cancer or it's treatment. This chapter will address these issues, to assist women with cancer through the menopausal transition.

Definitions

The accepted definition of menopause is 12 months of amenorrhea, in the absence of any attributable cause [1]. Many women with cancer experience ovarian failure before the age of 40, or experience an early menopause, occurring before the age of 45.

Premature Ovarian Failure

Premature ovarian failure (POF) is common amongst women of reproductive age treated for cancer. As diagnostic methods enable earlier diagnosis, and treatment permits longer survival, the number of women surviving with cancer is increasing. Estimates are that 62% of adult patients and 77% of children survive greater than 5 years post treatment [2]. Age is the most important individual risk factor; in older patients the onset of ovarian failure is more rapid, within 2-4 months, compared to 6- 16 months in younger patients, and it is much less likely to be reversible, it is permanent in 90% of women compared to approximately 50% of younger women [5]. In women with breast cancer treated, adjuvant chemotherapy with CMF (Cytoxan, Methotrexate and 5-fluorourqacil) is associated with menopause in 40% of those less than 40 years, and 70% of women over 40 years [3]. The incidence of menopause varied by type of disease and therapy. In women with lymphoma, the incidences of POF is as high as 90% of women two years post treatment for Non Hodgkin's Lymphoma and 50% in those with Hodgkin's Lymphoma [4].

Ionizing radiation can also induce menopause. With exposure to radiation, both the amount of radiation, and the age of the patient are critical. The LD 50 of the human oocyte has been estimated to be < 2 Gy [6]. The young ovary has a larger pool of oocytes, and is more tolerant of radiation; a predictive model has been developed for the immediate cessation of ovarian function from ovarian radiation. The effective sterilizing dose (ESD: dose of fractionated radiotherapy [Gy] at which premature ovarian failure occurs immediately after treatment in 97.5% of patients) has been calculated; ESD at birth is 20.3 Gy; at 10 years 18.4 Gy, at 20 years 16.5 Gy, and at 30 years 14.3 Gy. The time to ovarian failure after lesser doses of radiation has also been modeled. Young women exposed to radiation can expect an earlier cessation of ovarian function, and the same trend to increasing sensitivity with age is seen [7].

In gynecologic cancer, bilateral oopherectomy may be necessary, with surgical menopause an inevitable consequence. In women with simple hysterectomy, the age of menopause has been reported to be younger, occurring at a mean age of 49.5 years (p<0.001) [8] Women with hysterectomy and ovarian conservation report more severe menopausal symptoms than women with spontaneous menopause [9]. Women post-hysterectomy with ovarian conservation appear to be at higher risk of ovarian failure [10].

The ovarian histology in therapy induced ovarian failure has the same appearance as in natural menopause with depletion of primordial follicles. FSH levels are elevated, and estradiol levels low to low-normal. Unlike physiologic menopause, there is the potential with POF of spontaneous ovulation, many years after the onset of amenorrhea. The likelihood of spontaneous ovulation is greater in younger patients, but in all cases is unpredictable, and can occur even where ovarian biopsy indicates depletion of follicles [11,12].

Clinical Impact of Premature Ovarian Failure

Women undergoing an abrupt and premature menopausal transition experience increased severity of menopausal symptoms [13,14,15] and have specific health risks in consequence of early onset menopause. In young women experiencing surgical menopause there is the immediate issue of loss of fertility, with the added stress of severe menopausal symptoms and loss of libido.

Loss of fertility will have a profound impact on health and quality of life. It is more likely to have an adverse impact in women who have reproductive regret or in cultures that place a high value on fertility. Fertility options such as ovum donation or surrogacy may be helpful.

Bilateral oopherectomy results in an abrupt fall of estradiol to menopausal levels, without the gradual decline that characterizes natural menopause. Androgen levels in surgical oopherectomy are particularly low, only 37% of the levels in naturally menopausal women [16,17]. Testosterone levels gradually decline from mid reproductive life, with the post-menopausal ovary producing more testosterone than the pre-menopausal ovary. The abrupt and profound loss of testosterone in surgical or induced menopause results in significant symptoms, including profound loss of libido, and is particularly distressing in younger women. Young women are far more likely to be distressed by low libido or sexual function score. In a study of American women aged 20-65, 25% reported marked distress about their sexuality; younger women were more troubled than their older counterparts by a lack of sexual interest, p=0.01 [18].

Crandall found menopausal symptoms to be more severe in breast cancer patients who experience a menopausal transition during treatment [19]. A persistent increase in hot flash severity was noted. Adjustment for tamoxifen use did not alter the symptoms reported. Concerns about menopausal symptoms emerge once the focus on active treatment has passed. A qualitative study of 27 women post-chemotherapy for breast cancer [20] documented the progression of concerns. Initially concerns with cancer and its treatment overshadow any concerns about menopause, but as women move beyond that phase to survivorship, the reality of menopause and its difficulties emerged. Concerns were related both to typical symptoms, but also to the equating of menopause with premature aging, an interpretation that was felt irrespective of age. Women further felt that their oncologists tended to dismiss their concerns. Menopause appears to be a particularly laden term to describe the induced ovarian failure experienced by young women. Symptom management will be discussed later in this chapter.

Early onset of menopause impacts adversely on overall health. In an epidemiologic study of nearly 38,000 Norwegian women with natural menopause, the age of menopause was found to be inversely related to mortality, with increased mortality for every year of earlier onset [21]. Women with premature menopause are also at risk for degenerative diseases, notably osteoporosis and atherosclerosis.

Premature Ovarian Failure and Atherosclerosis

Premature atherosclerosis has long been suspected by the increased risk in postmenopausal women, and the ten-year apparent gap between the onset of CHD in women when compared to men. The Framingham study provided early evidence that women who were post menopausal had a higher risk for heart disease than did age matched pre-menopausal women, although there was no increase in metabolic risk factors [22]. In the Nurses' Health Study, there was no increase in risk in age matched women who had undergone natural menopause, but in women who had undergone bilateral oopherectomy and who had never taken estrogens after menopause they saw an increased risk of CHD (RR=2.2, 95% CI 1.2-4.2) [23]. In a population study of Dutch women, each year of advancement of menopausal; age was associated with a 2% increase in cardiovascular mortality [24]. Hormone replacement in younger menopausal women may reduce this resk. A recent meta-analysis of randomized trials of hormone therapy concluded that for women younger than 60 years of age there was a total reduction in cardiac events, odds ratio of 0.68 (95% CI 0.48-0.96)[25].

There is explanatory evidence that atherosclerosis is accelerated from the time of menopause, with changes noted over time from the onset of menopause in the intima media thickness of the coronary vessels [26] and evidence of an increase in carotid atherosclerosis [27]. The various lines of research evidence that point to early benefit and later harm associated with hormone therapy have been the subject of a recent review [28].

Premature Ovarian Failure and Osteoporosis

Osteoporosis and decreased bone density are also described in women with premature menopause, but appear as a particular risk factor for women with chemotherapy induced ovarian failure in cancer [29,30,31,32]. There are multiple reasons for this. There is a well known effect of hypo-estrogenism on bone metabolism, with rapid loss of bone density following menopause, and an increase in bone density with decreased risk of fracture associated with hormone replacement. For women with cancer, there are additional risk factors. There is an impact from chemotherapeutic drugs, and especially steroid use. Prolonged bed rest is a known risk factor for bone density loss, and will affect many women who have had a prolonged illness or treatment. Women who are fatigued and feeling unwell are less likely to be engaging in exercise, increasing risk of both bone loss and fracture. Adult survivors of pediatric cancer have been found to be at increased risk of osteopenia and osteoporosis, directly related to the number of courses of chemotherapy they received [33].

Finally, women with breast cancer appear to be at particular risk of osteoporosis [34,35]. In an longitudinal study, Kanis found the incidence of fracture over three years follow-up from diagnosis, to be increased nearly five fold in the cancer population. In women with soft tissue recurrence this increase rose to approximately 20 fold. When fracture risk was adjusted for age, duration of follow-up and prevalent fracture, the risk was 4.7 (95% CI, 2.3-9.9; P < 0.0001) in women newly diagnosed with breast cancer and 22.7 (95% CI, 9.1-57.1; P<0.0001) in the women with recurrent breast cancer [36].

Over and above the risks associated with chemotherapy agents and steroids, women with breast cancer frequently receive anti estrogen treatment in the form of selective estrogen receptor modulators, or aromatase inhibitors. Aromatase inhibitors have a direct adverse effect upon bone metabolism, but the clinical significance of this is not clear. In the ATAC study women treated with aromatase inhibitor had higher risk of osteoporosis and fracture than those treated with tamoxifen [37] with an incidence of 7.7 % in tamoxifen, vs 11% after 5 years, in women treated with anastrozole, translating into fracture rates per 1000 woman-years of 22·6 for anastrozole and 15·6 for tamoxifen (hazard ratio 1·44, 95% CI 1·21–1·68, p<0·0001). Fracture rates were not increased at the hip, although these were infrequent, and are more typically a fracture of the elderly. Vertebral fractures were increased (p<0.03).

Goss *et al* did not find an increase in fractures after 5 years of letrozole [38] Studies comparing aromatase inhibitors are clinically relevant, as tamoxifen has been the standard of hormonal therapy, but tamoxifen appears to reduce bone density in pre-menopausal women, but may be slightly beneficial in older post menopausal women [39].

Premature Ovarian Failure: Summary

Women with induced ovarian failure therapy experience loss of fertility, increased severity of menopausal symptoms, as well as specific health risks with respect to cardiovascular disease and osteoporosis. Women should be advised of their likelihood of ovarian failure, based on their age, risk factors and planned treatment, and the time-frame within which they may expect it. As there is an understandable focus on disease treatment, information about consequences may not be fully understood, but an openness to future discussions will have been established.

Loss of fertility will be particularly hard for women somen; consultation with infertility specialists to outline options in advance of treatment may be beneficial.

Baseline screening for risk factors for cardiac disease and osteoporosis, and testing including lipids and bone density testing establish a foundation for counseling and preventive care [40,41]. With survival increasing for women with cancer, and screening programmes enabling earlier diagnosis, preparation and planning for long-term survival are recommended. The American Society of Clinical Oncology noted, "Most women with newly diagnosed breast cancer are at risk of osteoporosis due to either their age or their breast cancer treatment. Oncology professionals, especially medical oncologists, need to take an expanded role in the routine and regular assessment of these women's bone health" [42]. In addition to appropriate dietary and exercise advice, there is a role for bis-phosphonates in prevention of osteoporosis in women at high risk of fracture.

Cardiovascular disease does appear to be accelerated in women with early menopause, for women in whom hormone therapy is not contraindicated, an early discussion with respect to the role of hormone therapy in premature ovarian failure is important, as women with this condition are likely to inappropriately apply the findings of the Women's Health Initiative study to their situation. Using the term premature ovarian failure may help to reduce confusion with physiologic menopause.

Menopausal Symptoms in Women with Cancer

Impact and Quality of Life in Cancer Survivors

Women with cancer and natural menopause may experience more severe symptoms and require specific considerations with respect to treatment. Symptoms of menopause are not generally specific to menopause, and may need to be distinguished from symptoms related to their disease or its treatment.

As commonplace as menopausal symptoms may be, their impact on quality of life can be easily underestimated. Daly *et al* assessed quality of life in a sample of menopausal women, using rating scales and utility values, where 0 is equivalent to death and 1.0 perfect health, found that menopausal women rated their quality of life with mild symptoms as .65, and with severe symptoms 0.3 [43]. These ratings confirm that women with symptoms do experience a substantial deterioration in quality of life, one that has lead to a search for safe and effective means of relief.

Schultz assessed menopausal symptoms in women who had a history of breast cancer and found that hot flashes, painful intercourse, inability to concentrate, fatigue, sleep disturbances and feeling unhappy impacted significantly on quality of life [44]. They found that numerous symptoms common in, but not specifically to menopause, were more severe in women who had undergone chemotherapy and radiotherapy as part of their treatment, including arthritis ($p<0.0007$), dizziness ($p<0.004$) and memory loss ($p<000003$), compared to women who had surgery alone.

Harris, in a case-control survey of 110 breast cancer survivors aged 16 to 69, found that menopausal symptoms were 5.3 times (95% CI 2.7-10.2) more common in breast cancer survivors than in the controls [45]. Gupta also found a very high prevalence of disruptive symptoms; 95% of two hundred women assessed reported symptoms, with significant impact on their quality of life. Severe hot flashes, night sweats and symptoms of vaginal dryness were particularly troublesome [46]. Older post-menopausal women on tamoxifen had somewhat less severe somatic symptoms, but no difference in vasomotor symptoms. Morales on the other hand, noted increase in the severity of vasomotor symptoms with both tamoxifen and with aromatase inhibitors ($p<0.0001$ and $p=0.014$) [47]. In this series of 184 patients, tamoxifen was also associated with decreased libido ($p< 0.0001$) , where aromatase inhibitors were associated with an increase in musculo-skeletal symptoms, and in vaginal dryness and dyspareunia ($p=0.0039$ and $p=0.001$).

Menopause Related Symptoms

Menopause is associated with a typical constellation of symptoms. Longitudinal community-based surveys in many countries all record increases in reports of disruptive symptoms, including hot flashes and sweats, depressed mood, sleep disturbances, sexual concerns or problems, cognitive symptoms, vaginal dryness, urinary incontinence, and somatic or bodily pain with menopause. The prevalence of specific symptoms varies somewhat between national and ethnic groups, but are universal phenomena. These observational studies have been well summarized in a recent review by Fugate-Woods [48].

Vasomotor Symptoms

The hot flash, or hot flush, is a subjective sensation of warmth, that maybe accompanied by other symptoms, including anxiety, irritability, sweating, palpitations, and panic. Hot flashes are the popular hallmark symptom of menopause, and are experienced by up to 80% of women, of whom 10-20% report severe symptoms [49]. In the general population the peak of symptoms occurs in the late menopausal transition, to the early postmenopausal years, but symptoms can persist for decades thereafter. Approximately 10% of women still complain of hot flushes into their seventies [50].

The hot flash can last from a few seconds, to several minutes (typically 3-5 minutes), but can last for hours [51]. Physiologic changes associated with the hot flash include blood flow increases to the skin, and there is an increase in skin temperature, sweating and skin conductance. A feeling of being chilled, and shivering may follow hot flashes [52]. Some women experience a sense of anxiety or apprehension with the hot flash.

The hot flash can be a nonspecific response to many physiologic challenges, but the menopausal hot flash, is only a part of the vaso-motor disturbance; women report as a difficulty maintaining a comfortable temperature, alternately feeling too hot, or shivering with cold. Increases in ambient temperature or exercise are able to provoke hot flashes. These symptoms are thought to be due to alteration in the CNS thermoregulatory set point located in the anterior portion of the hypothalamus. Freedman has observed that threshold between sweating and shivering (thermo neutral zone) is wider in asymptomatic menopausal women (0.4°) than in symptomatic and in women with severe symptoms is virtually absent, 0 ° [53]. Freedman has also documented the circadian rhythm that women report, demonstrating an increase frequency in hot flashes in the evening and night. Sweating is more commonly associated with nocturnal flashes, the reason for night sweats is not known.

Complementary and Alternative Management of Vasomotor Symptoms

Women with a history of cancer are likely to be interested in non-hormonal alternative treatments for vasomotor symptoms, Harris found breast cancer survivors were 25 (95% CI 8.3-100) times less likely to use estrogen, and 7.4 (95% CI 2.5-21.9) times more likely to use alternatives than non-affected women. Women with a history of breast cancer are seven times more likely to report the use of soy based phytoestrogens, vitamin E and herbal remedies [45,64].

The challenge becomes to find effective alternatives to offer. Assessment of effective therapies for hot flashes can only be made by placebo-controlled trials, as the placebo effect is considerable, and the natural spontaneous resolution of hot flashes is also substantial. A 58% reduction in hot flashes was noted for placebo in a recent Cochrane review [54], stressing the need for well-designed studies with sufficient power to accurately detect a treatment effect.

Much recent attention has been paid to environmental, lifestyle and behavioural techniques that can reduce the discomfort of hot flushes, and to herbal and botanical remedies.

Environmental factors Hot flashes can be provoked by high ambient temperature, leading to advice to dress in light clothing, and in layers. Moisture wicking material is commercially available in nightwear designed with cancer patients in mind [55]. The use a fan is also helpful, particularly for sleep, as is reducing room temperature.

Physical activity Women who are physically active tend to report fewer hot flashes, but exercise *per se* has not been found to be effective in reducing vasomotor symptoms [56], and in fact increased the frequency of hot flashes, presumable as a manifestation of the reduced thermo-neutral zone [52]. Women should be advised to exercise in moderation, and early in the day for maximum benefit to vasomotor symptoms. Women with cancer may be de-conditioned or less active with exercise because of fatigue, pain or complications of treatment. Maintaining some level of physical fitness may be helpful.

Paced respiration There is some evidence for the benefit of paced respiration [52,57,58,59]. Paced respiration reduced hot flashes by as much as 50%, and was more effective than relaxation therapy.

Herbal and botanical remedies have been the subject of popular interest and scientific study [60,61,62]. Six trials have found evidence for benefit of Black Cohosh; these studies have methodological flaws, but nonetheless have consistent results. There have been isolated case reports of hepatotoxicity with black cohosh [63]; a consideration of particular importance in women who may be receiving other medications with potential hepatotoxicity. Dong quai, vitamin E and Evening Primrose Oil have not been found to be effective [63]

The phytoestrogens Harris found greatly increased use of soy amongst breast cancer survivors, both for menopausal symptoms, and in hope of preventing recurrence [45]. The isoflavones (soy or red clover derived) have not proven to be as effective as might have been hoped; clinical outcomes have been modest, and studies have not shown consistent benefit [65,66]. In a recent meta-analysis by Nelson [67] a non-statistically significant benefit was noted for red clover siofalvones, of −0.44 hot flushes per day (95% CI, -1.47 to 0.58). A small benefit was noted for the soy isofalvones of − 0.97 after 6 weeks (95% CI, -1.82 to − 0.12). Findings were inconsistent, and drop out rates in some trials are quite substantial, due to bloating and gas. There is ongoing research and considerable individual variation in response to phyto-estrogens, so it is reasonable to give these alternatives a therapeutic trial [68].

Drug-Herb Interaction

The potential for drug-herb interactions is relevant. Recent reviews catalogue some of the potential interaction [69,70]. There are a number of herbal remedies that have potential interactions with warfarin, including several that are popular with menopausal women, including red clover, don quai, ginseng and vitamin, chamomile and green tea [69,70,71]. The potential for interaction with chemotherapeutic drugs is particularly important, as menopausal women use a variety of complementary and alternative remedies. Six of the top ten best-selling herbal preparations in the United States are frequently used by menopausal women, including ginseng, soy, black cohosh, St John's Wort and valerian [72]. Cancer patients are more likely than the general population to use complementary therapies. Most users do not inform their physicians of this. Because of the narrow therapeutic index of many chemotherapeutic agents, a subtle interaction may lead to a significant clinical effect. Many interactions are described in animal models, and their human impact remains potential. Thus women and their physicians need to be aware of these concerns.

Soy is commonly used by menopausal women, as a supplement, in the form of a phytoestrogenic extract, as well as a foodstuff. There is evidence of stimulation of breast tissue by phytoestrogens [73,74,75]. Moreover, there may be an interaction between phytoestrogens and the selective estrogen receptor modulator tamoxifen [76]. Safety data on the use of phytoestrogen supplements, in medicinal amounts, as opposed to their use as a dietary component, is needed. There is some basic science to suggest that some tumors may grow in response to Phytoestrogens [77]. Interactions *in vitro* have been observed that might impair the efficacy of adjuvant therapy [78,79]. Authors advise women to refrain from use of phytoestrogens, at least during active therapy. Prudence, and use of these compounds as a food rather than in pharmacologic doses should be advised.

Table 1. Top Selling Herbal Supplements in the United States

2002 Rank	Herb	Plant Name	Primary Clinical Indications	Retail Sales in 2002* ($US)	2001 Rank
1	Garlic	*Allium sativum*	Hypercholesterolemia	34,509,288	3
2	Ginkgo	*Ginkgo biloba*	Dementia, intermittent claudication	32,998,528	1
3	Echinacea	*Echinacea purpurea*†	Prevention of common cold	32,448,966	2
4	Soy	*Glycine max*	Menopausal symptoms	28,252,518	5
5	Saw palmetto	*Serenoa repens*	Benign prostate hyperplasia	23,053,036	6
6	Ginseng	*Panax ginseng*	Physical and mental fatigue	21,686,192	4
7	St. John's wort	*Hypericum perforatum*	Mild depression	14,969,575	7
8	Black cohosh	*Actaea racemosa*‡	Menopausal symptoms	12,333,188	10
9	Cranberry	*Vaccinium macrocarpon*	Urinary tract infection	11,857,782	9
10	Valerian	*Valeriana officinalis*	Insomnia, stress	8,120,329	8
11	Milk thistle	*Silybum marianum*	Alcoholic cirrhosis and hepatitis	7,762,350	12
12	Evening primrose	*Oenothera biennis*	Premenstrual syndrome	6,024,896	13
13	Kava	*Piper methysticum*	Anxiety	4,423,427	11
14	Bilberry	*Vaccinium myrtillus*	Diabetic retinopathy	3,381,351	15
15	Grape seed	*Vitis vinifera*	Allergic rhinitis	3,054,816	14

*Data obtained from Blumenthal[12].
†Other species include *E. angustifolia*, and *E. pallida*.
‡Formerly *Cimicifuga racemosa*.

Black Cohosh, one of the most frequently used preparations by menopausal women has no known drug interaction. A table listing herbal preparations with potential interaction is provided in Table 2.

Table 2. Specific Herbal Remedies to Avoid During Chemotherapy

Herb	Table 7. Specific Herbal Remedies to Discourage and Avoid During Chemotherapy Concurrent Chemotherapy/Condition (suspected effect)
Garlic	Avoid with decarbazine (CYP2E1 inhibition); caution with other concurrent chemotherapy (inconclusive data)
Ginkgo	Caution with camptothecins, cyclophosphamide, EGFR-TK inhibitors, epipodophyllotoxins, taxanes, and vinca alkaloids (CYP3A4 and CYP2C19 inhibition); discourage with alkylating agents, antitumor antibiotics, and platinum analogues (free-radical scavenging)
Echinacea	Avoid with camptothecins, cyclophosphamide, EGFR-TK inhibitors, epipodophyllotoxins, taxanes, and vinca alkaloids (CYP3A4 induction)
Soy	Avoid with tamoxifen (antagonism of tumor growth inhibition), and treatment of patients with estrogen-receptor positive breast cancer and endometrial cancer (stimulation of tumor growth)
Saw palmetto	No significant interactions expected
Ginseng	Caution with camptothecins, cyclophosphamide, EGFR-TK inhibitors, epipodophyllotoxins, taxanes, and Vinca alkaloids (CYP3A4 inhibition); discourage in patients with estrogen-receptor positive breast cancer and endometrial cancer (stimulation of tumor growth)
St. John's wort	Avoid with all concurrent chemotherapy (CYP2B6, CYP2C9, CYP2C19, CYP2E1, CYP3A4, and P-glycoprotein induction)
Black cohosh	No significant interactions expected
Cranberry	No significant interactions expected
Valerian	Caution with tamoxifen (CYP2C9 inhibition), cyclophosphamide, and teniposide (CYP2C19 inhibition), cyclophosphamide, and teniposide (CYP2C19 inhibition)
Milk thistle	No significant interactions expected
Evening primrose	No significant interactions expected, but caution with highly extracted drugs (serum-binding displacement)
Kava	Avoid in all patients with pre-existing liver disease, with evidence of hepatic injury (herb-induced hepatotoxicity), and/or in combination with hepatotoxic chemotherapy; caution with camptothecins, cyclophosphamide, EGFR-TK inhibitors, epipodophyllotoxins, taxanes, and vinca alkaloids (CYP3A4 induction)
Bilberry	No significant interactions expected
Grape seed	Caution with camptothecins, cyclophosphamide, EGFR-TK inhibitors, epipodophyllotoxins, taxanes, and vinca alkaloids (CYP3A4 induction), and with alkylating agents, antitumor antibiotics, and platinum analogues (free-radical scavenging)

Abbreviation: EGFR-TK, epidermal growth factor receptor tyrosine-kinase.

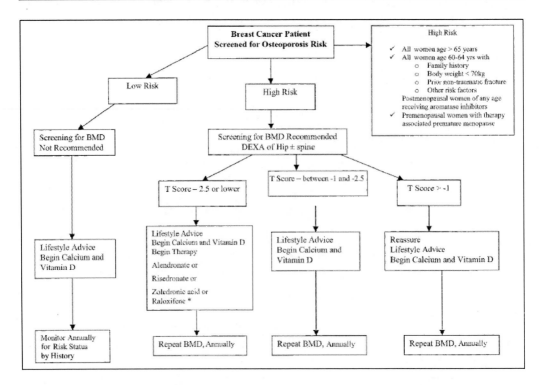

Figure 1. Recommended Management for patients diagnosed with Non metastatic Breast Cancer

Non-hormonal medical treatments

A variety of non-hormonal medical treatments have been evaluated, either for use in menopause, or more specifically, for use in women with a history of breast cancer [80,81]. Clonidine, a centrally acting α agonist, has been in use for the management of menopausal symptoms for many years [82]. Evidence for its use is derived from small trials with mixed result. It has been investigated in tamoxifen-induced hot flashes, where it showed a modest benefit, a 20 to 38% reduction with substantial placebo effect [83,84]. Sleeplessness, constipation drowsiness and dry mouth are common side effects. Goldberg noted that while statistically impressive, the results of a 20% reduction in symptoms were not clinically important, noting that patients did not prefer Clonidine over placebo because of adverse effects, and concluded that better means of relief were needed. In practice the clinical experience with Clonidine has not been particularly favourable. Freedman showed that Clonidine raised the sweating threshold in symptomatic, but not asymptomatic women [85]. This is consistent with the clinical observation that Clonidine seems particularly helpful to patients with the complaint of night sweats.

While Clonidine retains a place in the options available, Interest has turned to selective seratonin re-uptake inhibitors (SSRI's) paroxetine [86,87] and the seratonin and norepinephrine re-uptake inhibitors (SNRIS), Venlafaxine, both of which have RCT evidence of efficacy for VMS. Recent evidence that Paroxetine has the potential of reducing the levels of an active metabolite of tamoxifen [88,89] would favour the use of Venlafaxine, although there is no clinical data to suggest that this is clinically significant. Biglia used a lower dose of Venlafaxine, 37.5 mgm extended release formulation with good success. The benefit was gradual, with further improvement noted over eight weeks of treatment of up to a 59% improvement in the hot flush score (a composite of frequency and severity). Even with the low dose, 15% of women reported nausea and vomiting, though this subsided after the first week of treatment [90]. Other side effects include decreased appetite, decreased libido, dry mouth and constipation.

In Nelson's meta-analysis of SSRIs and SNRI's based on 6 trials, there was a significant reduction in hot flashes compared to placebo of −1.13 (95% CI −1.70 to -0.57) hot flashes/day [35]. When breast cancer patients who were treated with tamoxifen were considered separately, the reduction increased to −1.40 (95% CI -1.97 to −0.82). This may or may not be deemed clinically significant.

In a head to head trial with depo-medroxyprogesterone acetate (MPA), better control of symptoms with fewer side effects was achieved with MPA. However until the role of Progestin in breast caner is clarified, it is likely that a SNRI would be preferred over a Progestin [91].

There have been two trials of Gabapentin. The 300 mgm dose was not effective, while with 900 mgm day there was a significant reduction in hot flash frequency and severity by 67% [92,93]. Side effects include fatigue, dizziness, rash, palpitations, but overall drop outs on treatment were few. Reduction in pain was a positive side effect of treatment.

Hormone Therapy

For women able to use hormone therapy, it remains the single most effective modality for dealing with menopausal symptoms. Estrogen therapy has been used for hot flashes since the

1950's; its effectiveness has recently been reassessed and confirmed. The Cochrane review calculated a 75% reduction in hot flash frequency, and a significant decrease in symptom severity (OR 0.13, 95% CI 0.06-0.27).

All types of estrogen (conjugated oral estrogens, oral estradiol) and routes (oral vs. transdermal) have been found to be equally efficacious for relief of hot flashes [94] Transdermal estrogens are particularly appropriate for women who wish to avoid first pass- hepatic metabolism of estrogen, by smokers, and by women who prefer a transdermal to an oral route of administration. There is some evidence to suggest that they have a lesser impact on blood coagulability [95,96,97] and they appear to have a lesser impact on mammographic breast density [98].

After the publication of WHI there has been heightened interest in low dose hormone therapy. Lower doses for estrogen therapy to control hot flashes has been found to be less effective in reducing frequency and severity of hot flashes, but with fewer adverse effects than conventional doses. Recent reviews of data [99,100] have concluded that there is an approximately 65% reduction in hot flashes with low dose HT, against a 75-90% reduction with conventional, and a 35% reduction in placebo arms. The time to maximum effect is also much longer in lower dose therapy, taking 8-12 weeks for maximal effect, compared to four weeks with conventional doses.

Low dose HT has been found to be associated with fewer reported side effects, such as breast tenderness, and fewer adverse events, In the Nurse's Health Study long term use of Premarin 0.625mgm was associated with an increased risk of stroke (OR 1.35 95%CI 1.08-1.68). The risk was higher for higher doses of Premarin. This was not seen in women on low dose (0.3 mgm) of Premarin. Both groups had an equal reduction in cardiovascular disease risk [101]. There is, as yet, no evidence for increased safety with respect to breast cancer risk [102] Paganini- Hill recently reported on apparent benefit of low-dose, rather than moderate dose hormone therapy in a long-term follow-up of the Leisure World cohort.

Specific consideration: hormone replacement in women with cancer

There are two broad categories of women in whom consideration of hormones may arise, those with an early menopause induced by treatment, regardless of their symptomatology, and those with menopausal symptoms, regardless of their age at menopause [103]. Young women with induced menopause are at risk for premature atherosclerosis, osteoporosis, decreased libido and increased severity of menopausal symptoms. There is consensus that women with premature menopause, in the absence of contra-indication, should be offered physiologically appropriate hormone replacement. Controversy arises in management of women with a history of an estrogen dependent tumor. This has been the subject of several recent reviews, with authors expressing a range of opinion, from strongly advising against HT to others finding the evidence to be less compelling [104,105,106]. There have also been meta-analyses addressing this controversy [107,108].

In women with a history of early stage endometrial cancer, there is somewhat more consensus, as the cancer can be completely surgically removed, and epidemiological studies have consistently shown reduced, or no increased risk of recurrence [109,110,111,112]. There is an overall benefit in treated women. Unfortunately, there is no RCT data, and the trial that was underway was halted shortly after the release of the WHI findings. Thus, there is potential for selection bias to have affected the outcome. Since endometrial cancer is more common in older postmenopausal women in whom symptoms typically have abated, the question of use of hormones to manage symptoms is less likely to arise.

Breast cancer is often diagnosed in younger women, in whom the question of hormone therapy is more likely to arise. Since publication of WHI patients are themselves more likely to avoid the use of hormone therapy, and pursue alternative therapies [45]; however controversy remains. The concerns regarding use of hormone therapy is supported by the fact that, unlike endometrial cancer, breast cancer may not be completely surgically removed, with breast cancer patients having an ongoing risk of recurrence even twenty years or longer post diagnosis. As well, a reduced recurrence rate is seen in patients treated with tamoxifen or aromatase inhibitors. The studies of women treated with hormone therapy are less clear. The eight observational studies of women treated with hormone therapy include over 1200 breast cancer patients, and more than 2800 controls, and have shown a reduced recurrence risk with hormone therapy. In the meta-analysis by Col this RR was 0.64 (95% CI 0.50 –0.82) [107]. Treated women have tended to be younger and with less advanced disease, and the possibility of selection bias exists. There have been two randomized of hormone therapy, neither of which were completed, and which raise some further questions. The HABITS trial was halted prior to completion when an interim analysis found an increased risk of recurrence at 2.1 years; the RR was 3.3 (95% CI 1.5 -7.4)[113]. The Stockholm trial was halted shortly after HABITS, even though it had shown a reduced risk in women followed to 4.1 years (RH 0.82, 95% C! 0.35-1.9) [114]. Many fewer women in the HABITS trail used tamoxifen (21% vs. 52% in the Stockholm trial) The HABITS did not utilize a standard approach to hormone therapy, but randomized women to be treated according to local practice. An important difference between these two trials was the use of progestin. In the HABITS trail, the majority of women with an intact uterus were prescribed combined continuous HT. In the Stockholm trial the HT regimen was standardized, with a protocol designed to reduce exposure to progestin, and to administer it sequentially. Older women received a long cycle progestin, and all were prescribed a hormone free interval. Accumulating evidence on the increased risk of breast cancer associated with estrogen progestin, compared to estrogen alone is very consistent with the differences noted in these two trials [115], and is supported by our understanding of the biologic response of the breast vs. the endometrium to progestins. Progestins are classified on the basis of their ability to induce secretory change in estrogen primed (rabbit) endometrium, however the breast cells are known to be proliferating during the luteal phase. Apoptosis in breast tissue is maximal 48 hours after progestin withdrawal. Finally, progestational agents show differing profiles with respect to breast proliferation vs apoptosis in vitro, and clinical evidence will be helpful in providing clinical advice.

In the absence of unequivolcal evidence for safety, current practice is to avoid hormone therapy in women with a history of breast cancer. Individual consideration can be given to women whose symptoms are intractable, unresponsive to alternative approaches and impairing quality of life. In these cases, the lowest effective dose for the shortest time needed to manage symptoms is prudent. Currently there is no consensus that favours any particular hormone therapy regimen or progestational agent, however, it is an area of ongoing research, as clinicians seek to identify patients who would be at risk, and those who might benefit from the option of hormone therapy [116,117].

Sleep Disturbance

Sleep disturbances are a very common symptom in the menopausal transition, and are particularly common in survivors of cancer, in whom they are associated with a significantly decreased quality of life. Gupta found that 86% of women reported sleep disturbance, and 65% reported moderate to sever symptoms [46]. This contrasts with the SWAN study [118], which surveyed women in the community from early menopausal transition, through to post menopausal, and found sleep disturbance was reported by approximately 30%.

The most common complaints of menopausal women are of difficulty falling asleep, and of frequent awakenings, with difficulty falling back to sleep. The most symptomatic women were those with surgical menopause, 43.5% or those in the late transition, at 43.5%. In the early menopause 40.6% reported sleep disturbance. Hot flashes were strongly associated with sleep disturbance, as indicated by an OR 1.99 (95%CI 1.81–2.19). Physical activity was inversely associated with sleep disturbance, only 31.2% of active women, compared to 60.8% of the least active women reported symptoms [119].

Common sleep disturbances that increase with age include increased sleep latency, increased nocturnal awakening, and early awakening with difficulty returning to sleep. These disturbances are increased with poor health [120]. Although sleep disturbance is strongly associated with vasomotor flushes, insomnia can occur in the absence of any reported hot flushes, and may be the only menopausal complaint.

Sleep complaints cannot be assumed to be as a result of hot flashes, but deserve to be investigated for other factors. Potential contributors to sleep disruption are medical illness, such as hyperthyroidism or Cushing's, psychiatric illness, obstructive sleep apnea, medications or substances such as caffeine or alcohol, and restless leg syndrome. Behavioural and environmental factors include poor sleep hygiene, stress, disturbance by a spouse, and shift work. Poor sleep conditions include old mattresses, high ambient noise, light or temperature.

Management of sleep disturbances

Sleep disturbances are common, and are particularly common in cancer survivors, but should only be attributed to menopause after excluding other possible causes. Sleep hygiene and behavioural changes are the first strategy in managing sleep problems. While there has been some dispute as to the causative role of the hot flash in sleep disruption, there has been consistent evidence that hormone therapy does improve sleep quality

After ruling out other causes of sleep disruption, sleep hygiene and behavioural changes should be addressed. Education about normal changes in sleep, including the shift in circadian rhythm towards earlier awakening may be helpful in setting realistic expectations.

Basic sleep hygiene includes avoidance of heavy evening meals and stimulants, sleeping in a dark, quiet room, restricting the bedroom to sleep, relaxing activity or warm milk at bedtime. Behavioural therapy includes bedtime routines, relaxation therapy and cognitive behavioural therapy

Physical activity levels are associated with better sleep quality, and there is evidence that adopting a regular exercise habit may be beneficial. Both regular walking and stretching appear beneficial, but vigorous exercise should be avoided close to retiring, because of an increase in hot flashes associated with increases in core body temperature [121].

Hormone therapy has long been used for improvement of sleep at menopause, and the WHI has confirmed the beneficial effect [122] the improvement in sleep appears to be only partially associated with reduction in reported hot flashes [123,124]. Suggesting that estrogen may be acting through other neural means to improve sleep quality.

Depressed Mood

Feeling sad or blue is a commonly reported symptom of women in the menopausal transition; in population studies 19-29% of women report such feelings. There is little longitudinal follow-up data to track the resolution or persistence of these symptoms, but cross sectional studies indicate that reporting of sad feelings peaks in the transition, and is less frequent in older post menopausal women. Clinical depression is far less common affecting 4-6% of women [125,126,127]. Depression is not considered a normal part of menopause. In the SWAN study, depressive symptoms were far more common in women reporting sleep disturbance (39.7% of women with sleep problems, vs. 15.4% of those without) and a similar association was noted for vasomotor symptoms (36.6% vs. 18%) [128]. This study noted a peak of symptoms with 28.9% in the menopausal transition, vs. 22% in the post menopause, against a baseline of 20% pre-menopausal. Menopausal status (peri menopausal vs. post menopausal) was independently significantly associated with risk of psychological distress, independent of all co-variates, and race/ethnicity.

Risk factors for development of depression during the peri-menopausal period include a history of depressive disorders, poor physical heath and life stressors (lack of employment and social support), history of surgical menopause, and a long peri-menopausal transition [129]. Avis, in a longitudinal study of women in the state of Massachusetts, found no association between depressive symptoms and circulating estrogen levels. A definite association was found between the incidence of depression and reports of other menopausal symptoms, notably hot flushes and sleep disturbance [130]. This study supports the "domino" theory, which proposes that depression is a result of vasomotor symptoms leading to sleep disturbance, which in turn leads to irritability and depression. In the Melbourne study, negative mood was significantly predicted by a history of premenstrual complaints, negative attitudes towards menopause and aging, and low parity. Menopausal symptoms, poor self-health, negative feelings towards partner, smoking, stress and sedentary life style [131].

Management of mood symptoms

Women with predominantly mood complaints need to be carefully evaluated to rule out clinical depression, and managed accordingly. Conventional modalities for treatment of clinical depression, as in any other phase of life, include psychotherapy (cognitive behavioural therapy or interpersonal therapy), anti-depressant medication, and other therapies as indicated.

For women in whom there is no contra-indication, there may be a therapeutic role for estrogen therapy. The role of estrogen therapy in the management of mood disorders at menopause has been the subject of recent reviews [132,133,134]. Estrogen therapy has shown significant benefit for women with mild to moderate depressive symptoms in the late menopausal transition and early post menopause. A quantitative review of 26 studies examining the effect of hormones on mood using broad inclusion criteria and including non-placebo controls [132], found the overall mean effect size of hormone replacement therapy (HT) to improve mood was 0.68 (variance = 0.14, p< 0.00).

Hormone therapy appears of particular benefit to women in the transition or early post menopause. Women who were 5-10 years postmenopausal did not benefit from the administration of estrogen [135]. There is a placebo effect, and there may be an adverse impact on mood for women receiving MPA in addition to estrogen. Relief of depressive symptoms in peri-menopausal women treated with HT has been noted independent of a reduction in vasomotor symptoms, and benefits were observed in women with or without vasomotor symptoms, suggesting that the mechanism of action of estrogen is at multiple levels in the CNS [136]. Estradiol has also been found to be effective in treating peri-menopausal women meeting criteria for major depressive disorder [137].

Vulvo-vaginal Symptoms

Vulvo-vaginal symptoms are among the most commonly reported in menopausal women. Unlike vasomotor or mood symptoms, that spontaneously resolve, vaginal symptoms are progressive with prolonged hypo-estrogenism in menopause. Vulvo vagainl symptoms are more pronounced in women who are being treated with aromatase inhibitors, and in women who have had vaginal irradiation.

Vaginal dryness is reported by from 27% to 55% of healthy menopausal women [138], and dyspareunia from 32% to 41%. Women may complain of decreased sensitivity to touch, and decreased sensitivity has been objectively documented [139]. It is thought that only one fifth of women suffering from vulvo vaginal complaints will actually seek help from a physician [140], placing the onus on the physician to enquire into vaginal health. The detection and management changes associated with urogenital aging are the subject of recent reviews [141,142].

Estrogen is not the only contributor to the changes noted at menopause; aging in and of itself contributes to atrophy. Over time, the vagina undergoes shortening and narrowing, with loss of the vaginal fornices, and loses distensability. These progressive changes can culminate in a rigid and contracted vagina; the vaginal walls may become adherent with synechiae from chronic inflammation. In end stage atrophy, sexual intercourse becomes impossible. Women with irradiated vaginas or with surgical foreshortening and hypoestrogenism need to be monitored to avoid this complication.

Prevention

The risk of vaginal atrophy is higher in women who smoke, in women who are sexually inactive [143], and in women who have never had a vaginal birth [144]. Vaginal health is better maintained, in women with higher circulating levels of androgen, and in women who are more frequently sexually active [143].

Treatment of gynecologic cancer can affect vaginal health through reduction of vaginal length, surgical remodeling of the introitus, radiation changes to soft tissues and their blood supply, or surgical disruption of nerves or blood vessels. Early institution of vaginal estrogen, as a cream or ring, and teaching women to use dilators from an early stage in treatment is helpful.

If possible, regular sexual activity with intercourse will help to maintain vaginal health. In addition to the increased blood flow associated with sexual arousal, and the mechanical distension provided, the seminal fluid itself, rich in prostaglandins, sex steroids, and essential fatty acids, is postulated to benefit the vaginal epithelium [144].

Management of atrophic vaginitis

Atrophic vaginitis is most effectively treated with the use of exogenous estrogen, (particularly vaginal estrogen). For women in whom estrogen therapy is contra-indicated or not acceptable to all, symptomatic management can reduce the symptoms of dryness and irritation, or supply lubrications for vaginal intercourse.

Vaginal moisturizers, containing a non-hormonal moisturizing vaginal gel containing water, glycerin, mineral oil, polycarbophil, carbopol, hydrogenated palm oil glyceride and sorbic acid (Replens®) used three times a week has been found effective to relieve symptoms of atrophic vaginitis, by adhering to the vaginal epithelium and retaining moisture [145,146] but does not reverse atrophic changes. Water-soluble lubricants can improve comfort with intercourse.

Atrophic vaginitis can develop in women on low dose systemic therapy [147]. In these women, as well as women who have only vaginal symptoms, vaginal delivery systems of estrogen provide a low dose that effectively reverses atrophic change, and relieves symptoms [148].

A recent Cochrane review of sixteen studies, which involved a total of 2129 participants [149]. All formulations of local estrogen, cream, ring or low dose tablet, had efficacy in both relieving symptoms of dryness and pruritis or burning, as well as improving scores for vaginal moisture, vaginal elasticity, and fluid volume.

Vaginal estrogens in doses sufficient to relieve atrophic symptoms do not raise circulating levels of estrogen beyond post-menopausal levels making them available for women in whom estrogen replacement would be otherwise contra-indicated [150]. The comparative studies between the newer silicone impregnated rings or tablets and vaginal estrogen cream to employ higher doses of estrogen cream that are currently recommended, making comparison difficult. Low dose vaginal estrogen appears to have a safe endometrial profile [151,152,153,154].

In the Cochrane review no cases of endometrial cancer were reported, though rare cases of endometrial hyperplasia were noted with low dose vaginal estrogens. Johnston [155] has concluded that there is no evidence to support annual surveillance of women on low does of local vaginal therapy (estradiol 25 mcg tablet twice weekly, estradiol ring replaced q 3 monthly, or CEE 0.5 grams 3/week). Other authors have noted that there may still be a need for caution [156] as some women may exhibit a greater endometrial response than others. The reports are on a relatively small number of women. Thus it seems reasonable to individualize surveillance, taking into account endogenous estrogen production in heavier women, or increased absorption in women with a thin atrophic vaginal epithelium. In women in whom estrogens are contraindicated, using vaginal products strictly as prescribed is important. Part of the achievement of low circulating levels is believed to come from thickening of the vaginal epithelium, women who increase the interval between application of vaginal estrogen may theoretically increase their exposure. There are limited clinical studies looking at recurrence rates, but to date their appears to be no risk, or increased risk of breast cancer in women using vaginal estrogen [157].

Aches and Pain

One of the most troubling symptoms that women experience is of joint pain and stiffness, or generalized aches and pains; symptoms that make women 'feel old" and may hamper physical activity. Patients who have had chemotherapy appear to be at greatly increased risk of arthritis and joint pain; this common symptom is not specific to menopause [158].

Joint pain is among the most commonly reported symptoms of menopause, experienced by up to 67% of peri-menopausal women [159]. In the SWAN study the odds ratio of joint pain and stiffness in the menopausal transition was 1.48 (CI 1.35-1.62) and even higher in women who had undergone surgical menopause (OR 1.5, CI 1.33-1.69). Joint symptoms were the most commonly reported symptom in the Melbourne longitudinal study of the menopausal transition [160].

Management of joint pain and stiffness

Physical activity may help pain and stiffness, particularly exercise that promotes flexibility and stretching [161]. In the SWAN study, joint stiffness was much more common in women who reported little to no physical activity, compared to those reporting the highest level of activity, (73.1% vs. 46.8%). These were associations, and it is not possible to determine if increased pain and soreness contributed to being less physically active, or vice versa. In the Melbourne women associations between pain and lower mood, and higher BMI were noted, but the authors noted that it was not possible to tease out the relationship between these observations.

Menopausal hormone therapy appears to improve musculo-skeletal symptoms. In the WHI, women assigned to E+P were more likely than women assigned to placebo to report relief of joint pain and stiffness, and from generalized aches and pains (47.1 vs. 38.4%, OR 1.43, CI 1.24-1.64, p<0.01, and 49.3 vs. 43.7%, OR 1.25, CI 1.05-1.44, p=0.02 respectively). Women assigned to E+P were also less likely to develop new onset of joint pain (OR 0.68, CI 0.61-0.76, p<0.01), or general aches and pains (OR 0.73, CI 0.66-0.82, p<0.01).

There appears to be little known about how to mitigate these symptoms specifically in the cancer survivor.

Sexuality

Sexual concerns are among the most frequent in women attending menopause clinics [162] and the most common complaint amongst women in the menopausal transition is of decreased interest. Women with cancer, particularly cancers that have affected body image (the breast or genital tract) or who have undergone treatment that diminishes the blood supply or innervation of the genitals, or in whom estrogen therapy is contra indicated.

Changes in sexual function appear normal with age and menopause, and sexual concerns are very common. In the Melbourne study of women aged 45-55, the frequency of self-reported sexual dysfunction rose from 42% in the early menopausal transition, to 88% after 8 years, in the post-menopause. Sexual concerns included lowered interest, responsiveness, frequency, and change in feelings toward the partner. Vaginal dryness and discomfort increased with age.

Sexual function is affected by both age and estradiol levels. Dennerstien has conducted one of the few longitudinal studies of sexual function. The Melbourne Women's Midlife Health Project study involved a cohort of women aged 45-55 was followed for nine years [163]. In A decline in sexual function was noted with age, and duration of relationship, but an additional negative impact was associated with menopause, and the declining levels of estradiol (not androgens). The changes that women experience in their sexual function can impact their self-identity, their relationships, and their sense of connectedness to a highly sexualized society.

A decrease in sexual function that is not distressing to the woman is not classified as a dysfunction. In a study of American women aged 20-65, 25% reported marked distress about their sexuality, with younger women being more troubled than older women by a lack of sexual interest, p=0.01 [163].It is important that clinicians obtain a sexual history, and determine what the impact is to the patient. In the WISHes study, hypoactive sexual desire disorder was accompanied by significant psychological, emotional and interpersonal distress, lower sexual and partner satisfaction, and decreased general health status, both mental and physical health [165].Basson notes that mental well being, health and feelings towards one's partner are the most important predictors of sexual function, with biological factors modulating the response. She further notes that in women with distressing loss of sexual function in menopause, both menopausal interest and response tend to be suppressed [166]. Lack of interest is experienced as an absence of sexual thoughts and fantasies, little attraction to others, and rare initiation of any sexual activity.

Management

Anticipation of changes in sexuality, and letting women know help is available should issues arise is very helpful. Women with body image concerns after cancer surgery or treatment may require counseling to re-discover their sexual identity. Relationship issues and past sexual concerns need to be addressed. Fatigue may be a particular concern for women who have undergone treatment for cancer. Improved physical conditioning, achieved by an exercise program and healthy diet may ameliorate some of the fatigue. Behavioural changes in patterns of sexual activity, to avoid times when fatigue may be more pronounced, may be effective.

Vaginal estrogen and moisturizers can improve sexual satisfaction, and lubricants can assist with dryness. Androgen replacement has been shown to be effective for women who have undergone surgical menopause, however, these trials have not included women with breast cancer. The potential for testosterone being metabolized to estrogen is an unresolved concern.

Conclusion

With increasing numbers of cancer survivors, and earlier diagnosis, unprecedented number of women are going through menopause with a history of cancer. Menopause poses unique challenges to these women and to their health care providers. There are specific considerations for younger women, related both to the implications of a premature "menopause", with loss of fertility, psychosexual impact, and significant health risks for cardiovascular disease and osteoporosis. Women going through the menopausal transition in association with cancer treatment, particularly women who are treated with radiation or chemotherapy in addition to surgery, appear to be at increased risk of severe menopausal symptoms. The more severe symptoms are particularly difficult to manage in women in whom hormone therapy is contraindicate, but a variety of non-hormonal options do offer some relief. The role of hormone therapy in women with a history of an estrogen sensitive breast cancer remains controversial. Hormones are only offered for the most severely symptomatic women if other approaches have failed.

References

[1]   World Health Organization Research on the Menopause in the 1990s. *Technical report.*, 866, Geneva, Switzerland. 1996.

[2]   Meister, LA; Meadows, AT. Late effects of childhood cancer. *Curr Probl Pediatr* 1993, 23, 102-31.

[3]   Goodwin, PJ; Ennis, M; Pritchard, KI; Trudeau, M; Hood, N. Risk of menopause during the first year after breast cancer diagnosis. *J Clin Oncol.*, 1999, Aug;17(8), 2365-70.

[4]   Bokemeyer, C; Schmoll HJ; van Rhee J; Kuczyk M; Schuppert F; Poliwoda H. ong-term gonadal toxicity after therapy for Hodgkin's and non-Hodgkin's lymphoma. *Ann Hematol.* 1994 Mar;68(3), 105-10.

[5]   Shapiro, CL; Recht, A. Side Effects of Adjuvant Treatment of Breast Cancer. *N. Engl. J. Med., June,* 28, 2001, 344(26), 1997-2008.

[6]   Wallace, WH; Thomson, AB; Kelsey, TW. The radiosensitivity of the human oocyte. *Hum Reprod.*, 2003 Jan;18(1), 117-21.

[7]   Wallace, WH; Thomson, AB; Saran, F; Kelsey, TW. Predicting age of ovarian failure after radiation to a field that includes the ovaries. *Int J Radiat Oncol Biol Phys.*, 2005 Jul 1; 62(3), 738-44.

[8]   Hendrix, SL. Bilateral oophorectomy and premature menopause. *Am J Med.*, 2005, Dec 9, 118(12 Suppl 2), 131-5.

[9]   Oldenhave, A; Jaszmann, LJ; Everaerd, WT; Haspels, AA. Hysterectomized women with ovarian conservation report more severe climacteric complaints than do normal climacteric women of similar age. *Am J Obstet Gynecol.*, 1993, Mar;168(3 Pt 1), 765-71.

[10]   Riedel, HH; Lehmann-Willenbrock, E; Semm, K. Ovarian failure phenomena after hysterectomy. *J Reprod Med.*, 1986, Jul;31(7), 597-600.

[11]   Szlachter, BN; Nachtigall, LE; Epstein, J; et al. Premature ovarian failure: A reversible entity? *Obstet Gynecol,* 1979, 54, 396-398.

[12]   Rebar, RW; Connolly, HV. Clinical features of young women with hypergonadotropic amenorrhea. *Fertil Steril,* 1990, 53, 804-810.

[13]   Elit, L; Esplen, MJ; Butler, K; Narod, S. Quality of life and psychosexual adjustment after prophylactic oophorectomy for a family history of ovarian cancer. *Fam Cancer.*, 2001, 1(3-4), 149-56.

[14]   Ganz, PA. Menopause and breast cancer: symptoms, late effects, and their management. *Semin Oncol.*, 2001 Jun, 28(3), 274-83. Review.

[15]   Berg, G; Gottwall, T; Hammar, M; Lindgren, R. Climacteric symptoms among women aged 60-62 in Linkoping, Sweden, in 1986.Maturitas. 1988 Oct;10(3), 193-9. Erratum in: *Maturitas,* 1988 Dec;10(4), 363. Gottgall T [corrected to Gottwall T.

[16]   Judd, HL; Lucas, WE; Yen, SS. Serum 17 beta-estradiol and estrone levels in postmenopausal women with and without endometrial cancer. *J Clin Endocrinol Metab.*, 1976 Aug; 43(2), 272-8.

[17]   Laughlin, GA; Barrett-Connor, E; Kritz-Silverstein, D; von Muhlen, D. Hysterectomy, oophorectomy, and endogenous sex hormone levels in older women: the Rancho Bernardo Study. *J Clin Endocrinol Metab.*, 2000, Feb, 85(2), 645-51.

[18]   Bancroft, J; Loftus, J; Long, JS. Distress about sex: a national survey of women in heterosexual relationships. *Arch Sex Behav.*, 2003, Jun; 32(3), 193-208.

[19]   Crandall, C; Petersen, L; Ganz, PA; Greendale, GA. Association of breast cancer and its therapy with menopause-related symptoms. *Menopause.*, 2004, Sep-Oct;11(5), 519-30.

[20]   Knobf, MT. Carrying on: the experience of premature menopause in women with early stage breast cancer. *Nurs Res.*, 2002, Jan-Feb;51(1), 9- 17.

[21]   Jacobsen, BK; Heuch, I; Kvale, G. Age at natural menopause and all-cause mortality: a 37-year follow-up of 19,731 Norwegian women. *Am J Epidemiol.*, 2003, 157, 923-929.

[22]   Kannel, WB; Hjortland, MC; McNamara, PM; Gordon, T. Menopause and risk of cardiovascular disease: the Framingham study. *Ann Intern Med.*, 1976 Oct;85(4), 447-52.

[23]   Colditz, GA; Willett, WC; Stampfer, MJ; Rosner, B; Speizer, FE; Hennekens, CH. Menopause and the risk of coronary heart disease in women. *N Engl J Med.*, 1987, Apr 30, 316(18), 1105-10.

[24]   van der Schouw, YT; van der Graaf, Y; Steyerberg, EW; Eijkemans, JC; Banga, JD. Age at menopause as a risk factor for cardiovascular mortality. *Lancet.*, 1996 Mar 16, 347(9003), 714-8.

[25] BRIEF REPORT: Coronary Heart Disease Events Associated with Hormone Therapy
      in Younger and Older Women. A Meta-Analysis Shelley, R; Salpeter, MD; Judith ME
      Walsh, MD; MPH, Elizabeth, Greyber, MD; Edwin, E; Salpeter, PhD *Journal of
      General Internal Medicine,* 2006, 21, 4 363.

[26] Mack, WJ; Slater, CC; Xiang, M; Shoupe, D; Lobo, RA; Hodis, HN. Elevated
      subclinical atherosclerosis associated with oophorectomy is related to time since
      menopause rather than type of menopause. *Fertil Steril.,* 2004, Aug; 82(2), 391-7.

[27] Joakimsen, O; Bonaa, KH; Stensland-Bugge, E; Jacobsen, BK. Population-based study
      of age at menopause and ultrasound assessed carotid atherosclerosis: The Tromso
      Study. *J Clin Epidemiol.,* 2000 May; 53(5), 525-30.

[28] Ouyang, P; Michos, ED; Karas, RH. Hormone replacement therapy and the
      cardiovascular system lessons learned and unanswered questions. *J Am Coll Cardiol.,*
      2006, May 2, 47(9), 1741-53. Epub, 2006, Apr 17. Review.

[29] Molina, JR; Barton, DL; Loprinzi, CL. Chemotherapy-induced ovarian failure:
      manifestations and management. *Drug Saf.,* 2005, 28(5), 401-16. Review.

[30] Ramaswamy, B; Shapiro, CL. Osteopenia and osteoporosis in women with breast
      cancer. *Semin Oncol.,* 2003, Dec, 30(6), 763-75. Review.

[31] Chlebowski, RT. Bone health in women with early-stage breast cancer. *Clin Breast
      Cancer.,* 2005, Feb, 5 Suppl(2), S35-40. Review.

[32] Mackey, JR; Joy, AA. Skeletal health in postmenopausal survivors of early breast
      cancer. *Int J Cancer.,* 2005 May, 10, 114(6), 1010-5. Review.

[33] Kelly, J; Damron, T; Grant, W; Anker, C; Holdridge, S; Shaw, S; Horton, J; Cherrick,
      I; Spadaro, J. Cross-sectional study of bone mineral density in adult survivors of solid
      pediatric cancers. *J Pediatr Hematol Oncol.,* 2005, May; 27(5), 248-53.

[34] Shapiro, CL; Manola, J; Leboff, M. Ovarian failure after adjuvant chemotherapy is
      associated with rapid bone loss in women with early-stage breast cancer. *J Clin Oncol.,*
      2001, Jul 15, 19(14), 3306-11.

[35] Lester, J; Dodwell, D; McCloskey, E; Coleman, R. The causes and treatment of bone
      loss associated with carcinoma of the breast. *Cancer Treat Rev.,* 2005, Apr;31(2), 115-
      42. Review.

[36] Kanis, JA; McCloskey, EV; Powles, T; et al. A high incidence of vertebral fracture in
      women with breast cancer. *Br J Cancer,* 1999, 79, 1179-81.

[37] Howell, A; Cuzick, J; Baum, M; Buzdar, A; Dowsett, M; Forbes, JF; Hoctin-Boes, G;
      Houghton, J; Locker, GY; Tobias, JS; ATAC Trialists' Group. Results of the ATAC
      (Arimidex, Tamoxifen, Alone or in Combination) trial after completion of 5 years'
      adjuvant treatment for breast cancer. *Lancet.,* 2005, Jan 1-7, 365(9453), 60-2.

[38] Goss, PE; Ingle, JN; Martino, S; Robert, NJ; Muss, HB; Piccart, MJ; Castiglione, M;
      Tu, D; Shepherd, LE; Pritchard, KI; Livingston, RB; Davidson, NE; Norton, L; Perez,
      EA; Abrams, JS; Cameron, DA; Palmer, MJ; Pater, JL. Randomized trial of letrozole
      following tamoxifen as extended adjuvant therapy in receptor-positive breast cancer:
      updated findings from NCIC CTG MA.17. *J Natl Cancer Inst.,* 2005, Sep 7, 97(17),
      1262-71.

[39] Early Breast Cancer Trialists' Collaborative Group. Tamoxifen benefits of estrogen plus progestin in healthy postmenopausal for early breast cancer: an overview of the randomized trials. *Lancet,* 1998, 351, 1451-67.

[40] McCune, JS; Games, DM; Espirito, JL. Assessment of ovarian failure and osteoporosis in premenopausal breast cancer survivors. *J Oncol Pharm Pract.,* 2005, Jun;11(2), 37-43.

[41] McCune, JS; Games, DM; Espirito, JL. Assessment of ovarian failure and osteoporosis in premenopausal breast cancer survivors. *J Oncol Pharm Pract.,* 2005, Jun, 11(2), 37-43.

[42] Hillner, BE; Ingle, JN; Chlebowski, RT; Gralow, J; Yee, GC; Janjan, NA; Cauley, JA; Blumenstein, BA; Albain, KS; Lipton, A; Brown, S. American Society of Clinical Oncology. American Society of Clinical Oncology 2003 update on the role of bisphosphonates and bone health issues in women with breast cancer. *J Clin Oncol.,* 2003 Nov 1, 21(21), 4042-57. Epub 2003 Sep 8. Erratum in: *J Clin Oncol.,* 2004 Apr 1;22(7), 1351.

[43] Daly, E; Gray, A; Barlow, D; McPherson, K; Roche, M; Vessey, M. Measuring the impact of menopausal symptoms on quality of life. *BMJ.,* 1993, Oct 2, 307(6908), 836-40.

[44] Schultz, PN; Klein, MJ; Beck, ML; Stava, C; Sellin, RV. Breast cancer: relationship between menopausal symptoms, physiologic health effects of cancer treatment and physical constraints on quality of life in long-term survivors. *J Clin Nurs.,* 2005, Feb, 14(2), 204-11.

[45] Harris, PF; Remington, PL; Trentham-Dietz, A; Allen, CI; Newcomb, PA. Prevalence and treatment of menopausal symptoms among breast cancer survivors. *J Pain Symptom Manage.,* 2002, Jun, 23(6), 501-9.

[46] Gupta, P; Sturdee, DW; Palin, SL; Majumder, K; Fear, R; Marshall, T; Paterson, I. Menopausal symptoms in women treated for breast cancer: the prevalence and severity of symptoms and their perceived effects on quality of life. *Climacteric.,* 2006, Feb, 9(1), 49-58.

[47] Morales, L; Neven, P; Timmerman, D; Christiaens, MR; Vergote, I; Van Limbergen, E; Carbonez, A; Van Huffel, S; Ameye, L; Paridaens, R. Acute effects of tamoxifen and third-generation aromatase inhibitors on menopausal symptoms of breast cancer patients. *Anticancer Drugs.,* 2004, Sep;15(8), 753-60.

[48] Nancy Fugate Woods, PhD, RN; Ellen Sullivan Mitchell, PhD, RN; Symptoms during the menopausal transition: prevalence, severity, trajectory, and significance in women's lives. *The American Journal of Medicine,* 2005, Vol 118, (12B), 14S-24S.

[49] Stearns, V; Ullmer, L; Lopez, JF; Smith, Y; Isaacs, C; Hayes, D. Hot flushes. *Lancet.* 2002, Dec, 360(9348), 1851-61.

[50] Rodstrom, K; Bengtsson, C; Lissner, L; Milsom, I; Sundh, V; Bjorkelund, C. A longitudinal study of the treatment of hot flushes: the population study of women in Gothenburg during a quarter of a century. *Menopause.,* 2002, May-Jun, 9(3), 156-61.

[51] Freedman, RR. Physiology of hot flashes. *Am J Hum Biol.,* 2001, 13, 453-64.

[52] Freedman, RR. Hot flashes: behavioral treatments, mechanisms, and relation to sleep. *Am J Med.,* 2005, Dec 19, 118(12 Suppl 2), 124-30.

[53] Freedman, RR; Krell, W. Reduced thermoregulatory null zone in postmenopausal women with hot flashes. *Am J Obstet Gynecol.,* 1999, 181, 66-70.

[54] MacLennan, AH; Broadbent, JL; Lester, S; Moore, V. Oral oestrogen and combined oestrogen/progestogen therapy versus placebo for hot flushes. The Cochrane Database of Systematic Reviews 2004, Issue 4. Art. No.: CD002978. DOI: 10.1002/14651858. CD002978.pub2 http://www.coolfemme.ca

[55] Wilbur, J; Miller, AM; McDevitt, J; Wang, E; Miller, J. Menopausal status, moderate-intensity walking, and symptoms in midlife women. *Res Theory Nurs Pract.*, 2005 Summer; 19(2), 163-80.

[56] Germaine, LM; Freedman, RR. Behavioral treatment of menopausal hot flashes: evaluation by objective methods. *J Consult Clin Psychol.*, 1984, 52, 1072-1079.

[57] Freedman, RR; Woodward, S. Behavioral treatment of menopausal hot flushes: evaluation by ambulatory monitoring. *Am J Obstet Gynecol.*, 1992, 167, 436-439.

[58] Freedman, RR; Woodward, S; Brown, B; Javaid, JI; Pandey, GN. Biochemical and thermoregulatory effects of behavioral treatment for menopausal hot flashes. *Menopause.*, 1995, 2, 211-218.

[59] Low Dog; Tieraona Menopause: a review of botanical dietary supplements. *Amer. J Med.,* 2005 118 (12) Suppl Dec, 98-108.

[60] Desindes, S; Belisle, S; Graves, G. SOGC Consensus on Menopause JOGC, 2006 *in press*

[61] Geller, SE; Studee, L. Botanical and dietary supplements for menopausal symptoms: what works, what does not. *J Womens Health.*, 2005, Sep, 14(7), 634-49.

[62] Whiting, PW; Clouston, A; Kerlin, P. Black cohosh and other herbal remedies associated with acute hepatitis. *Med J Aust.,* 2002, Oct 21, 177(8), 440-3.

[63] Newton, KM; Buist, DS; Keenan, NL; Anderson, LA; LaCroix, AZ. Use of alternative therapies for menopause symptoms: results of a population-based survey. Obstet Gynecol. 2002 Jul;100(1), 18-25. Erratum in: *Obstet Gynecol.,* 2003, Jan, 101(1), 205.

[64] Krebs, EE; Ensrud, KE; MacDonald, R; Wilt, TJ. Phytoestrogens for treatment of menopausal symptoms: a systematic review. *Obstet Gynecol.*, 2004, Oct;104(4), 824-36.

[65] Phipps, WR; Duncan, AM; Kurzer, MS. Isoflavones and postmenopausal women: a critical review. *Treat Endocrinol.*, 2002, 1(5), 293-311.

[66] Nelson, HD; Vesco, KK; Haney, E; Fu, R; Nedrow, A; Miller, J; Nicolaidis, C; Walker, M; Humphrey, L. Nonhormonal therapies for menopausal hot flashes: systematic review and meta-analysis. *JAMA.,* 2006 May 3, 295(17), 2057-71.

[67] Barentsen, R. Red clover isoflavones and menopausal health. *J Br Menopause Soc.,* 2004, Mar;10 Suppl 1, 4-7.

[68] Huntley, A. Drug-herb interactions with herbal medicines for menopause. *J Br Menopause Soc.,* 2004, Dec;10(4), 162-5.

[69] Woodward, KN. The potential impact of the use of homeopathic and herbal remedies on monitoring the safety of prescription products. *Hum Exp Toxicol.*, 2005, May, 24(5), 219-33.

[70] Heck, AM; DeWitt, BA; Lukes, AL. Potential interactions between alternative therapies and warfarin *Am J Health Syst Pharm.*, 2000, Jul 1, 57(13), 1221-7.

[71] Sparreboom, A; Cox, MC; Acharya, MR; Figg, WD. Herbal remedies in the United States: potential adverse interactions with anticancer agents. *J Clin Oncol.*, 2004, Jun 15, 22(12), 2489-503.

[72] Petrakis, NL; Barnes, S; King, EB; et al: Stimulatory influence of soy protein isolate on breast secretion in pre- and postmenopausal women. *Cancer Epidemiol Biomarkers Prev,*1996, 5, 785-794.

[73] Hargreaves, DF; Potten, CS; Harding, C; et al: Two-week dietary soy supplementation has an estrogenic effect on normal premenopausal breast. *J Clin Endocrinol Metab,* 1999, 84, 4017-4024,.

[74] Allred, CD; Allred, KF; Ju, YH; et al: Soy diets containing varying amounts of genistein stimulate growth of estrogen-dependent (MCF-7) tumors in a dose-dependent manner. *Cancer Res,* 2001, 61, 5045-5050,.

[75] Ju, YH; Doerge, DR; Allred, KF; et al: Dietary genistein negates the inhibitory effects of tamoxifen on growth of estrogen-dependent human breast cancer (MCF-7) cells in athymic mice. *Cancer Res,* 2002, 62, 2474-2477.

[76] Limer, JL; Parkes, AT; Speirs, V. Differential response to phytoestrogens in endocrine sensitive and resistant breast cancer cells in vitro.*Int J Cancer.*, 2006, Aug 1, 119(3), 515-21.

[77] Ju, YH; Doerge, DR; Allred, KF; Allred, CD; Helferich, WG. Dietary genistein negates the inhibitory effect of tamoxifen on growth of estrogen-dependent human breast cancer (MCF-7) cells implanted in athymic mice. *Cancer Res.*, 2002, May 1, 62(9), 2474-7

[78] Wesierska-Gadek, J; Schreiner, T; Gueorguieva, M; Ranftler, C. Phenol red reduces ROSC mediated cell cycle arrest and apoptosis in human MCF-7 cells. *J Cell Biochem.*, 2006, Jun 1; [Epub ahead of print].

[79] Loprinzi, CL; Stearns, V; Barton, D. Centrally active nonhormonal hot flash therapies. *Am J Med.*, 2005, Dec 19, 118(12 Suppl 2), 118-23.

[80] Fugate, SE; Church, CO. Nonestrogen treatment modalities for vasomotor symptoms associated with menopause. *Ann Pharmacother.*, 2004 Sep, 38(9), 1482-99. Epub Aug 3.

[81] Nagamani, M; Kelver, ME; Smith, ER. Treatment of menopausal hot flashes with transdermal administration of clonidine. *Am J Obstet Gynecol.*, 1987 Mar, 156(3), 561-5.

[82] Pandya, KJ; Raubertas, RF; Flynn, PJ; Hynes, HE; Rosenbluth, RJ; Kirshner, JJ; Pierce, HI; Dragalin, V; Morrow, GR. Oral clonidine in postmenopausal patients with breast cancer experiencing tamoxifen-induced hot flashes: a University of Rochester Cancer Center Community Clinical Oncology Program study. *Ann Intern Med.* 2000, May, 16, 132(10), 788-93.

[83] Goldberg, RM; Loprinzi, CL; O'Fallon, JR; Veeder, MH; Miser, AW; Mailliard, JA; Michalak, JC; Dose, AM; Rowland, KM; Jr; Burnham, NL. Transdermal clonidine for ameliorating tamoxifen-induced hot flashes. *J Clin Oncol.* 1994 Jan;12(1), 155-8. Erratum in: *J Clin Oncol.*, 1996, Aug;14(8), 2411.

[84] Freedman, RR; Dinsay, R. Clonidine raises the sweating threshold in symptomatic but not in asymptomatic postmenopausal women. *Fertil Steril.*, 2000, Jul, 74(1), 20-3.

[85] Stearns, V; Beebe, KL; Iyengar, M; Dube, E. Paroxetine controlled release in the treatment of menopausal hot flashes: a randomized controlled trial. *JAMA,* 2003, 289, 2827-34.

[86] Weitzner, MA; Moncello, J; Jacobsen, PB; Minton, S. A pilot trial of paroxetine for the treatment of hot flashes and associated symptoms in women with breast cancer. *J Pain Symptom Manage,* 2002, 23, 337- 45.

[87] Stearns, V; Johnson, MD; Rae, JM; Morocho, A; Novielli, A; Bhargava, P; Hayes, DF; Desta, Z; Flockhart, DA. Active tamoxifen metabolite plasma concentrations after coadministration of tamoxifen and the selective serotonin reuptake inhibitor paroxetine. *J Natl Cancer Inst.,* 2003, Dec 3, 95(23), 1758-64.

[88] Jin, Y; Desta, Z; Stearns, V; Ward, B; Ho, H; Lee, KH; Skaar, T; Storniolo, AM; Li, L; Araba, A; Blanchard, R; Nguyen, A; Ullmer, L; Hayden, J; Lemler, S; Weinshilboum, RM; Rae, JM; Hayes, DF; Flockhart, DA. CYP2D6 genotype, antidepressant use, and tamoxifen metabolism during adjuvant breast cancer treatment. *J Natl Cancer Inst.,* 2005, Jan 5, 97(1), 30-9.

[89] Biglia, N; Torta, R; Roagna, R; Maggiorotto, F; Cacciari, F; Ponzone, R; Kubatzki, F; Sismondi, P. Evaluation of low-dose venlafaxine hydrochloride for the therapy of hot flushes in breast cancer survivors. *Maturitas.,* 2005, Sep 16, 52(1), 78-85

[90] Loprinzi, CL; Levitt, R; Barton, D; Sloan, JA; Dakhil, SR; Nikcevich, DA; Bearden, JD. 3rd, Mailliard JA; Tschetter LK; Fitch TR; Kugler JW. Phase III comparison of depomedroxyprogesterone acetate to venlafaxine for managing hot flashes: North Central Cancer Treatment Group Trial N99C7. *J Clin Oncol.,* 2006, Mar 20, 24(9), 1409-14. Epub 2006, Feb 27.

[91] Guttuso, T; Jr; Kurlan, R; McDermott, MP; Kieburtz, K. Gabapentin's effects on hot flashes in postmenopausal women: a randomized controlled trial. *Obstet Gynecol.,* 2003, Feb;101(2), 337-45.

[92] Pandya, KJ; Morrow, GR; Roscoe, JA; Zhao, H; Hickok, JT; Pajon, E; Sweeney, TJ; Banerjee, TK; Flynn, PJ. Gabapentin for hot flashes in 420 women with breast cancer: a randomised double-blind placebo-controlled trial. *Lancet.,* 2005, Sep 3-9;366(9488), 818-24.

[93] Nelson, HD. Commonly used types of postmenopausal estrogen for treatment of hot flashes: scientific review. *JAMA.,* 2004, Apr 7, 291(13), 1610-20.

[94] Post, MS; van der Mooren, MJ; van Baal, WM; Blankenstein, MA; Merkus, HM; Kroeks, MV; Franke, HR; Kenemans, P; Stehouwer, CD. Effects of low-dose oral and transdermal estrogen replacement therapy on hemostatic factors in healthy postmenopausal women: a randomized placebo-controlled study. *Am J Obstet Gynecol.,* 2003, Nov;189(5), 1221-7.

[95] Scarabin, PY; Oger, E; Plu-Bureau, G. EStrogen and THromboEmbolism Risk Study Group. Differential association of oral and transdermal oestrogen-replacement therapy with venous thromboembolism risk. *Lancet.,* 2003, Aug 9;362(9382), 428-32.

[96] Eilertsen, AL; Hoibraaten, E; Os, I; Andersen, TO; Sandvik, L; Sandset, PM. The effects of oral and transdermal hormone replacement therapy on C-reactive protein levels and other inflammatory markers in women with high risk of thrombosis. *Maturitas.,* 2005, Oct 16, 52(2), 111-8.

[97] Harvey, J; Scheurer, C; Kawakami, FT; Quebe-Fehling, E; de Palacios, PI; Ragavan, VV. ormone replacement therapy and breast density changes. *Climacteric.*, 2005, Jun; 8(2), 185-92.

[98] Ettinger, B. Vasomotor symptom relief versus unwanted effects: role of estrogen dosage. *Am J Med.*, 2005, Dec 19, 118(12 Suppl 2), 74-8.

[99] Crandall, C. Low-dose estrogen therapy for menopausal women: a review of efficacy and safety. *J Womens Health (Larchmt).,* 2003, Oct;12(8), 723-47.

[100] Grodstein, F; Manson, JE; Colditz, GA; Willett, WC; Speizer, FE; Stampfer, MJ. A prospective, observational study of postmenopausal hormone therapy and primary prevention of cardiovascular disease. *Ann Intern Med.*, 2000, Dec 19, 133(12), 933-41.

[101] Collins, JA; Blake, JM; Crosignani, PG. Breast cancer risk with postmenopausal hormonal treatment. *Hum Reprod Update.*, 2005, Nov-Dec, 11(6), 545-60. Epub 2005 Sep 8.

[102] Clemons, M; Clamp, A; Anderson, B. Management of the menopause in cancer survivors. *Cancer Treat Rev.*, 2002, Dec, 28(6), 321-33. Review.

[103] Pritchard, KI; Khan, H; Levine, M. Steering Committee on Clinical Practice Guidelines for the Care and Treatment of Breast Cancer. Clinical practice guidelines for the care and treatment of breast cancer: 14. The role of hormone replacement therapy in women with a previous diagnosis of breast cancer. *CMAJ.*, 2002, Apr 16;166(8), 1017-22. Review

[104] Creasman, WT. Hormone replacement therapy after cancers. *Curr Opin Oncol.*, 2005 Sep, 17(5), 493-9. Review.

[105] Biglia, N; Gadducci, A; Ponzone, R; Roagna, R; Sismondi, P. Hormone replacement therapy in cancer survivors. *Maturitas.*, 2004, Aug 20, 48(4), 333-46. Review.

[106] Col, NF; Kim, JA; Chlebowski, RT. Menopausal hormone therapy after breast cancer: a meta-analysis and critical appraisal of the evidence. *Breast Cancer Res.*, 2005, 7(4), R535-40. Epub 2005, May 19.

[107] Meurer, LN; Lena, S. Cancer recurrence and mortality in women using hormone replacement therapy: meta-analysis. *J Fam Pract.*, 2002, Dec, 51(12), 1056-62.

[108] Suriano, KA; McHale M; McLaren, CE; Li, KT; Re, A; DiSaia, PJ. Estrogen replacement therapy in endometrial cancer patients: a matched control study.*Obstet Gynecol.*, 2001, Apr, 97(4), 555-60.

[109] Chapman, JA; DiSaia, PJ; Osann, K; Roth, PD; Gillotte, DL; Berman, ML. Estrogen replacement in surgical stage I and II endometrial cancer survivors. *Am J Obstet Gynecol.*, 1996, Nov; 175(5), 1195-200.

[110] Lee, RB; Burke, TW; Park, RC. Estrogen replacement therapy following treatment for stage I endometrial carcinoma. *Gynecol Oncol.*, 1990, Feb, 36(2), 189-91.

[111] Creasman, WT; Henderson, D; Hinshaw, W; Clarke-Pearson, DL. Estrogen replacement therapy in the patient treated for endometrial cancer. *Obstet Gynecol.*, 1986, Mar;67(3), 326-30.

[112] Holmberg, L; Anderson, H. HABITS steering and data monitoring committees. ABITS (hormonal replacement therapy after breast cancer--is it safe?), a randomised comparison: trial stopped. *Lancet.*, 2004, Feb 7, 363(9407), 453-5.

[113] von Schoultz, E; Rutqvist, LE; Stockholm Breast Cancer Study Group. Menopausal hormone therapy after breast cancer: the Stockholm randomized trial. *J Natl Cancer Inst.*, 2005, Apr 6, 97(7), 533-5.

[114] Chlebowski, RT; Anderson, GL. Progestins and recurrence in breast cancer survivors. *J Natl Cancer Inst.*, 2005, Apr 6, 97(7), 471-2.

[115] Kwan, K; Ward, C; Marsden, J. Is there a role for hormone replacement therapy after breast cancer? *J Br Menopause Soc.*, 2005, Dec;11(4), 140-4. Review.

[116] Batur, P; Blixen, CE; Moore, HC; Thacker, HL; Xu, M. Menopausal hormone therapy (HT) in patients with breast cancer. *Maturitas.*, 2006, Jan 20, 53(2), 123-32. Review.

[117] Gold, EB; Sternfeld, B; Kelsey, JL; et al. Relation of demographic and lifestyle factors to symptoms in a multi-racial/ethnic population of women 40-55 years of age. *Am J Epidemiol.*, 2000, 152, 463-473.

[118] Moe, KE. Hot flashes and sleep in women. *Sleep Med Rev.*, 2004, Dec;8(6), 487-97

[119] Dzaja, A; Arber, S; Hislop, J; Kerkhofs, M; Kopp, C; Pollmacher, T; Polo-Kantola, P; Skene, DJ; Stenuit, P; Tobler, I; Porkka-Heiskanen, T. Women's sleep in health and disease. *J Psychiatr Res.*, 2005 Jan; 39(1), 55-76.

[120] Tworoger, SS; Yasui, Y; Vitiello, MV; Schwartz, RS; Ulrich, CM; Aiello, EJ; Irwin, ML; Bowen, D; Potter, JD; McTiernan, A. Effects of a yearlong moderate-intensity exercise and a stretching intervention on sleep quality in postmenopausal women. *Sleep.*, 2003, Nov 1, 26(7), 830-6

[121] Brunner, RL; Gass, M; Aragaki, A; Hays, J; Granek, I; Woods, N; Mason, E; Brzyski, R; Ockene, J; Assaf, A; LaCroix, A; Matthews, K; Wallace, R. Women's Health Initiative Investigators. Effects of conjugated equine estrogen on health-related quality of life in postmenopausal women with hysterectomy: results from the Women's Health Initiative Randomized Clinical. *Arch Intern Med.*, 2005, Sep 26, 165(17), 1976-86

[122] Polo-Kantola, P; Erkkola, R; Helenius, H; Irjala, K; Polo, O. When does estrogen replacement therapy improve sleep quality? *Am J Obstet Gynecol.* 1998 May;178(5), 1002-9.

[123] Gambacciani, M; Ciaponi, M; Cappagli, B; Monteleone, P; Benussi, C; Bevilacqua, G; Vacca, F; Genazzani, AR. Effects of low-dose, continuous combined hormone replacement therapy on sleep in symptomatic postmenopausal women. *Maturitas.* 2005 Feb 14;50(2), 91-7.

[124] Kaufert, PA; Gilbert, P; Tate, R. The Manitoba Project: a re-examination of the link between menopause and depression. *Maturitas.*, 1992, 14, 143-155

[125] Avis, NE; Crawford, S; Stellato, R; et al. Longitudinal study of hormone levels and depression among women transitioning through menopause.Climacteric., 2001, 4, 243-249

[126] Woods, NF; Mariella, A; Mitchell, E. Patterns of depressed mood across the MT: approaches to studying patterns in longitudinal data. *Acta Obstet Gynecol Scand.*, 2002, 81, 623-632.

[127] Brornberger, Joyce, T. Meyer, Peter, M; Kravitz, Howard, M. Sommer, Barbara Cordal, Adriana Powell, Lynda Ganz, Patricia A. Sutton-Tyrrell, Kim, Psychologic Distress and Natural Menopause. *American Journal of Public Health.*; Sep 2001, 91, (9), p1435-43

[128] Avis, NE; Brambilla, D; McKinlay, SM; Vass, K. A longitudinal analysis of the association between menopause and depression: results from the Massachusetts women's health survey. *Ann Epidemiol.*, 1994, 4, 214-2.

[129] Avis, NE; Crawford, S; Stellato, R; Longcope, C. Longitudinal study of hormone levels and depression among women transitioning through menopause. *Climacteric.* 2001 Sep;4(3), 243-9.

[130] Guthrie, JR; Dennerstein, L; Taffe, JR; Lehert, P; Burger, HG. The menopausal transition: a 9-year prospective population-based study. The Melbourne Women's Midlife Health Project. *Climacteric.*, 2004 Dec, 7(4), 375-89.

[131] Zweifel, JE; O'Brien, WH. A meta-analysis of the effect of hormone replacement therapy upon depressed mood. Psychoneuroendocrinology., 1997, Apr;22(3), 189-212. Erratum in: *Psychoneuroendocrinology.*, 1997, Nov;22(8), 655

[132] Schmidt, Peter, J. Mood, depression, and reproductive hormones in the menopausal transition. *The American Journal of Medicine* 2005 Volume: 118, Issue: 12, Supplement 2 December, 19, 54-58

[133] Grigoriadis, S; Sherwin, B. Mood and Memory Disorders *JOGC.*, 2006, *in press*

[134] Morrison, MF; Kallan, MJ; Ten Have, T; Katz, I; Tweedy, K; Battistini, M. Lack of efficacy of estradiol for depression in postmenopausal women: a randomized, controlled. *Biol Psychiatry.*, 2004, Feb 15;55(4), 406-12

[135] Schmidt, PJ; Nieman, L; Danaceau, MA; Tobin, MB; Roca, CA; Murphy, JH; et al. Estrogen replacement in perimenopause-related depression: A preliminary report. *Am J Obstet Gynecol.*, 2000, 183, 414-20

[136] De Noaves Soares, C; Almeida, OP; Joffee, H; Cohen, LS. Efficacy of estradiol for the treatment of depressive disorders in perimenopausal women. *Arch Gen Psychiatry.*, 2001, 58, 529-34.

[137] Stenberg, A; Heimer, G; Ulmsten, U; Cnattingus, S. Prevalence of genitourinary and other climacteric symptoms in 61-year-old women. *Maturitas.*, 1996, 24, 31-6

[138] Romanzi, LJ; Groutz, A; Feroz, F; Blaivas, JG. Evaluation of female external genitalia sensitivity to pressure/touch: a preliminary prospective study using Semmes-Weinstein monofilaments. *Urology.*, 2001, 57(6), 1145-50.

[139] Berg, G; Gottqall, T; Hammar, M; Lindgren, R. Climacteric symptoms among women aged 60-62 in Linkoping, Sweden in 1986. *Maturitas.*, 1988, 10, 193-9

[140] Johnston, SL; Farrell, SA; Bouchard, C. et al SOGC Joint Committee - Clinical Practice Gynaecology and Urogynaecology. Detection and management of urogenital atrophy. *JOGC.*, 2004, 26 (%), 503-15

[141] Castelo-Branco, C; Cancelo, MJ; Villero, J; Nohales, F; Julia, MD. Management of post-menopausal vaginal atrophy and atrophic vaginitis. *Maturitas.*, 2005, Nov 15;52 Suppl 1, S46-52. Epub 2005 Sep 1.

[142] Leiblum, S; Bachmann, G; Kemmann, E; Colburn, D; Swartzman, L. Vaginal atrophy in the postmenopausal woman. The importance of sexual activity and hormones. *JAMA.*, 1983, Apr 22-29, 249(16), 2195-8

[143] Pandit, L; Ouslander, JG. Postmenopausal vaginal atrophy and atrophic vaginitis. *Am J Med Sci.*, 1997 Oct;314(4), 228-31.

[144] Bygdeman, M; Swah, ML. Replens versus dlienoestrol cream in symptomatic treatment of vaginal atrophy in postmenopausal women. *Maturitas.,* 1996, 23, 259-63.

[145] Nachtigall, LE. Comparative study: Replens versus local estrogen in menopausal women. *Fertil Steril.,* 1994, 61, 178-80.

[146] Palacios, S; Castelo-Branco, C; Cancelo, MJ; Vazquez, F. Low-dose, vaginally administered estrogens may enhance local benefits of systemic therapy in the treatment of urogenital atrophy in postmenopausal women on hormone therapy. *Maturitas.,* 2005, Feb, 14, 50(2), 98-104.

[147] Cardozo, L; Bachmann, G; McClish, D; Fonda, D; Birgerson, L. Meta-analysis of estrogen therapy in the management of urogenital atrophy in postmenopausal women: second report of the Hormones and Urogenital Therapy Committee. *Obstet Gynecol.,* 1998, Oct, 92(4 Pt 2), 722-7.

[148] Suckling, J; Lethaby, A; Kennedy, R. Local oestrogen for vaginal atrophy in postmenopausal women. *Cochrane Database Syst Rev.,* 2003, (4), CD001500.

[149] Weisberg, E; Ayton, R; Darling, G; Farrell, E; Murkies, A; O'Neill, S; Kirkegard, Y; Fraser, IS. Endometrial and vaginal effects of low-dose estradiol delivered by vaginal ring or vaginal tablet. *Climacteric.,* 2005, Mar, 8(1), 83-92.

[150] Gabrielsson, Johan, Wallenbeck, Ingrid, Larsson, Gregor; Birgerson, Lars; Heimer, Gun Studies of the low dose ring have shown negligible serum levels New kinetic data on estradiol in light of the vaginal ring concept. *Maturitas.,* S35-S39 and have not showm any endometrial response.

[151] Bachmann, G. The estradiol vaginal ring--a study of existing clinical data. *Maturitas.,* 1995, Dec, 22, Suppl, S21-9.

[152] Bakos, O; Smith, P; Heimer, G; Ulmsten, U. Transvaginal sonography of the internal genital organs in postmenopausal women on low-dose estrogen treatment. *Ultrasound Obstet Gynecol.,* 1994, Jul 1, 4(4), 326-9.

[153] Rioux, JE; Devlin, C; Gelfand, MM; Steinberg, WM; Hepburn, DS. 17beta-estradiol vaginal tablet versus conjugated equine estrogen vaginal cream to relieve menopausal atrophic vaginitis. *Menopause.,* 2000, May-Jun;7(3), 156-61.

[154] Johnston, S. SOGC *Canadian Consensus on Menopause, 2006, JOGC in press.*

[155] Ballagh, SA. Vaginal hormone therapy for urogenital and menopausal symptoms. *Semin Reprod Med.,* 2005, May, 23(2), 126-40.

[156] Dew, JE; Wren, BG; Eden, JA. A cohort study of topical vaginal estrogen therapy in women previously treated for breast cancer. *Climacteric.,* 2003, Mar;6(1), 45-52.

[157] Maccormick, RE. Possible acceleration of aging by adjuvant chemotherapy: A cause of early onset frailty? *Med Hypotheses.,* 2006, 67(2), 212-5. Epub Mar 20.

[158] Xu, J; Bartoces, M; Neale, AV; Dailey, RK; Northrup, J; Schwartz, KL. Natural history of menopause symptoms in primary care patients: a MetroNet study. *J Am Board Fam Pract.,* 2005, Sep-Oct; 18(5), 374-82.

[159] Szoeke, CE; Cicuttini, F; Guthrie, J; Dennerstein, L. Self-reported arthritis and the menopause. *Climacteric.,* 2005, Mar;8(1), 49-55.

[160] Sherman, KJ; Cherkin, DC; Erro, J; Miglioretti, DL; Deyo, RA. Comparing yoga, exercise, and a self-care book for chronic low back pain: a randomized, controlled trial. *Ann Intern Med.,* 2005, Dec 20, 143(12), 849-56.

[161] Dennerstein, L; Alexander, JL; Kotz, K. The menopause and sexual functioning: a review of the population-based studies. *Annu Rev Sex Res*. 2003, 14, 64-82.

[162] Lorraine Dennerstein, PhD, Philippe Lehert, PhD, Henry Burger, MD; Janet Guthrie, PhD Sexuality. *The American Journal of Medicine,* 2005, Vol 118 (12B), 59S-63S.

[163] Bancroft, J; Loftus, J; Long, JS. Distress about sex: a national survey of women in heterosexual relationships. *Arch Sex Behav.*, 2003, Jun;32(3), 193-208.

[164] Leiblum, Sandra, R; PhD Koochaki, Patricia, E; PhD ; Rodenberg, Cynthia, A; PhD Barton, Ian P; BSc Rosen, Raymond, C. PhD Hypoactive sexual desire disorder in postmenopausal women: US results from the Women's International Study of Health and Sexuality (WISHeS). *Menopause*. 13(1), 46-56, January/February 2006.

[165] Basson, R; Graves, G, Johnston, S. SOGC Canadian Consensus on Menopause. *JOGC* 2006, in press.

In: Menopause: Vasomotor Symptoms, Systematic...   ISBN: 978-1-60876-930-8
Editors: J. Michalski, I. Nowak, pp. 165-191   © 2010 Nova Science Publishers, Inc.

Chapter VII

Consequences and Management of Menopause in Women with Breast Cancer*

C. Simmons,[1] S. Verma and M. Clemons[2]

[1] Internal Medicine Resident McMaster University
[2] Division of Medical Oncology, Toronto-Sunnybrook Regional Cancer Centre,
2075 Bayview Avenue, Toronto, Ontario, M4N 3M5, Canada

Abstract

Breast cancer is a common malignancy and remains a major health issue with significant morbitiy and mortality. Surveillance, Epidemiology and End Results (SEER) data shows that white women in the US have a 13.1% lifetime risk of developing breast cancer, while African American women have a 9.6% lifetime incidence. The lifetime risk of dying of breast cancer is 3.4% in both groups [1]. It has been known for over 100 years that breast tissue is sensitive to endogenous hormones. However, it has only become clear in recent decades that prolonged exposure to endogenous and exogenous sex steroids, particularly estrogens can lead to the development of breast cancer [2,3].

In view of the hormone dependent nature of breast cancers, issues around the management of cancer treatment related menopausal symptoms are particularly pertinent. The reasons that women with breast cancer are more prone to both the short and long term consequences of menopause are as follows:

- The average age of diagnosis with breast cancer in women is 62, making most women peri- or post-menopausal at the time of their diagnosis.
- At diagnosis, many women are taking an estrogen replacement which they are conventionally instructed to discontinue. This may result in an abrupt recurrence of menopause-associated symptoms.

---

* A version of this chapter was also published in *Trends in Breast Cancer Research*, edited by Andrew P. Yao, published by Nova Science Publishers, Inc. It was submitted for appropriate modifications in an effort to encourage wider dissemination of research.

- For post-menopausal women, therapeutic hormonal manipulation with agents such as tamoxifen and the aromatase inhibitors, leads to an adjustment of a woman's endogenous estrogen state and consequently menopausal symptoms are a common consequence.
- For pre-menopausal women receiving either endocrine or chemotherapy premature and permanent menopause is common [2] Chemotherapy and endocrine therapy with aromatase inhibitors also have additional adverse effects on bone health.
- As a consequence of improved therapy and/or earlier detection more women are surviving breast cancer and living longer [3]. As a result patients are living longer with their menopausal symptoms.

Based on the above factors, the management of menopause and its complications in breast cancer survivors is becoming an increasingly concerning issue – both in the short and long term. While estrogens and hormone replacement therapy has been studied extensively for the treatment and prevention of post-menopausal symptoms, their use in breast cancer patients is questionable. Current guidelines state that the use of hormone replacement therapies in breast cancer patients is not recommended [4]. Alternatives to this therapy include several non-hormonal agents and lifestyle modifications which will be discussed further. These therapies and recommendations may help improve the general health and quality of life in post-menopausal women with breast cancer.

Introduction

Earlier detection and better treatment have both contributed to an improved prognosis in women diagnosed with breast cancer. Of the 180,000 women diagnosed with invasive breast cancer in the United States each year, more than 80% can now expect to live at least 5 years [5]. Evidence from the Surveillance, Epidemiology, and End Results (SEER) program of the National Cancer Institute suggests that the incidence of hormone positive breast cancer is rising which may partly be due to increased use of hormone therapy. As a result, many women are left to contend with the long-lasting effects of their cancer therapy, including either natural or chemotherapy induced menopause. This brings about unique problems for this group of women as they face the symptoms and health issues not only about their cancer but also those associated with menopause and aging. The breast is an estrogen sensitive tissue and the use of estrogen to manage menopausal symptoms and associated disease states has been discouraged in breast cancer survivors. This paper will discuss the effect of estrogen on breast tissue, as well as the symptoms, consequences, and management of menopausal symptoms and complications, in breast cancer patients.

Hormones and Breast Tissue

It has been know for over 100 years that the breast tissue is sensitive to the production of endogenous hormones. This was initially shown by Beatson who demonstrated that bilateral oopherectomy resulted in remission of breast cancer in a proportion of pre-menopausal women [6]. However it has become clearer in recent decades that prolonged exposure to endogenous and exogenous sex steroids, and estrogens in particular lead to the development of the majority of breast cancers. Paradoxically, estrogen is the most frequently prescribed drug in the world, with 38% of postmenopausal American women using it [7].

Estrogen: Mechanism of Action

The mechanism of action of estrogen has been studied extensively. In the classic model for estrogen action, estrogen receptors (ER) located in the nuclei of target cells are activated by the binding of estradiol. This stimulates dimerization of the alpha and beta isoforms of the estrogen receptor which then allows interaction with specific DNA sequences within the promoters of response genes. The DNA-bound estrogen receptor then regulates target gene transcription either positively or negatively [8].

Estrogen: Breast Tissue Effects

Estradiol acts locally on the mammary gland to stimulate DNA synthesis and promote mammary bud formation [9]. It is thought that this activity is predominantly mediated by the nuclear estrogen receptor alpha. The importance of this isoform of the estrogen receptor in the development of mammary tissue is evidenced in the poor development of the mammary glands of knockout mice who are ER-alpha-null but ER-beta positive [10] The content of ER-alpha and progesterone receptors in the lobular structures of the breast is directly proportional to the rate of cellular proliferation [11]. There are 3 different types of lobular structures, with different proportions of ER and progesterone receptor (PgR) positive cells. These structures are named Lob 1 through 3 sequentially. Lob 1 contains the least differentiated cells and has the highest proportion of ER and PgR positive cells. The highest level of proliferative activity is observed in the undifferentiated lobular structures of these Lob 1 structures present in the breast of young nulliparous females [12]. Under the hormonal influences of the menstrual cycle, there is progressive differentiation into Lob 2 and Lob 3. Compared to the cells comprising Lob 1, the rate of cellular proliferation is decreased three-fold in Lob 2, and ten-fold in Lob 3 cells [13]. Lob 1 cells contain a higher percentage of ER and PgR positive cells than Lob 2 or 3, indicating a progressive decrease in the number of receptor-positive cells as the breast structure becomes more differentiated.

The biologic differences in the lobular structures of mammary tissue may have a profound implication for cancer risk. It has been found that the cells in Lob 1 are more susceptible to being transformed by chemical carcinogenesis in vitro and in experimental animals [12]. These cells are also the site of origin for ductal carcinomas. The proliferative cells differ from those that are receptor-positive, suggesting that the proliferative influence of estrogen on the breast epithelium is indirect [11].

Several factors related to reproductive development appear to predispose women to breast cancer. For example, women with early onset of menarche (before age 12 years) or late menopause (after age 55 years) have an increased risk of developing breast cancer [14]. This is felt to be due to prolonged exposure to estrogen.

The actual mechanism by which estrogen leads to the development of breast cancer is not completely understood. Generally, it is felt that estrogen promotes growth of existing malignancies in the breast. However, estrogens and their metabolic products are also shown to induce direct and indirect changes in DNA structure, such as free radical-mediated DNA damage, genetic instability, and mutations in cells in culture and in vivo, suggesting a role for estrogens in cancer initiation [15]. Estrogens may also have a pre-initiation effect in the development of breast cancer. An elevated level of estrogen detected in utero has been associated with an increased risk of breast cancer in animal models [16]. There has been indirect evidence of this in human models also. Elevated fetal estrogen levels have also been shown to permanently alter the morphology of mammary gland causing a persistent presence of epithelial structures known to be sites of malignant growth [15]. Virtually all mouse mammary tumor models and mouse xenograft models as well as many in vitro cell lines are dependent on estrogen for their growth and spread [4].

Symptoms of Menopause and Their Management

Hot Flashes

The vasomotor symptoms of a hot flash are described as a sudden transient sensation of internal heat and redness of the face and upper body. It is often accompanied by sweating and dizziness, and may be followed by a chill. In some cases it may also be accompanied by a feeling of anxiety and palpitations. Objective findings include peripheral vasodilatation, tachycardia, and large skin-conduction changes. Core body temperature is not elevated but may drop shortly after the hot flash [17]

The hot flash is the most frequent menopausal symptom. The prevalence of hot flashes in studies of naturally post-menopausal North American women ranges from 30-80%, with most symptoms decreasing over 4-5 years [18]. International studies have found that black, white, and Hispanic women report more vasomotor symptoms in menopause than Japanese or Chinese women [19]. The variation between individual women in frequency, intensity, and impact on quality of life is also substantial. Some women suffer from hot flashes as frequently as every 20 minutes, while others are barely affected at all. It is evident that the impact of hot flashes can range from minor nuisance to severe disruption of mental and physical quality of life. The reasons for this wide variability are not well understood.

Etiology

Hot flashes are due to vasomotor instability and lead to thermoregulatory changes. The thermoregulatory center in the hypothalamus is a key factor in the understanding of the cause of hot flashes. Even though core body temperature does not change, all mechanisms to promote heat loss are triggered: vasodilatation, sweating, and behavioural adjustments [17]. This triggering of heat loss mechanisms suggest that they are precipitated by a transient downward resetting of the body's thermoregulatory set point. Yet it is not clear how this happens. However, the association between a drop in circulating levels of estrogen and hot flashes has been well documented [20]. It seems that the sudden change in estrogen levels, not simply the lack of estrogen, is linked to the cause of hot flashes [21].

Breast cancer survivors report higher levels of frequency and intensity of hot flashes than age matched controls. [22]. This may be for a number of reasons:

- The average age of diagnosis with breast cancer in women is 62, making most women peri- or post-menopausal at the time of their diagnosis.
- Breast cancer is primarily a disease of postmenopausal females, and at diagnosis many women are taking estrogen replacement which they are conventionally instructed to discontinue, resulting in an abrupt recurrence of menopause-associated symptoms.
- In addition hormonal therapy (including both surgical and chemical castration) and chemotherapy can also lead to additional treatment-related side effects [23]. An example of this is tamoxifen, which is commonly associated with hot flashes [24]. Randomised trials have shown that women who receive tamoxifen have more frequent and intense hot flashes than women receiving placebo resulting in significantly more fatigue, poorer sleep quality and poorer physical health [25] For patients starting tamoxifen the pattern of hot flashes is typically one of a gradual increase over the first 2 to 3 months followed by a plateau phase and then slow dissipation [26].
- For pre-menopausal women receiving either endocrine or chemotherapy premature and permanent menopause is common [2]. Chemotherapy and endocrine therapy with aromatase inhibitors also have additional adverse effects on bone health.
- As a consequence of improved therapy and/or earlier detection more women are surviving breast cancer and living longer [27]. As a result patients are living longer with their menopausal symptoms.

Most women tolerate hot flashes and are able to remain active. However, others find them distressing and some may become less compliant with and even consider discontinuing therapy. These problems have become more pronounced as long-term tamoxifen therapy is now advocated not only for early-stage breast cancer but also for breast cancer prevention. There is therefore a continuing need for safe, effective treatments for hot flashes.

Non-Pharmacological Treatments for Hot Flashes

The conventional approach to the non-pharmacological treatment of hot flashes includes keeping a cool ambient temperature, avoiding precipitants (e.g. spicy food, coffee and alcohol), wearing loosely woven "breathable" cotton fabric, and layering clothing so that pieces can be removed [28]. Some have also suggested that regular aerobic exercise decreases the frequency and severity of hot flashes. Two surveys (one involving 1500 women), found that those who exercise regularly were less troubled by vasomotor symptoms than women who exercise sporadically [29]. Behavioural approaches such as paced respiration, progressive muscle-relaxation training and other biofeedback techniques have been found to lower the rate of hot flashes in some women [30]. A Swedish study found that acupuncture administered once or twice per week in 30 minute sessions for 8 weeks reduced the number of hot flashes [31].

It has been demonstrated that patients can benefit from a structured, often nurse led, care plan [32]. Even relatively simple symptom assessment, education, counseling and, as appropriate, specific pharmacological and behavioural interventions have been shown to lead to a statistically significant improvement in menopausal symptoms and sexual functioning. These approaches may also be combined with pharmacological therapy to improve outcome.

Pharmacological Treatments for Hot Flashes

When evaluating the efficacy of pharmacological treatment in the management of hot flashes, the placebo effect must be considered. Multiple placebo-controlled trials have shown a 25% decrease in symptoms with 4 weeks of placebo therapy [17]. There is also the suggestion that the placebo effect can account for up to a 75% reduction in symptoms in several of these studies, [33, 34 35 36 37]. This should be considered especially in the cases of anecdotal evidence and non-controlled studies of agents for the treatment of hot flashes.

Hormonal Therapy

Estrogen

Estrogen has been the most studied and most prescribed hormonal medication for the treatment of menopausal symptoms. It has a dose response effect for relieving hot flashes, and the dose can be titrated to symptomatic relief [38]. More than 40 randomized controlled trials have compared the effects of estrogen versus placebo and the effects of different estrogen preparations [39]. Most of these studies show that estrogen reliably decreases vasomotor symptoms. It has been shown to reduce the symptoms of hot flashes by 80 to 90% and effectively does this regardless of whether menopause is induced by natural cause, chemotherapy, surgery, tamoxifen use or androgen ablation therapy [17].

The Women's Health Initiative found that while long term estrogen use was beneficial to bone mineral density, it has a deleterious effect with regards to increasing the risk of breast cancer, stroke, venous thrombo-embolism and coronary artery disease [40]. The safety of short term use is not clear, and study results in this setting are pending.

Indirect evidence for the use of estrogen replacement in women with a previous breast cancer diagnosis comes from case series and cohort studies [41, 42, 43] In these, women had early stage breast cancer and were given HRT to relieve menopausal symptoms. None of these small studies showed any obvious increase in risk of breast cancer recurrence related to HRT. However, these studies were flawed in that they were non-randomized, non-controlled, and patients were likely highly selected to receive HRT. Data available at this point is preliminary and further studies are needed.

Part of the difficulty in designing clinical trials for HRT use in breast cancer survivors, it that this patient population will not accept much increased risk in recurrence of their breast cancer in order to take HRT [44] Three randomized trials are now underway. The HABITS study which opened in 1996, is an open randomized clinical study designed to assess the safety of use of hormone replacement therapy in women with radically treated in situ, stage I or early stage II breast cancer. Accrual aim is for 1300 women, currently 434 are enrolled [45]. A second Swedish study (opened in 1998) and a British study (opened in 2001) are each assigning women with breast cancer to HRT or no HRT for 2 years [4]. Until results from these randomized trials are available increased risk related to HRT for women with a prior diagnosis of breast cancer cannot be ruled out. In the interim, national guidelines recommend that clinicians should remain cautious about using estrogen replacement therapy in women with a previous diagnosis of breast cancer and particularly so in those with estrogen receptor positive disease [4]. In reality less than 5% of breast cancer patients are actually treated with HRT [23].

Progesterone

Megestrol acetate is a progestational agent that relieves hot flashes. Placebo-controlled, double-blind, randomised crossover trials in both male and female cancer patients have shown that patients assigned megestrol acetate had a 75-80% reduction in their hot flashes compared with a 20-25% reduction seen in those assigned placebo [46]. Minimal adverse effects were noted in the 4 week treatment period; however, 31% of women did experience withdrawal bleeding at 1 to 4 weeks after cessation of therapy. Megestrol acetate appears to be equally effective for women receiving concurrent tamoxifen. Interestingly in this setting there was a marked increase in hot flashes for a few days after initiation of megestrol acetate, before a gradual reduction of hot flashes over 2-3 weeks.

DMPA is a long acting intramuscularly administered progestin that has also been used in the treatment of hot flashes [47]. It is given once every two weeks intramuscularly. One study described a series of patients treated with DMPA who reported a 90% decrease in hot flashes in women treated with 3 DMPA infections at 2 week intervals, with control of hot flashes lasting up to 6 months in some patients. There is a large phase 3 study currently being conducted by the North Central Cancer Treatment Group. Transdermal progestin has also been studied and shown to have an 83% reduction in the symptoms of hot flashes [48].

While progestagens are clearly efficacious and work as well as an estrogen to control hot flashes, their use has potential drawbacks. Their side effects include vaginal spotting, withdrawal bleeding, cramping, weight gain, increased appetite and depression. There is also an increased risk of thromboembolic events, in particular when used concurrently with tamoxifen [23]. In breast cancer patients there are also no conclusive data as to whether or not progestins have a detrimental effect on breast related prognosis, although higher doses are already established in the treatment of metastatic breast cancer. Clinical trials addressing this issue are ongoing [49].

Tibolone

Tibolone is a synthetic derivative of a C-19 nortestosterone compound [50]. It is administered orally and is converted into active metabolites with estrogenic, progestagenic, and androgenic properties. Developed as an alternative to combined estrogen/progestagen replacement therapy, it has weak estrogenic, progestogenic and androgenic properties. It has been found to reduce symptoms of hot flashes significantly more than placebo in randomized controlled trials, and has been found to be as effective as combined HRT in the short-term [51]

The main unwanted side effect of Tibolone is breakthrough bleeding. There is also some speculation about an increase in cardiovascular disease based upon its effect on lipid profile and reduction in HDL [52].

No long term data exists on tibolone and risk of breast cancer. Data from most in vitro experiments show that tibolone inhibits sulfatases that convert endogenous estrogens to their active form and suggests a prevention role in the development of breast cancer cell lines [53] Animal experiments have shown that tibolone is at least as effective as tamoxifen in preventing development and growth of breast tumours in the rat model [54]. However, one in vitro study actually found that tibolone increased the proliferation of breast cancer cell lines [55].

Studies with short term tibolone use show that there is no increase in breast density, as opposed to HRT which does induce an increase in breast density [56]. This suggests that tibolone has no proliferative effect on normal mammary epithelium in humans. In addition, it has been shown to have an inhibitory effect on endometrial cells which suggests a decrease in endometrial carcinoma.

In summary, tibolone is an effective alternative to HRT for the short-term management of menopausal symptoms, and although there is no data on breast cancer risk in humans, surrogate markers suggest that it may be safer than HRT. Its overall safety has yet to be determined.

Non-Hormonal Therapy

Serotonin reuptake inhibitors

Serotonin may be one of several neurotransmitters involved in the development of hot flashes and its potential role in the mechanism of hot flashes has been studied extensively [57]. Estrogen withdrawal is associated with decreased levels of circulating serotonin, as well as an up-regulation in serotonin receptors in the hypothalamus. Activation of certain serotonin receptors has been shown to mediate heat loss [58]. However, the role of serotonin in central regulatory pathways is complex, as activation of some receptors induces a negative feedback and inhibition of other serotonin receptors. Therefore, the effect of a change in serotonin level varies depending on the type of receptor activated.

In the 1990s, some clinicians anecdotally observed a decrease in hot flashes in post-menopausal women being treated for depression with selective serotonin reuptake inhibitors and other newer antidepressants. Studies were then developed to assess the role of these agents for treatment of hot flashes.

The first agent to undergo investigation for its role in management of hot flashes was venlafaxine [59]. In an open-label nonrandomized series of 28 breast cancer survivors there was a 50% reduction in the combined end point of hot flash frequency and severity with the use of venlafaxine [59]. Researchers then performed a double blind placebo controlled trial of 191 women with either a history of breast cancer or reluctance to take hormonal treatment because of fear of breast cancer, randomized to placebo versus one of three venlafaxine doses (37.5mg, 75 mg, or 150 mg). After four weeks of therapy, the placebo group reported a 27% reduction in hot flash scores, whereas the treatment groups had a 37%, 61%, and 61% reduction at the three different dose levels respectively [60]. The side effects of dry mouth, decreased appetite, nausea, and constipation were found more frequently in the venlafaxine group than in the placebo group. Overall improvement in quality of life was statistically significant in the venlafaxine groups over placebo.

Fluoxetine has been shown to decrease hot flashes in a randomized, double-blinded placebo controlled crossover trial [61]. Similar to the venlafaxine trail, the women enrolled had either previous diagnosis of breast cancer or concerns about taking hormonal therapy. Some patients were also taking tamoxifen or raloxifene during the study period. The patients randomized to receive Fluoxetine experienced a 50% reduction in hot flashes compared with a 36% reduction for those using placebo.

Likewise, the SSRI paroxetine has been studied in an open label pilot study in 30 breast cancer survivors. After 4 weeks of therapy patients experienced a 67% reduction in the frequency of hot flashes experienced [62] Side effects include somnolence that necessitated cessation of therapy or dose reduction. Currently double-blind placebo controlled trials are underway [57].

These newer antidepressants are therefore effective for the non-hormonal treatment of hot flashes and they have the added benefit of early efficacy in a number of days within onset of therapy. They are also efficacious in patients receiving Tamoxifen. They were initially developed as antidepressants and therefore also improve anxiety, insomnia, and irritability, and, of course, depression which may affect many women diagnosed with breast cancer.

Clonidine

Clonidine hydrochloride is an anti-hypertensive agent. It is a centrally active adrenergic agonist that reduces vascular reactivity. Placebo trials of oral clonidine found it effective to varying degrees in controlling hot flashes caused by natural or surgical menopause [23]. Studies of oral and transdermal clonidine in breast cancer survivors have shown a statistically significant (P < 0.0001), but clinically moderate (20% reduction form baseline) reduction in hot flashes p63, 64 65]

Unfortunately, the side effects of Clonidine for many patients include postural hypotension, difficulty sleeping, constipation, dry mouth and drowsiness [23]. At this point the drug-related toxicities seem to outweigh the modest benefits of this agent.

Vitamin E

Vitamin E (Tocopherol) has also been reported as an agent that improves hot flash symptoms. Despite a lack of prospective evidence, it has been recommended for many years. A recent NCCTG study examined the benefit of moderate dose vitamin E (800 IU/d) in a randomized placebo-controlled crossover trail in 120 women with a history of breast cancer [66]. A slight decrease in hot flash frequency (1 less hot flash per day) was found in the vitamin E group.

Vitamin E is a non-toxic agent with no hormonal properties. It is also inexpensive and is widely available. For these reasons there are advantages to recommending the use of vitamin E as it allows patients to get the well described placebo effect. However, recent concerns have been raised about the use of high dose vitamin E.

Herbal

Many herbal remedies and alternative medicines are marketed to women for the management of hot flashes and other menopausal symptoms. Many of these substances have real physiologic effects but are largely untested and totally unregulated by laws governing other pharmaceutical agents. Some of the herbal treatments will be discussed below.

Black cohosh

Black cohosh is a perennial herb in the buttercup family and is commonly known in rural areas as black snakeroot, rattleweed, bugbane, bugwort, and sometimes squaw root. [67]. Black cohosh is widely used in Europe to treat menopausal symptoms [68]. It appears to be free of significant side effects and drug interactions, however, long-term effects of its use are unknown. In Germany, where the herb is approved for use in treating menopausal symptoms, it is recommended only for short-term (fewer than six months) use [69].

Most clinical trials have been conducted black cohosh root extract developed in Germany and standardized to contain (20 mg) of black cohosh extract per tablet. [70] The general experience suggested from the herbal literature is that black cohosh is a safe and effective agent for the relief of menopausal symptoms, including vasomotor instability. Research by the German manufacturer has shown that black cohosh supplements have no effect on follicle-stimulating hormone, leutinizing hormone, estrone and estradiol, progesterone, sex hormone binding globulin, the vaginal maturation index, or endometrial thickness [71]. Therefore, in spite of the fact that black cohosh is said to be estrogenic, it in fact does not appear to act as an estrogen.

One recent publication on black cohosh was done in 85 breast cancer survivors. Subjects received placebo or black cohosh, 20 mg twice daily. Both treatment and placebo groups had significant declines in number and intensity of hot flashes over time, but the differences between the groups were not statistically significant [72]. This study may not be universally applicable, as fifty-nine of the 85 women were on tamoxifen. Only nine women who took black cohosh were not also taking tamoxifen, and these nine women had very marked reduction in symptoms. Unfortunately the subset was too small for independent statistical analysis. These findings do not completely negate the use of black cohosh for the management of hot flashes, as it may be that tamoxifen dampens the effectiveness of black cohosh. Further trials are needed.

Dong quai

This root, which has vasodilatory and antispasmodic effects, has been used in Chinese medicine for more than 2,000 years [73]. In one double-blind randomized, placebo-controlled study, 71 women with menopausal symptoms, including hot flushes or night sweats, were assigned to receive dong quai or placebo for 24 weeks. The results showed no significant difference in relief of menopausal vasomotor symptoms between the two groups [74]. The study also showed no difference in endometrial thickness, maturation of vaginal cells, serum estradiol, or estrone levels. The authors concluded that dong quai, when used alone, was no more useful than placebo in the treatment of menopausal symptoms.

Traditional Chinese herbalists have faulted this study because dong quai is not usually used as solo therapy, but is used in conjunction with other herbs. They maintain that the synergistic effect of dong quai acting with other herbs accounts for the beneficial effects. To date, however, it can only be concluded that dong quai used alone is no better than placebo in reducing menopausal vasomotor symptoms.

Nonetheless, dong quai is promoted and sold as a single botanical, often in very low doses, (far lower than the 7 to 12 g used by some traditional Chinese medicine practitioners). One branded product of dong quai, Rejuvex, also contains bovine ovarian, uterine, mammary, and pituitary tissues. The ingestion of bovine brain and spinal cord tissue imposes a potential risk for development of new variant Creutzfeldt-Jakob disease, also known as bovine spongiform encephalopathy or mad cow disease [75]. Considering an absence of proved efficacy, adulteration with animal tissues, and potential for photosensitization, neoplasia, coagulopathy, and herb-drug interactions, the use of Dong Quai is not recommended.

Phytoestrogens

Asian women have fewer menopausal symptoms, and report fewer hot flashes [76]. This has led to interest in dietary differences, in particular the consumption of phytoestrogens. Phytoestrogens are plant-derived estrogens that are found principally in soybeans and soy-based dishes. They can bind to estrogen receptors and have weak estrogen-like effects which could alleviate hot flashes. Soybeans also contain proteins called isoflavones which share many of the properties of endogenous estrogens and compete with these by binding to estrogen receptors causing both estrogen agonist and/or antagonist effects [77]. Based on anecdotal evidence of hot flash relief with soy extracts, several clinical trials have been conducted to determine the efficacy of phytoestrogens in the treatment of menopausal symptoms.

A recent randomised trial in 123 breast cancer survivors showed no benefit for a soy beverage containing 90 mg of isoflavones over placebo [78]. Another double-blind, randomized trial assessed 155 breast cancer survivors in the United States with substantial hot flashes [79]. Subjects were given a soy product formulated in 600-mg tablets each containing 50 mg of soy isoflavones; dosage was 1 tablet 3 times a day (equal to 150 mg/d of isoflavones). Results showed that the soy product was no more effective than placebo in relieving vasomotor symptoms.

Another double-blind, parallel, multicenter, randomized, placebo-controlled trial assessed the effect of daily dietary supplementation with soy protein on hot flashes in postmenopausal Italian women [80]. Eligible women were experiencing at least 7 moderate-to-severe hot flashes per 24 hours during at least 2 of the 4 weeks before the study. For 12 weeks, 51 women received 60 g of isolated soy protein containing 40 g of proteins and 76 mg of isoflavones (aglycone units); 53 women received 60 g of casein (placebo) containing 40 g of proteins but no isoflavones. By the end of the study the women taking soy protein had a

45% reduction in hot flashes compared with a 30% reduction in women taking placebo ($P <$ .01).

Most clinical trials performed with phytoestrogens do not show a clinically or statistically significant improvement of hot flashes over placebo [81]. However, it is theoretically possible that concentrated phytoestrogen and red clover supplements may have estrogenic actions in the breast and endometrium [82] and the presence of coumarins in some clover species may also affect coagulation [83]. In clinical practice therefore it would seem prudent to encourage patients to consume foods rich in phytoestrogens, such as vegetables, grains and legumes; which are also excellent sources of fibre, unsaturated protein, vitamins and minerals instead of concentrated supplements [23].

Other pharmacological interventions

Several other drugs have been tested in the treatment of hot flashes. Some agents have been shown to be no more effective than placebo, such as propranolol and gamolenic acid [84]. Others were effective but limited by toxicities, such as methyldopa. For others there is little available long-term data, for example gabapentin [85].

It is important that patients are aware that some women experience no benefit from one hot flash therapy while others may report a substantial improvement with placebo. In addition it should be emphasized that each therapy should be tried for at least a month as some take time to work [84].

Urogenital Symptoms

In addition to the above mentioned thermoregulatory changes, urogenital changes can occur in postmenopausal women. These can be divided into those resulting in vulvovaginal symptoms, such as vaginal itching, discomfort, and dyspareunia, and those resulting in lower urinary tract symptoms, such as frequency, urgency, recurrent urinary tract infections (UTIs), and incontinence. These characteristic changes are caused by a combination of physiologic aging and the effects of decreased estrogen levels. The effects of estrogen deprivation on vulvovaginal tissue have been well established [86]. As women go through menopause, the vaginal and urethral epithelium becomes progressively deprived of estrogen and the tissue loses epithelial thickness, rogation, moisture, vascularity, and elasticity. These changes result in thin, flat vulvar tissue. In addition, the vagina shortens and narrows, with a resulting change in the angle of the urethral meatus relative to the symthysis pubis from 90° to 180°. This decreased distance between the urethra and introitus increases the chance of urethral symptomatology with any type of vaginal manipulation [20].

In addition to these physical changes, vaginal cytology also changes with menopause, from primarily superficial cells to primarily parabasal cells. This accounts for the loss of rogation, elasticity, and vascularity. Decreased elasticity and thinness leads to increased susceptibility to trauma, resulting in bleeding, fine petechiae, and ulcerations. There is also a decrease in vaginal blood flow, vaginal secretions and vaginal lubrication in response to sexual stimulation, which may lead to dyspareunia.

Alkalinization of the vaginal environment (a major natural defense mechanism) is lost in the postmenopausal state. This is caused by a decrease in cellular glycogen levels, which in turn causes a decrease in the amount of lactobacilli found in the vagina. This leads to a decrease in the amount of lactic acid present and subsequently an increase in the vaginal pH. The loss of this natural defense mechanism allows the vagina to become colonized with pathogenic bacteria and enteric flora, which can predispose women to urinary tract infections.

The true prevalence of urogenital atrophy is unknown because many women view symptoms of vaginal dryness, dyspareunia, incontinence, and nocturia as an inevitable part of the aging process. Also, some women are embarrassed by these symptoms and only about 25% will seek any form of treatment, either from an urologist or a gynecologist [87].

These problems are more prevalent in cancer survivors undergoing premature menopause as a result of both age-related loss of endogenous estrogens and the effects of their cancer therapy [23]. Tamoxifen in particular is known to increase the frequency of gynecological symptoms in both pre- and postmenopausal women [88]

Non-pharmacological

Non-hormonal, drug free bio-adhesive vaginal moisturizers have been shown to be efficacious alternatives to estrogen therapy. These moisturizers (such as Replens, and K-Y jelly) substantially reduce vaginal dryness and dyspareunia in breast cancer survivors [89]. The water soluble lubricants are usually found to be more effective as they do not become as viscous after application. However, these lubricants do not relieve all vaginal symptoms and do not alter urinary symptoms.

Pharmacological treatment

The standard treatment for atrophic vulvovaginitis and urogenital symptoms in menopausal women has been estrogen replacement therapy. Estrogen replacement increases urethral tone and sensitivity to neurotransmitters and relaxes the bladder smooth muscle [90]. It also results in a change in vaginal cytology from predominantly parabasal to superficial cells, a decrease in the vaginal pH, and an increase in the vaginal blood flow [91]. Many routes of estrogen administration have been studied, including oral, transdermal, and vaginal.

The vaginal route has been the most explored for the treating of atrophic vulvovaginitis, because this route allows delivery directly to the urogenital tissues, avoids the enterohepatic first-pass effect, and results in a more rapid local response. It may also have a beneficial effect on the urethra, as it increases urethral resistance, thickens the vaginal and urethral walls, and improves the underlying connective tissue and vascular supply.

In addition, lower doses of vaginally administered estradiol-releasing vaginal rings and estriol pessaries are as efficacious as topical creams in alleviating lower urinary tract symptoms [92]. Plasma levels of estrogen remain virtually unchanged with use of the vaginal ring, whereas topically administered estrogen tablets have been shown to cause a rise in systemic plasma estrogen levels to pre-menopausal range [93]. However, there is no data to assess the risk of vaginal estrogen use in patients with breast cancer.

It must be noted, however, that the reduction of symptoms related to the urogenital system will be gradual, as urogenital atrophy is a chronic condition subject to relapse if treatment is discontinued. An alternative to ERT is tibolone (a weak estrogenic compound mentioned above).

Bone Complications of Menopause

Another consequence of the menopause is the development of osteoporosis. Peak bone mass is attained in women between the ages of 25-35, then gradually declines until menopause, when the rate of decline in bone mass decreases at a faster rate. This is the result of increases in the rate of bone remodelling and an imbalance between osteoblast and osteoclast activity [94]. Irreversible bone loss occurs primarily in trabecular bone. There are two phases to bone loss – a rapid phase which lasts approximately 5 years and produces a loss of 3% per year in the spine, and a slower phase of bone loss that begins at age 55. The exact mechanism of this is not known, however it is felt to be hormone independent, as it is also observed in men.

Estrogen has a direct effect on bone cells to promote mineral density and reduce bone resorption by osteoclasts. Estrogen is also believed to act on bone through its effects on bone marrow stromal and mononuclear cells. These cells produce lower amounts of interleukins and tumour necrosis factor when an adequate amount of estrogen is present, and more amounts are produced in the absence of estrogen. The net result of loss of estrogen in menopause is a dramatic acceleration in bone loss.

The effects of estrogen in preserving bone mineral density and in increasing the risk of breast cancer should mean that survivors of breast cancer are at lower risk for osteoporosis than the general population [95]. However, the decline in estrogen during the perimenopausal transition caused by adjuvant chemotherapy can accelerate the normal age-related decline in bone density even further than expected [96].

Long term data on fractures in women with chemotherapy induced menopause are unavailable. It is known that osteoporosis causes an increase risk of bone fractures. The morbidity and mortality associated with hip fracture, (most common fracture caused by falls), is substantial. It is therefore recommended that those diagnosed with this condition receive treatment to decrease the risk of fractures.

The risk factors for the development of osteoporosis, as outlined by the Royal College of Physicians, include the following: premature menopause (before age 40); family history of osteoporosis; taken steroids for more than 6 months; premenopausal amenorrhea for more than 6 months; liver, thyroid, or renal disease; history of excess alcohol intake; taken GnRH analogues for more than 6 months. Anyone with these risk factors should be offered bone density screening, and those with low bone mass should be considered for therapy.

Non-pharmacological

Osteoporosis can now be prevented and treated with a number of approaches that do not involve estrogen or progesterone. Diet, exercise, and an appropriate intake of calcium (1-1.5gm per day) and vitamin D (400-800IU per day), are important factors in the prevention of osteoporosis [97]. In addition, certain risk factors may be modified. For example, smoking cessation, weight bearing exercise, and treatment of any metabolic or endocrine disorders will decrease the risk of bone loss.

Pharmacological

Estrogen

While the above mentioned strategies may decrease the risk of bone loss, none are as effective in decreasing bone resorption as estrogen. Thus estrogen should be considered to prevent further bone loss not only in women with established osteoporosis, but also in those with accelerated bone loss. Therapeutic measures for osteoporosis have traditionally included HRT. Estrogens play a key role in the activation of osteoblast and osteoclast activity, and preserve bone mineral density and reduce bone resorption by osteoclasts. This has been evidenced in various studies, which have shown HRT to decrease the incidence of vertebral fractures in postmenopausal women [98, 99]. In addition, the recent Women's Health Initiative study found that women taking HRT had fewer fractures than women not taking HRT [100] The associated side effects of HRT are well documented, and have been mentioned previously in this chapter. It is unclear if bone density loss is accelerated after withdrawal of estrogen replacement. A recent study has suggested that at 10 years post discontinuation of HRT bone mineral density and fracture risk were similar to patients who had not received estrogens [101].

Bisphosphonates

Alternative agents are available for the management of osteoporosis. The Early Postmenopausal Intervention Cohort (EPIC) has show bisphosphonates to be almost as effective as HRT in increasing bone density by the and also to prevent the loss of bone density normally seen when given either during or after adjuvant chemotherapy [96], [102]. Alendronate, a bisphosphonate has effects comparable to those of estrogen for both the treatment of osteoporosis (10 mg/day or 70 mg once a week) and for its prevention (5 mg/day). Other agents, such as risendronate and etidronate have similar effects to alendronate and increase in bone density and a decrease in fractures. Zolendronate is another option for osteoporosis prevention as it has been shown to produce effects on bone turnover and bone density with once yearly dosing that are as great as those achieved with daily bisphosphonate dosing [103]. Indeed, a yearly intravenous bisphosphonate could easily be incorporated into cancer follow-up clinics.

The side effect profiles of the oral bisphosphonates are related primarily to pill esophagitis. Therefore oral bisphosphonate usage is complicated by their need to be administered on an empty stomach and in an upright position to decrease the gastrointestinal side effects.

The safety and efficacy of long-term alendronate (5 and 10 mg/day) was demonstrated in a seven year study of postmenopausal women with osteoporosis. The benefits of bisphosphonates were found to be similar to HRT in women to treat or prevent osteoporosis, making these agents an appropriate non-hormonal alternative to HRT in women with a previous breast cancer diagnosis or other contraindications to HRT.

Tamoxifen

Tamoxifen maintains bone density in postmenopausal women and is another alternative to HRT in women with breast cancer [104]. Although it has antiestrogen effects on breast tissue, it has a weak estrogenic effect on bone. In a two-year study, tamoxifen 20mg daily caused a 1.7% increase in radial bone density and a 1.2% increase in lumbar spine density, compared to a decrease in bone density in the placebo group. Also, in the Breast Cancer Prevention Trial (NSABP-P1), there were slightly fewer fractures of the hip, radius, and spine in women receiving tamoxifen versus those receiving placebo (RR 0.81, 95% CI 0.63 to 1.05) [105].

In premenopausal women, however, tamoxifen may result in bone loss. In a British study of the effect of tamoxifen on bone mineral density (BMD), it was found that in premenopausal women, BMD decreased progressively in the lumbar spine (P < .001) and in the hip (P < .05) for women on tamoxifen compared to the placebo group [104]. The mean annual loss in lumbar BMD per year in the tamoxifen-treated women who remained premenopausal throughout the study period was 1.44% over the three year study period, (1.88% calculated on an intent-to-treat basis). This should be considered in treatment of premenopausal women for prevention of breast cancer. In premenopausal women, other alternate choices for the management of osteoporosis should be made.

The side effect profile of tamoxifen must also be considered, as its estrogenic effects on the uterus can precipitate endometrial hyperplasia and occasionally neoplasia. Tamoxifen may also increase a woman's risk of deep vein thrombosis. Other side effects are also related to its anti-estrogenic effects, which include a worsening of hot flushes.

Raloxifene

Raloxifene is a selective estrogen receptor modulator (SERM) and it is currently the only SERM licensed for use in osteoporosis. As part of the MORE study, post-menopausal women with osteoporosis were randomized to receive either Raloxifene (60mg or 120mg) or placebo, in addition to calcium and vitamin D. At 2 years, there was a 38% reduction in vertebral fractures in women with a previous history of fractures and a 52% reduction in those without a history of prior fractures for the women who took Raloxifene compared to placebo [106]. It was also shown that bone density increased by 2.4% in the lumbar spine and hip which is slightly less than with estrogen. Further data comparing tamoxifen with Raloxifene will be available from the ongoing STAR trial [107].

In contrast to estrogen and tamoxifen, raloxifene does not appear to cause endometrial hyperplasia. Raloxifene's exact role in the menopausal management is not clear, but it is a reasonable option for prevention of osteoporosis, in particular because of the diminishing role of estrogen. However concern has been raised about increased relapse rates in women given raloxifene after 5 years of tamoxifen [108].

Calcitonin

Calcitonin is a natural hormone which causes a brief inhibition of bone resorption by osteoclasts. It is not deficient in patients with osteoporosis, but additional calcitonin has been shown to enhance the inhibitory effect on osteoclastic activity. It is given either by subcutaneous injection or intranasally, and is effective therapy for osteoporosis and particularly for bone pain associated with fractures. Nasal calcitonin has been found to increase bone density (by 2.5 percent over a three year period in some reports) [109], and reduce fracture rates (by 48 to 77 percent in various studies). This improvement in BMD may be less than that observed with estrogen or bisphosphonates. One study has suggested that calcitonin may not protect the hip as well as the spine, however this was not found in other reports [110].

Side effects are related to local nasal irritation and occasional systemic effects such as flushing or nausea and long term use of calcitonin can lead to the development of antibodies and resistance. This has been observed in the treatment of Paget's disease, and is usually preceded by a rise in serum alkaline phosphatase. However, such a warning system does not exist in osteoporosis [111] and has led to some reluctance in the use of calcitonin for long-term treatment of osteoporosis. However, some studies have shown that nasal calcitonin maintains efficacy in preventing perimenopausal bone loss after as long as five years of continuous use.

Cardiovascular Complications

Cardiovascular disease remains the number one killer of women and men in North America. Women have a decreased risk compared to men until they reach menopause, at which point their risk equals that of men. The protective effects of estrogen on cardiovascular disease risk have been studied extensively. Estrogen modulates serum cholesterol by decreasing serum levels of low density lipoprotein (LDL) cholesterol and elevating levels of high density lipoprotein (HDL) cholesterol. Estrogen also has a direct effect on vasomotor tone and vascular wall cholesterol uptake and metabolism. In postmenopausal women, cholesterol levels gradually rise and the risk of atherosclerotic disease increases substantially. There is concern, therefore, that prolonged estrogen deprivation may put survivors of breast cancer at higher risk for heart disease. There is as yet no clinical data on the importance of estrogen deprivation in such women.

Non-pharmacological

Conventional cardiovascular disease prevention strategies should not be denied to cancer survivors. These include the management of known risk factors for heart disease, such as hypertension, diabetes and elevated lipid levels, as well as the encouragement of smoking cessation [112]. A recent prospective observational study found that exercise and increased physical activity had a strong, graded, inverse association with the risk of coronary events and total cardiovascular events. This data indicates that walking and vigorous exercise is associated with substantial reduction in the incidence of cardiovascular events among postmenopausal women, irrespective of race or ethnic group, age, or body mass index. In contrast, prolonged sitting was found to predict increase in cardiovascular risk [113].

Pharmacological

Estrogen

Traditionally, estrogen replacement therapy was felt to be of cardio-protective benefit in menopausal women because of its positive effects on lipid profile. However, with increasing evidence to indicate that HRT increases the risk of cardiovascular disease, it is now not recommended for primary or secondary prevention of heart disease in postmenopausal women.

This data comes from several studies, including the Heart and Estrogen/Progestin Replacement Study (HERS), a randomized placebo-controlled trial of HRT in women at high risk for cardiac events. No significant benefit of HRT was seen, and despite favorable changes in serum lipid profiles, there was an increase in cardiac events in patients treated with HRT during the first year of the trial. Thromboembolic event rates also increased in the treatment arm to a level that was comparable to Tamoxifen therapy.

The Women's Health Initiative also studied the effect of HRT on cardiovascular risk and found no benefit. The study was stopped early after a median of 5.2 years follow-up due to significant increased incidences of coronary heart disease (Hazard Ratio (HR) 1.29), stroke (HR 1.41), pulmonary embolism (HR2.13) and breast cancer (HR 1.26). Decreases in the risks of colorectal cancer and hip fractures were also found. Of note, the concurrent Women's Health Initiative study of ERT in hysterectomised women is still ongoing.

Currently, the American Heart Association (AHA) guidelines for estrogen therapy suggest that estrogen should not be prescribed for the primary or secondary prevention of CHD, and that it should be discontinued if an acute CHD event occurs and should not be resumed as a secondary prevention strategy.

Statins

Statins have well-established efficacy in both primary and secondary prevention of ischemic heart disease [114]. Studies comparing the use of statins with estrogen replacement have also shown the statins to be more effective in improving LDL cholesterol, triglyceride and HDL cholesterol profiles [115] The HPS(?) study was a large, multicenter, randomized placebo-controlled study of statin therapy in patients at high risk for cardiovascular events. It found that statin therapy taken over 5 years safely reduces the risk of heart attack, stroke, and death in high-risk patients. These findings were irrespective of lipid levels, age, sex or additional treatments. To this end, all women (and men) at high risk for heart disease should be considered for statin therapy [116]

In addition to cardioprotective benefits, statins have recently been evaluated as chemopreventitive agents for several types of cancer, including breast cancer. They offer a theoretical benefit through down regulation of Ras, up-regulation of p27, and alteration in estrogen levels. Recent in vitro studies also showed inhibition of the human breast cancer cell line MCF-7 by several commonly used statins [117]. However, findings from the Sentara Health Plan presented at American Society of Clinical Oncology (ASCO) 2003 showed no preventative benefit in women taking statin therapy, and in fact an increase in the prevalence of breast cancer in women under 50 years of age who were taking this medication [118].

While further studies are indicated to evaluate the role of statins in chemoprevention of breast cancer, they do remain an effective way of reducing cardiovascular risk in high risk patients.

Tamoxifen

Tamoxifen has been shown to lower the levels of total and low-density lipoprotein cholesterol in postmenopausal women without affecting the high density lipoprotein cholesterol. In contrast, it has minimal effects on the lipid profile of premenopausal women [119]. It has also been shown to reduce levels of CRP and other markers of inflammation which have been found to play a crucial role in the development of atherosclerosis, further showing a theoretical preventative benefit [120].

An increase in risk of DVT with Tamoxifen use has been shown in many studies. This increase in coagulation may have negative effects on cardiac risk, promoting clot formation in the coronary system as well as the peripheral vasculature.

The impact of the above changes in terms of development of cardiovascular disease in patients with breast cancer is not clear. Some studies have suggested a slight reduction in the incidence of coronary events with Tamoxifen; however, the National Surgical Adjuvant Breast and Bowel Project prevention trial (P-1) did not find a reduction in the risk of coronary events associated with use of tamoxifen.

Raloxifene

Like tamoxifen, raloxifene also lowers serum low-density lipoprotein (LDL) cholesterol concentrations but does not raise serum high-density lipoprotein (HDL) cholesterol concentrations [119]. The effect of raloxifene on the prevention of heart disease is currently being studied (RUTH study). Previous animal studies have shown that whereas estrogen therapy resulted in a 70% reduction in coronary artery plaque in monkeys, raloxifene had no effect. In fact, these monkeys treated with raloxifene had two to three times more atherosclerosis than those receiving estrogen. The results of further studies in humans have yet to be seen.

Summary

Menopause and its complications is becoming a greater concern for breast cancer survivors, as earlier detection and advances in therapy are leading to prolonged survival rates. At this point, estrogen therapy is not recommended for breast cancer survivors, due to its effects on breast tissue and role in the development of breast cancer itself. Nevertheless, the symptoms and health complications that may arise during and after menopause are concerning and have been shown to have a significant impact on quality of life.

This chapter has summarized some of the treatment options for the symptoms of hot flashes and urogenital symptoms associated with menopause. It should be emphasized that the appropriateness of each of these should be assessed on an individual basis. Many patients are reassured when caregivers address their symptoms. Some women may also find that using a treatment algorithm will give them a degree of control over these particularly distressing symptoms. General approaches to improving overall health (smoking cessation, exercise, diet and modifying alcohol consumption) should also be promoted as aids and adjunctive methods of improving quality of life.

With regards to health risks associated with menopause, it is becoming increasingly evident that estrogens may not be the optimal therapy to decrease risks of cardiovascular disease, and results from the women's health initiative actually implicate estrogens as increasing the risk of cardiovascular events. It should be remembered that cardiovascular disease is still the number one cause of mortality in North American women, and that preventative measures should be used in high risk individuals, including statin therapy, blood pressure modification, optimization of diabetes control and smoking cessation. The effects of selective estrogen receptor modulators on cardiac risk are still under assessment but may provide alternatives in the future.

Concerns about the development of osteoporosis are also evident in this patient population. At this point estrogens still provide excellent effects on the prevention of bone resorption, but alternatives including bisphosphonates may be more appropriate in breast cancer patients. In addition, some selective estrogen receptors may also offer preventative benefits in both the development of osteoporosis and breast cancer recurrence.

While breast cancer continues to be a prominent disease in women, our treatments are improving, and the age of breast cancer patients and survivors is increasing. While our ability to fight this disease improves, we still face challenges in the treatment and prevention of age and menopause related illnesses. The above has been a summary of medications and approaches that may be used by health professionals to help patients deal with menopausal symptoms and complications.

References

[1]   DeVita, et al. *Cancer principles and practice of oncology 16th edition*. Section 2, malignant tumors of the breast. 2001, Lippincott Williams and Wilkins, 1651.

[2]   Byrne, J; Fears, TR; Gail, MH; Pee, D; Connelly, RR; Austin, DF; Holmes, GF; Holmes, FF; Latourette, HB; Meigs, JW. Early menopause in long- term survivors of cancer during adolescence. *Am J Obstet Gynecol* 1992, 166, 788- 793.

[3]   www.cancer.gov/cancer_information/cancer_type/breast

[4]   Pritchard, et al. Clinical practice guidelines for the care and treatment of breast cancer: 14. The role of hormone replacement therapy in women with a previous diagnosis of breast cancer. *Canadian Medical Association Journal*, Volume 166, Number, 8, 2002.

[5]   Burstein, JH; et al. Primary care for survivors of breast cancer. *N Engl J Med,*, Vol. 343, No. 15, October 12, 2002. pp 1086-1094.

[6]   Beatson, GT. On the treatment of inoperable cases of carcinoma of themamma: suggestions for a new method of treatment, with illustrative cases. *Lancet*. 1896, 2, 104-7.

[7]   Keating, NL; Cleary, PD; Rossi, AS; Zaslavsky, AM; Ayanian, JZ. Use of hormone replacement therapy by postmenopausal women in the United States. *Ann Intern Med*. 1999, 130, 545-53.

[8]   Gruber, C; et al. Production and actions of estrogens. *N Engl J Med.*, Vol. 346, No. 5, January., 31, 2002.

[9]   Clemons, M; et al. Estrogen and the risk of breast cancer. *N Engl J Med.*, 2001, Vol. 344, No. 4, January 25,

[10]   Couse, JF; Korach, JS. Estrogen receptor-null mice *Endocr Rev.*, 1999, 20, 358.

[11]   Russo, J; Ao, X; Grill, C; Russo, IH. Pattern of distribution of cells poitive for estrogen receptor alpha and progesterone receptor in relation to proliferating cells in the mammary gland. *Breast Cancer Res Treat.*, 1999, 53, 217.

[12]   Russo, J. Up To Date Online version 11 2 Breast development and Anatomy, in www.uptodate.com.

[13]   Russo, J; Hu, YF; Silva, ID. Cancer risk related to mammary. *Microsc Res Tech.* 2001 52, 204.

[14]   Hulka, BS; Stark, AT. Breast cancer: cause and prevention. *Lancet* 1995, *346* 883-887,.

[15]   Hilakivi-Clarke, L. Estrogens, BRCA1 and Breast Cancer. *Cancer Research* 2000, 60, 4993-5001, September 15,.

[16]   Hilakivi-Clarke, L; Clarke, R; Onojafe, I; Raygada, M; Cho, E; Lippman, ME. A maternal diet high in n-6 polyunsaturated fats alters mammary gland development, puberty onset, and breast cancer risk among female rat offspring. *Proc Natl Acad Sci. USA*, 1997, *94* 9372–9377.

[17]   Shanafelt, TD; et al. Pathophysiology and Treatment of Hot Flashes. *Mayo Clin Proc.*, 2002, 77, 1207-1218.

[18]   Daly, E; Gray, A; Barlow, D; McPherson, K; Roche, M; Vessey, M. Measuring the impact of menopausal symptoms on quality of life. *BMJ.* 1993, 307, 836-840.

[19]   Obermeyer, CM: Menopause across cultures. *Menopause.* 2000, 7, 184-192,.

[20]   Leclair, DM; et al. Effects of Estrogen Deprivation: vasomotor symptoms, urogenital atrophy, and phsycobiologic effects. *Clinics in Family Practice.* Volume 4, Number 1, March, 2002.

[21]   Kronenberg, F: Hot flashes. *In* Lobo RA (ed): Treatment of the Postmenopausal Woman: Basic and Clinical Aspects. New York, Raven Press, 1994.

[22]   Carpenter, JS; Andrykowski, MA; Cordova, M; et al. Hot flashes in postmenopausal women treated for breast carcinoma: prevalence, severity, correlates, management, and relation to quality of life. *Cancer.*, 1998, 82, 1682-1691.

[23]   Clemons, M; Clamp, A; Anderson, B. Management of the menopause in cancer survivors. *Cancer Treat Rev.*, 2002, Dec, 28 (6), 321-33.

[24]   Love, RR; Camern, L; Connell, BL; et al. Symptoms associated with tamoxifen treatment in postmenopausal women. *Arch Intern Med* 1991, 151, 1842-7.

[25]   Fisher, B; Costantino, J; Redmond, C; Poisson, R; Bowman, D; Couture, J; Dimitrov, NV; Wolmark, N; Wickerham, DL; Fisher, ER; et al. A randomized clinical trial evaluating tamoxifen in the treatment of patients with node-negative breast cancer who have estrogen-receptor-positive tumors. *N Engl J Med.* 1989, 320, 479-484.

[26]   Loprinzi, CL; Zahasky, KM; Sloan, JA; et al. Tamoxifen-induced hot flashes. *Clin Breast Cancer.* 2000, 1, 52-56.

[27]   www.cancer.gov/cancer_information/cancer_type/breast.

[28] Management of hot flushes in breast cancer patients. Loprinzi et al *Lancet Oncology.* 2001, vol 2 April, 199-204.

[29] Ivarsson, T; et al. Physical exercise and vasomotor symptoms in postmenopausal women. *Maturitas.*, 29(2), 139-46 Jun 3 1998.

[30] Germaine, LM; Freedman, RR. Behavioral treatment of menopausal hot flashes: evaluation by objective methods .*J Consult Clin Psychol.* 1984, 52, 1072-1079.

[31] Wyon, Y; et al. Acupuncture against climacteric disorders? Lower number of symptoms after menopause. *Lakartidningen* 91(23), 2318-22, Jun 8, 1994.

[32] Carpenter, JS. Hot flashes and their management in breast cancer. *Semin Oncol Nurs.* 2000, 16, 214-225.

[33] Loprinzi, CL; Goldberg, RM; O'Fallon, JR; et al. Transdermal clonidine for ameliorating post orchiectomy hot flashes. *J Urol.*, 1994, 151, 634-636.

[34] Loprinzi, CL; Michalak, JC; Quella, SK; et al. Megestrol acetate for the prevention of hot flashes. *N Engl J Med.*, 1994, 331, 347-352.

[35] Barton, DL; Loprinzi, CL; Quella, SK; et al. Prospective evaluation of vitamin E for hot flashes in breast cancer survivors. *J Clin Oncol.*, 1998, 16, 495-500.

[36] Quella, SK; Loprinzi, CL; Barton, DL; et al. Evaluation of soy phytoestrogens for the treatment of hot flashes in breast cancer survivors: a North Central Cancer Treatment Group Trial. *J Clin Oncol.*, 2000, 18, 1068-1074.

[37] Loprinzi, CL; Kugler, JW; Sloan, JA; et al. Venlafaxine in management of hot flashes in survivors of breast cancer: a randomized controlled trial. *Lancet.* 2000, 356, 2059-2063.

[38] Greendale, GA; Reboussin, BA; Hogan, P; et al. Symptom relief and side effects of postmenopausal hormones: results from the Postmenopausal Estrogen/Progestin Interventions Trial. *Obstet Gynecol.*, 1998, 92, 982-988.

[39] Rymer, J; Morris, E. Menopausal Symptoms. *BMJ Vol.*, 321, No. 16, December 2000.

[40] Risks and Benefits of Estrogen Plus Progestin in Healthy Postmenopausal Women Principal Results From the Women's Health Initiative Randomized Controlled Trial Writing Group for the Women's Health Initiative Investigators *JAMA* 2002, 288, 321-333.

[41] Wile, AG; Opfell, RW; Margileth, DA; Anton-Culver, H. Hormone replacement therapy does not affect breast cancer outcome [abstract]. *Proc Am Soc Clin Oncol* 1991, 10, 58.

[42] Wile, AG; Opfell, RW; Magileth, DA. Hormone replacement therapy in previously treated breast cancer patients. *Am J Surg.* 1993, 165, 372-5.

[43] Eden, JA. A case controlled study of combined continuous estrogen-progestin replacement therapy among women with a personal history of breast cancer. *Menopause.* 1995, 2, 67-72.

[44] Pritchard, K; Llewellyn-Thomas, HA; Lewis, J; Sawka, CA; Franssen, E; Del Guidice, L; et al. The use of a probability trade-off task (PT-OT) to assess maximal acceptable increment in risk of breast cancer recurrence (MAIRR) in order to estimate sample size for a randomized clinical trial of hormone replacement therapy (HRT) in women with a previous diagnosis of breast cancer. *Proc Am Soc Clin Oncol.* 1996, 15, 213.

[45]   Holmberg, L. Hormonal replacement therapy after breast cancer diagnosis – is it safe? *ROC Uppsala*. March 11 1997.

[46]   Loprinzi; et al. Megestrol Acetate for the *Prevention of Hot Flashes.*, 331(6), 347-352. August 11, 1994.

[47]   Lobo, RA; McCormick, W; Singer, F; Roy S. Depo-medroxyprogesterone acetate compared with conjugated estrogens for the treatment of postmenopausal women. *Obstet Gynecol.*, 1984, 63, 1-5.

[48]   Leonetti, HB; Longo, S; Anasti, JN. Transdermal progesterone cream for vasomotor symptoms and postmenopausal bone loss. *Obstet Gynecol.*, 1999, 94, 225-228.

[49]   Hormonal replacement therapy after breast cancer – is it safe? [HABITS/BIG 03-97], *Southwest Oncology Group protocol* 9626.

[50]   Estrogen deprivation. *Clinics in Family Practice*. Volume 4, Number 1, March, 2002.

[51]   Kicovic, PM; Cortes-Prieto, J; Luisi, M; Milojevic, S; Franchi, F. Placebo-controlled cross-over study of effects of Org OD14 in menopausal women. *Reproduccion* 1982, 6, 81-91.

[52]   Bjarnason, NH; Bjarnason K; Haarbo, J; Bennink, HJTC; Christiansen, C. Tibolone: influence on markers of cardiovascular disease. *J Clin Endocrinol Metab*. 1997, 82, 1752–1756.

[53]   Kloosterboer, HJ. Tibolone: a steroid with a tissue-specific mode of action. *J Steroid Biochem Mol Biol*. 2001, 76, 231-238.

[54]   Lippert, C; Seeger, H; Wallwiener, D; Mueck, AO. Tibolone versus 17beta-estradiol/ norethisterone: effects on the proliferation of human breast cancer cells. *Eur J Gynecol Oncol* 2002, 23, 127- 130.

[55]   Kloosterboer, HJ; Schoonen, WGEJ; Deckers, GH; Klijn, JGM. Effect of progestagens and Org OD14 in in vitro and in vivo tumor models. *J Steroid Biochem Mol Biol* 1994, 49, 311- 318.

[56]   Lundstrom, E; Christow, A; Kersemaekers, W; Sbane, G; Azavedo, E; Solderqvist, G; Mol-Arts, M; Barkfeldt, J; von Schoultz, B. Effects of tibolone and continuous combined hormone replacement therapy on mammographic breast density. *Am J Obstet Gynecol*. 2002 186, 717- 722.

[57]   Tait, D; et al. Mayo Clin Proc, November, 2002, Vol 77 Pathophysiology and Treatment of Hot Flashes. 1207-1218.

[58]   Berendsen, HH. The role of serotonin in hot flushes. *Maturitas.*, 2000, 36, 155-164.

[59]   Loprinzi, CL; Pisansky, TM; Fonseca, R; et al. Pilot evaluation of venlafaxine hydrochloride for the therapy of hot flashes in cancer survivors. *J Clin Oncol*. 1998, 16, 2377-2381.

[60]   Loprinzi, CL; Kugler, JW; Sloan, JA; et al. Venlafaxine in management of hot flashes in survivors of breast cancer: a randomized controlled trial. *Lancet*. 2000, 356, 2059-2063.

[61]   Loprinzi, CL; Sloan, JA; Perez, EA; et al. Phase III evaluation of fluoxetine for treatment of hot flashes. *J Clin Oncol.*, 2002, 20, 1578-1583.

[62]   Stearns, V; Isaacs, C; Rowland, J; et al. A pilot trial assessing the efficacy of paroxetine hydrochloride (Paxil) in controlling hot flashes in breast cancer survivors. *Ann Oncol*. 2000, 11, 17-22.

[63] Goldberg, RM; Loprinzi, CL; O'Fallon, JR; Veeder, MH; Miser, AW; Mailliard, JA; Michalak, JC; Dose, AM; Rowland, KM; Jr, Burnham NL.Transdermal clonidine for ameliorating tamoxifen-induced hot flashes. *J Clin Oncol.* 1994, 12, 155-158.

[64] Pandya, KJ; Loughner, J; Raubertas, R; Bennett, JM. A double blind placebo controlled trial of clonidine for vasomotor symptoms in breast cancer patients on tamoxifen. *Proc Am Soc Clin Onc* 1990, 9, 340.

[65] Pandya, KJ; Raubertas, RF; Flynn, PJ; Hynes, HE; Rosenbluth, RJ; Kirshner, JJ; Pierce, HI; Dragalin, V; Morrow, GR. Oral clonidine in postmenopausal patients with breast cancer experiencing tamoxifen-induced hot flashes: a University of Rochester Cancer Center Community Clinical Oncology Program study. *Ann Intern Med.* 2000, 132, 788-793.

[66] Barton, DL; Loprinzi, CL; Quella, SK; et al. Prospective evaluation of vitamin E for hot flashes in breast cancer survivors. *J Clin Oncol.*, 1998, 16, 495-500.

[67] Thacker, HL; Booher, DL. Management of perimenopause: focus on alternative therapies. *Cleveland Clinic Journal Of Medicine*, Vol. 66, No. 4, April 1999, 213-218

[68] Foster, S. Black cohosh: Eimicifuga racemosa: a literature review. *Herbalgram.* 1999, winter, 35-49.

[69] Lieberman, S. A review of the effectiveness of *cimicifuga racemosa* (black cohosh) for the symptoms of menopause. *J Women's Health.* 1998, 7, 525-29.

[70] Gass, M; et al. Alternatives for women through menopause. American Journal of Obstetrics and Gynecology Volume 185, Number 2, August 2001.

[71] Schaper Brummer GmbH Co. KG. *Remifemin scientific brochure.* Salzgitter: Schaper & Brummer, 1997.

[72] Jacobson, JS; Troxel, AB; Evans, J; et al. Randomized trial of black cohosh for the treatment of hot flashes among women with a history of breast cancer. *J Clin Oncol.* 2001, 19, 2739-45.

[73] Morelli, V. Alternative therapies for traditional disease states: Menopause. *American Family Physician.* Volume 66, Number 1, July 1, 2002.

[74] Hirata, JD; Swiersz, LM; Zell, B; Small, R; Ettinger, B. Does dong quai have estrogenic effects in postmenopausal women? *Fertil Steril.* 1997, 68, 981-6.

[75] Taylor, M. Alternative medicine and the perimenopause an evidence-based review. *Obstet Gynecol Clin North Am* 01-Sep-2002, 29(3), 555-73.

[76] Oddens, BJ. The climacteric cross-culturally: the International Health Foundation South-east Asia study. *Maturitas.* 1994, 19, 155-156.

[77] Tham, DM; Gardner, CD; Haskell, WL. Clinical review 97, Potential health benefits of dietary phytoestrogens: a review of the clinical, epidemiological, and mechanistic evidence. *J Clin Endocrinol Metab.* 1998, 83, 2223-2235.

[78] Van Patten, CVL; Olivotto, IA; Chambers, K; Gelman, KA; Hislop, G; Templeton, E; Wattie, A; Prior, JC. Effect of soy phytoestrogen on hot flashes in postmenopausal women with breast cancer: a randomized controlled clinical trial. *J Clin Oncol* 2002, 20, 1449- 1455.

[79] Quella, SK; Loprinzi, CL; Barton, DL; Knost, JA; Sloan, JA; LaVasseur, BI; et al. Evaluation of soy phytoestrogens for the treatment of hot flashes in breast cancer

survivors: a North Central Cancer Treatment Group trial. *J Clin Oncol.* 2000, 18, 1068-74.

[80] Albertazzi, P; Pansini, F; Bonaccorsi, G; Zanotti, L; Forini, E; De Aloysio, D. The effect of dietary soy supplementation on hot flushes. *Obstet Gynecol.* 1998, 91, 6-11.

[81] Krebs, EE; Ensrud, KE; MacDonald, R; Wilt, TJ. Phytoestrogens for treatment of menopausal symptoms: a systematic review. *Obstet Gynecol.* 2004, 104(4), 824-36.

[82] Ginsburg, J; Prelevic, GM. Lack of significant hormonal effects and controlled trials of phyto-oestrogens. *Lancet.* 2000, 355, 163-164

[83] Fugh-Berman, A; Kronenberg, F. Red clover (Trifolium pratense) for menopausal women: current state of knowledge. *Menopause.* 2001, 8, 333-337

[84] Loprinzi, CL; Barton, DL; Rhodes, D. Management of hot flashes in breast cancer survivors. *Lancet Oncology*, April., 2001, 2, 199-204.

[85] Guttuso, T. Gabapentin's effects on hot flashes and hypothermia. *Neurol.* 2000, 54, 2161-2163.

[86] Pandit, L; Ouslander, JG. Postmenopausal vaginal atrophy and atrophic vaginitis. *The American Journal of Medical Science.* 314, 228–231, 1997.

[87] Johnston, SL; Farrell, SA; Bouchard, C; Farrell, SA; Beckerson, LA; Comeau, M; Johnston, SL; Lefebvre, G; Papaioannou, A. The detection and management of vaginal atrophy. *J Obstet Gynaecol Can* 2004, 26(5), 503-15.

[88] Day, R; Ganz, PA; Costantino, JP; Cronin, WM; Wickerham, DL; Fisher, B. Health-related quality of life and tamoxifen in breast cancer prevention: a report from the National Surgical Adjuvant Breast and Bowel Project P-1 Study. *J Clin Oncol.* 1999, **17**, 2659-2669

[89] Loprinzi, CL; Abu-Ghazaleh, S; Sloan, JA; vanHaelst-Pisani, C; Hammer, AM; Rowland, KM; Jr; Law, M; Windschitl, HE; Kaur, JS; Ellison, N. Phase III randomized double-blind study to evaluate the efficacy of a polycarbophil-based vaginal moisturizer in women with breast cancer. *J Clin Oncol.* 1997, 15, 969-973.

[90] Palacios, S; Castelo-Branco, C; Cancelo, MJ; Vazquez, F. Low-dose, vaginally administered estrogens may enhance local benefits of systemic therapy in the treatment of urogenital atrophy in postmenopausal women on hormone therapy. *Maturitas* 2005, 50(2), 98-104.

[91] Semmens, J; Wagner, G: Estrogen deprivation and vaginal function in postmenopausal women. *JAMA.* 248, 445, 1982

[92] Pandit, L; Ouslander, JG. Postmenopausal vaginal atrophy and atrophic vaginitis. *The American Journal of Medical Science.* 314, 228-231, 1997

[93] Sitruk-Ware, R. Estrogen therapy during menopause. Practical treatment recommendations. *Drugs.* 1990, 39, 203-217.

[94] Gruber; et al. Production and Action of Estrogens. *N Engl J Med.*, Vol. 346, No. 5 · January, 31, 2002. 340-352.

[95] Zhang, Y; Kiel, DP; Kreger, BE, et al. Bone mass and the risk of breast cancer among postmenopausal women. *N Engl J Med* 1997, 336, 611-7.

[96] Saarto, T; Blomqvist, C; Valimaki, M; Makela, P; Sarna, S; Elomaa, I. Chemical castration induced by adjuvant cyclophosphamide, methotrexate, and fluorouracil

chemotherapy causes rapid bone loss that is reduced by clodronate: a randomized study in premenopausal breast cancer patients. *J Clin Oncol.* 1997, 15, 1341-1347.

[97] Burstein, HJ; Winer, EP. Primary care for survivors of breast cancer. *N Engl J Med.* 2000, 343, 1086-1094.

[98] Lufkin, EG; Wahner, HW; O'Fallon, WM; Hodgson, SF; Kotowicz, MA; Lane, AW; Judd, HL; Caplan, RH; Riggs, BL. Treatment of postmenopausal osteoporosis with transdermal estrogen. *Ann Intern Med.* 1992, 117, 1-9

[99] Schneider, Dl; Barrett-Connor, EL; Morton, DJ. Timing of postmenopausal estrogen for optimal bone mineral density. The Rancho Bernando Study. *JAMA.* 1997, 277, 543-547

[100] Lindsay, R. Hormones and bone health in postmenopausal women. *Endocrine.* 2004, 24(3), 223-30.

[101] Hosking, D; Chilvers, CE; Christiansen, C; Ravn, P; Wasnich, R; Ross, P. Prevention of bone loss with alendronate in postmenopausal women under 60 years of age- Early Postmenopausal Intervention Cohort Study Group *N Engl J Med.* 1998, 338, 485- 492.

[102] Powles, TJ; McCloskey, E; Paterson, AH; Ashley, S; Tidy, VA; Nevantaus, A; Rosenqvist, K; Kanis, J. Oral clodronate and reduction in loss of bone mineral density in women with operable primary breast cancer.*J Natl Cancer Inst.* 1998, 90, 704-708.

[103] Reid et al. Intravenous Zoledronic acid in postmenopausal women with low bone mineral density. *New England Journal of Medicine* 2002, 346, 653-61.

[104] Powles, TJ; et al. Effect of tamoxifen on bone mineral density measured by dual-energy x-ray absorptiometry in healthy premenopausal and postmenopausal women. *J Clin Oncol* 1996, Jan, 14(1), 78-84.

[105] Fisher, B; Costantino, JP; Wickerham, DL; et al. Tamoxifen for prevention of breast cancer: report of the National Surgical Adjuvant Breast and Bowel Project P-1 Study. *J Natl Cancer Inst* 1998, 90, 1371-88.

[106] Ettinger, B; Black, DM; Mitlak, BH; Knickerbocker, RK; Nickelsen, T; Genant, HK; Christiansen, C; Delmas, PD; Zanchetta, JR; Stakkestad, J; Gluer, CC; Krueger, K; Cohen, FJ; Eckert, S; Ensrud, KE; Avioli, LV; Lips, P; Cummings, SR. Reduction of vertebral fracture risk in postmenopausal women with osteoporosis treated with raloxifene. *JAMA* 1999, 282, 637-645

[107] http://www.cancer.gov/clinicaltrials/digestpage/STAR

[108] O'Regan et al. Effects of Raloxifene after tamoxifen on breast and endometrial tumor growth in athymic mice. *Jounal of the National Cancer Institute*, 2002, Vol 94, no 4, 274-83. Feb 20,.

[109] Montemurro, L; et al. Prevention of corticosteroid induced osteoporosis with salmon calcitonin in sarcoid patients. *Calcif Tissue Int.*, 1991, 49, 71.

[110] Downs, RW; Bell, NH; Ettinger, MP; et al. Comparison of alendronate and intranasal calcitonin for the treatment of osteoporosis in postmenopausal women. *J Clin Endocrinol Metab* 200, 85, 1783.

[111] Overgaard, k; Riis, BJ; Christiansen, C; et al. Effect of salcatonin given intranasally on early postmenopausal bone loss. *BMJ* 1989, 299, 477.

[112] Ramsay, LE; Williams, B; Johnston, GD; MacGregor, GA; Poston, L; Potter, JF; Poulter, NR; Russell, G. British Hypertension Society guidelines for hypertension management 1999: summary *BMJ* 1999, 319, 630-635

[113] Manson, JE; et al. Walking Compared with Vigorous Exercise for the Prevention of Cardiovascular Events in Women. *N Engl J Med* 2002, 347, 716-25.

[114] The LIPID group. Prevention of cardiovascular events and death with pravastatin in patients with coronary heart disease and a broad range of initial cholesterol. *NEJM* 1998, 339, 1349-1357

[115] Darling, GM; Jowns, JA; McCloud, PI; Davis, SR. Estrogen and progestin compared with simvastatin for hypercholesterolemia in postmenopausal women *NEJM* 1997, 337, 595- 601

[116] Heart Protection Study Collaborative group. MRC/BHF Heart Protection Study of cholesterol lowering with simvastatin in 20 536 high-risk individuals: a randomised placebo-controlled trial. *Lancet* 2002, Vol 360 July 6, 7-22.

[117] Seeger, h; Wallweiner, D; Mueck, AO. Statins can inhibit proliferation of human breast cancer cells in vitro. *Exp Clin Endocrinol Diabetes.*, 2003, Vol 111(1), 47-48, Feb.

[118] Mortimer, JE; et al. Effect of statins on breast cancer incidence: Finding from the Sentara Health Plan. *Abstract No* 2003, 373.

[119] Delmas, PD; Bjarnason, NH; Mitlak, BH; Ravoux, AC; Shah, AS; Huster, WJ; Draper, M; Christiassen, C. Effects of raloxifeneon bone mineral density, serum cholesterol concentrations, and uterine endometrium in postmenopausal women. *N Engl J Med.* 1997, 337, 1641-1647.

[120] Cushman, M. Effects of hormone replacement therapy and estrogen receptor modulators on markers of inflammation and coagulation. *Am J Cardiol* 3-Jul-2002, 90(1A), 7F-10F

Index

B

C

E

F

G

I

J

K

L

N

O